OSCEsmart

Medical student OSCEs
The complete series

Dr. Sam Thenabadu

MBBS MRCP DRCOG DCH MA Clin Ed FRCEM MSc (Paed) FHEA FAcadMEd

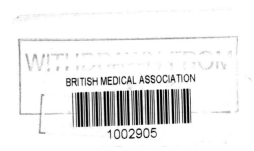

Ordering Information: Quantity sales. Special discounts are available on quantity purchases by corporations, associations, and others. For details, contact the publisher at the address above.

Orders by UK trade bookstores and wholesalers please visit www.scowenpublishing.com

Although every effort has been made to check this text, it is possible that errors have been made, readers are urged to check with the most up to date guidelines and safety regulations.

The authors and the publishers do not accept responsibility or legal liability for any errors in the text, or for the misuse of the material in this book.

Publisher's Cataloging-in-Publication data : OSCEsmart - Medical student OSCEs – The complete series.

Copyright © 2017 Simon Cowen Publishing

ISBN-10:0-9985267-5-4

ISBN-13:978-0-9985267-5-1

Message from the author

Doctors of all seniorities can remember the stress of the OSCE but even more so the stress of trying to study and practice for the OSCEs. A multitude of generic undergraduate and postgraduate resources can be found on line but quality, quantity, and completeness of content can vary. The aim of the OSCESmart editorial team is to bring together specialty focused books that have identified 50 core stations encompassing the essential categories of history taking, examinations, emergency moulages, clinical skills and data interpretation with a strong theme of communications running through all the stations.

The combined experience of consultants, registrars and junior doctors to write, edit and quality check these stations, promises to deliver content that is appropriate to reach a standard we would expect of new junior doctors entering their foundation internship years and into core training. It is important to know that these stations are all newly written and based at the level of clinical competencies we would expect from these grades of doctors. Learning objectives exist for undergraduate curricula and for the foundation years, and the scenarios are based and written around these. What they are not, are scenarios that have been 'borrowed' from any medical school.

Preparation is the key to success in most things, but never more so than for the OSCEs and a candidate that hasn't practised will soon be found out. These books will allow you to practice relevant scenarios with verified checklists to learn both content and the generic approach. The format will allow you to practice in groups with one person being the candidate, one the actor and one the examiner. Each scenario finishes with three learning points. Picture these as are three core learning tips that we would want you to take away if you had only a couple of days left to the exam. These OSCE scenarios promise to be a robust revision aide for the student looking to recap and consolidate for their exams, but equally importantly prepare them for life in clinical practice.

I am immensely proud of this OSCESmart series. I have had the pleasure of working with some of the brightest and most dynamic young clinicians and educators I know, and I am sure you will find this series covering the essential clinical specialties a truly robust and invaluable companion in those stressful times of revision. I must take this opportunity to thank my colleagues for all their hard work but most of all to thank my wonderful wife Molly for her unerring love and support and my sons Reuben and Rafael for all the joy they bring me.

Despite the challenging times the health service finds itself in, being a doctor remains a huge privilege. We hope that this OSCESmart series goes some way to help you achieve the excellence you and your patients deserve.

Best of luck, Dr Sam Thenabadu

About the author

Dr Sam Thenabadu

MBBS MRCP DRCOG DCH MA Clin Ed FRCEM MSc (Paed) FHEA FAcadMEd

Consultant Adult & Paediatric Emergency Medicine
Honorary Senior Lecturer & Associate Director of Medical Education

Sam Thenabadu graduated from King's College Medical School in 2001 and dual trained in Adult and Paediatric Emergency Medicine in London before being appointed a consultant in 2011 at the Princess Royal University Hospital. He has Masters degrees in Clinical Medical Education and Advanced Paediatrics.

He is undergraduate director of medical education at the King's College NHS Trust and the Deputy Head of Stage 3 at King's College School of Medicine. At postgraduate level he has been the Pan London Health Education England lead for CT3 paediatric emergency medicine trainees since 2011. Academically he has previously written two textbooks and has published in peer review journals and given numerous oral and poster presentations at national conferences in emergency medicine, paediatrics, medical education and patient quality and safety.

He has an unashamed passion for medical education and strives to achieve excellence for himself, his colleagues and his patients, hoping to always deliver this through an enjoyable learning environment. Service delivery and educational need not be two separate entities, and he hopes that those who have had great teachers will take it upon themselves to do the same for others in the future.

Co-Authors

ENT

Mr Agbolahan Sofela
BSc(Hons) MBBS MRCS (Eng)
Specialty Trainee in Neurosurgery, UK

Dr Christopher Ashton MBBS MSc.
Ophthalmology ST1 KSS

Mr Mihiar Sami Atfeh - MRCSed, DOHNS, MD.
Specialty Doctor & Honorary University Fellow –
Plymouth Hospitals NHS Trust & Plymouth University.

Mr Kush Bhatt MBBS Bsc MRCS.
ST3 Neurosurgery South West Peninsula Deanery
Dr. Neil Bowley MChem (hons), BMBS, PhD.
ST3 Ophthalmology South West Peninsula Deanery
Mr Gareth Lloyd BMBS BMedSci (Hons) MRCS DOHNS.
Specialty Registrar (StR) Otorhinolaryngology, London

Dr Pedro Santos Jorge MBBS LMD MMedEd.
Foundation trainee 2, London

Anaesthetics & Critical Care

Dr Joe Lipton
BSc (Hons) MBBS MRCP FRCA
Speciality Registrar ST5, Anaesthetics
South London School of Anaesthesia

Dr Sarah Jane Muldoon
MBChB MRCP FRCA
Speciality Registrar ST5, Anaesthetics
South London School of Anaesthesia

Dr Michael Shaw
MBChB FRCA EDIC
Speciality Registrar ST7, Anaesthetics
South London School of Anaesthesia

Dr Toby Winterbottom
MBBS BSc (Hons) MRCEM FRCA
Speciality Registrar ST5, Anaesthetics
Kent, Surrey & Sussex School of Anaesthesia

Dr Folasade Onakoya
BSc (Hons) MBBS

Dr Marilyn Boampomaa
MBBS BSc (Hons)
Junior Clinical Fellow, Anaesthetics
Princess Alexandra Hospital

With original illustrations by Anushka Athique

Orthopaedics & Rheumatology

Mr Dominic Davenport MBBS BSc MRCS
Specialist Registrar Trauma & Orthopaedic Surgery

Mr Alastair G Dick BSc MRCS MBBS
Specialist Registrar Trauma & Orthopaedic Surgery

Mr William Nash MBBS MRCS BEng
Specialist Registrar Trauma & Orthopaedic Surgery

Mr Amit S Patel MBBS BSc MRCS
Specialist Registrar Trauma & Orthopaedic Surgery

Dr Andrew Rutherford MBBS MSc MRCP
Senior Clinical Fellow in Rheumatology

Dr Sujith Subesinghe BSc (Hons) MBBS MRCP MSc (Dist.)
Specialist Registrar in Rheumatology and General Internal
Medicine

Psychiatry

Dr Esha Abrol
MBBS BSc PgCert (Medical Education)

Dr Michael Webb
MBBS BSc PgCert (MedEd)

Dr Priya Abrol MBBS BSc
Foundation Year 1 Doctor (FY1) - St Peter's Hospital,
London

Dr Golnar Aref-Adib MBBS BMedSci PGDipCAT MRCPsych
Specialist Trainee (ST4) General Adult Psychiatry & NIHR
Academic Clinical Fellow - UCL Division of Psychiatry,
London and Camden & Islington NHS Foundation Trust,
London

Dr Juliet Davidson MBBS BSc
Foundation Year 2 Doctor (FY2) - Brighton

Dr Sian L Holdridge MBBS BSc
Core Psychiatry Trainee (CT1) - London

Dr Melanie Knowles MBBS BSc
Core Psychiatry Trainee (CT2) - Barnet, Enfield and
Haringey Mental Health Trust, London

Dr Matthew Loughran MBChB BSc (Hons)
Core Psychiatry Trainee (CT2) - Royal Free London NHS
Foundation Trust, London

Dr Matthew L Naylor MBBS BSc
Foundation Year 2 Doctor (FY2) - Tunbridge Wells
Hospital, Royal Tunbridge Wells

Dr Shivanthi Sathanandan MBBS BSc MRCPsych
Specialist Trainee (ST6) General Adult Psychiatry and
Fellow at Practitioners' Health Programme - UCL
Partners, London

Dr Elizabeth Templeton MBCHB (Hons)
Core Psychiatry Trainee (CT3) - Camden & Islington NHS
Foundation Trust, London

Dr Chloe Wilkes BMBS BMedSci
Foundation Year 2 Doctor (FY2) - East Sussex

Surgery

Mr Nabeel Merali
MBBS MRCS MSc

Dr. Debo Adebayo BMBS, MClinEd,
Foundation Year 2, London

Dr. Adam Garland MBBS, BSc,
Foundation Year 2, London

Dr. Frederick Hartley, MBBS, MRCS,
Core Surgical Trainee Year 2, London

Major Max Marsden MBBS BSc DMCC DOHNS MRCS,
Clinical Research Fellow, General Surgery Registrar,
Military Deanery

Dr Sarah Schneider, MBChB, BMedSci Hons,
Emergency Medicine trainee (ACCS) CT1, London

Dr Daniel Thompson MBBS, BAHons,
Anatomy Demonstrator King's College London

Dr. Thomas Thompson, MBBS, BSc,
Foundation Year 2, London

Emergency medicine

Dr Dilhan Perusinghe MBBS MEng
CT3 Emergency Medicine

Dr Amy Attwater MBChB (Hons) BSc (Hons)
Staff Grade Clinical fellow in Emergency Medicine,
University Hospital Coventry and Warwickshire

Dr Thomas Peter Fox MBBS MRCEM

ST3 Emergency Medicine, University Hospital Lewisham,
London

Dr Yannic N.P. Graichen, BMBS, BMedSci,
ST3 Emergency medicine, Guy's and St Thomas' Hospital,
London

Dr Atul Kapoor MBChB
ST3 Emergency Medicine, Guy's and St Thomas' Hospital,
London

Dr Claire Kilbride MBChB
CT2 Emergency Medicine, Guy's and St Thomas' Hospital,
London

Dr Marthani Maheswaran MBBS BSc MRCEM
ST3 Emergency Medicine Homerton University Hospital

Dr Alexander C E Robertson, MBChB BSc MRCEM
ST3 Emergency Medicine, The Royal London Hospital

Dr Siobhan Roche, MBChB
CT2 Emergency medicine, Guy's and St Thomas' Hospital,
London

Dr Sarah Schneider, MBChB, BMedSci Hons,
CT1 Emergency Medicine trainee, Princess Royal
University Hospital

Dr Amy Servante, Bsc(Hons) MBBS
ST3 Emergency Medicine, King's College Hospital, London

Obstetrics & Gynaecology

Dr Rochelle Brainerd MBBS BSc (Hons)

Dr. Nadir Chowdhury MBBS BSc (Hons)
ST1 Paediatrics, London
Honorary Clinical Teaching Fellow, UCL Medical School

Dr. Melania Ishak MBBS BSc (Hons)
Obstetrics & Gynaecology Trust SHO, London

Dr. Rumana Lasker MBBS BSc (Hons)
GPST1, London

Dr. Amisha Mehta MBBS BSc (Hons)
GPST2, Oxford

Dr. Shreya Morzeria MBBS BSc (Hons)
GPST1, London

Dr. Anna Rosen MBChB DRCOG
GPST1, London

Dr. Kavita Shapriya MBBS BSc (Hons) MRCP
Core Medical Trainee Year 2, London

Dr. Surenthini Suntharalingam MBBS BSc (Hons) MRCP
Speciality Registrar in Haematology, Bristol

Medicine

**Dr Cathryn Mainwaring BM BS (Hons.) BMedsci (Hons.)
MRCP (UK)**

Dr Rebekah Davis MBChB BMedSci, GP Specialist Trainee
Year 1

Dr Samantha Fleury BMBS, Foundation Year Two Doctor

Dr Erin Kamp MBBS, Foundation Year Two Doctor

Dr Rupinder Kaur Gill MBBS, Foundation Year Two Doctor

Dr Daniella Osaghae MBBS BSc. (Hons.), Foundation Year
Two Doctor

Dr Radhika Patel MBBS BSc. (Hons.), Foundation Year
Two Doctor

Dr Saranya Ravindran MBBS BSc. (Hons.), Foundation
Year Two Doctor

Dr Aarthi Ravishankar MBBS BSc. (Hons.), Foundation
Year Two Doctor

Dr Chloe Wilkes, BMBS BMedSci, Foundation Year Two
Doctor

Paediatrics

**Dr Kunal Babla BSc(Hons) MBBS MSc MRCPCH
MAcadMEd**
ST6 Neonatal Medicine, London

Dr Morium Akthar BSc (Hons) MBBS MSc (Paed) MRCPCH
ST8 Paediatrics, London

Dr Eleanor Bond BSc (Hons) MBBS MRCPCH
ST8 Paediatrics, London

Dr Sarah Davies BM (Hons) MA (Oxon) Experimental
Psychology, MRCPCH
ST4 Paediatrics, London

Dr Charlotte Doyle BSc (Hons) MBBS
ST1 Paediatrics, London

Dr Dionysios N. Grigoratos BSc(Hons) MBBS(Lon)
MRCPCH
Paediatric Registrar, London

Dr Emily Haseler BM BCh MRCPCH
ST3 Paediatrics, London

Dr Sarah Hewett BSc(Hons) MBBS
ST2 Paediatrics, London

Dr Kathryn Smith MBChB MSc MRCPCH
ST5 Paediatrics, London

Dr Kirsten Thompson MBChB BMedSci
ST1 Paediatrics, London

Dr Lyndon Wells BMedSc (Hons) MBChB
ST2 Paediatrics, London

General practice

**Dr Nisha Patel MBBS BSc (Hons)
ST1 Paediatrics**

Dr Dugald Brown BSc, MBBS

Dr Yee-Teng Chon BSc (Hons), MBBS

Dr Malaz Elsaddig BSc MBBS
Clinical Teaching Fellow, University of Bristol, Swindon
Academy at Great Western Hospital

Dr Rhiannon Jones MBBS, MA (Cantab)
Emergency Department, Senior Resident Medical Officer,
Australia

Dr Balrik Kailey MBBS, BA
Core Medical Trainee, London

Dr Vishal Kumar MBBS
Cardio-Respiratory CT1, Leicester

Dr Kristina Nanthagopan BSc (Hons), MBBS
GPST2, London

Dr Christiana Page MBChB
Intensive Care Clinical Fellow, London

Dr Naim Slim BSc MBBS
Anatomy Demonstrator & Junior Clinical Fellow (General
Surgery), University of Cambridge

Table of Contents

Candidates instructions   1

    ENT   2

    Anaesthetics & Critical Care   5

    Orthopaedics & Rheumatology   11

    Psychiatry   17

    Surgery   21

    Emergency medicine   27

    Obstetrics & Gynaecology   31

    Medicine   34

    Paediatrics   39

    General Practice   43

Examiner's instructions   46

    ENT   47

    Anaesthetics & Critical Care   53

    Orthopaedics & Rheumatology   62

    Psychiatry   69

    Surgery   74

    Emergency medicine   79

    Obstetrics & Gynaecology   88

    Medicine   91

    Paediatrics   97

    General Practice   103

Actors instructions — 107

    ENT — 108

    Anaesthetics & Critical Care — 114

    Orthopaedics & Rheumatology — 124

    Psychiatry — 131

    Surgery — 145

    Emergency medicine — 151

    Obstetrics & Gynaecology — 160

    Medicine — 168

    Paediatrics — 174

    General Practice — 181

Marksheets + Learning points — 189

    ENT — 190

    Anaesthetics & Critical Care — 210

    Orthopaedics & Rheumatology — 235

    Psychiatry — 260

    Surgery — 281

    Emergency medicine — 306

    Obstetrics & Gynaecology — 331

    Medicine — 351

    Paediatrics — 376

    General Practice — 401

Candidates instructions

ENT — 2

Anaesthetics & Critical Care — 5

Orthopaedics & Rheumatology — 11

Psychiatry — 17

Surgery — 21

Emergency medicine — 27

Obstetrics & Gynaecology — 31

Medicine — 34

Paediatrics — 39

General Practice — 43

ENT

Case 1

You are the Emergency Department Foundation doctor and have been asked to take the initial history from a 6 year old boy presenting with 'muffled' hearing. Take a history and summarize your findings as you would when referring to the ENT registrar on-call.

After 6 minutes the examiner will stop you and ask you to summarise back your findings, suggest your management plan and answer some direct questions.

Case 2

You are a Foundation doctor doing a rotation at a GP practice. The next patient is complaining of a left sided otorrhoea. Please take a concise history and summarise your findings.

After 6 minutes the examiner will stop you and ask you to summarise back your findings, suggest your management plan and answer some direct questions.

Case 3

You are a Foundation doctor doing a rotation in the emergency department. The next patient is a 6 year old boy who has been sent to hospital by the school nurse with a bleeding left ear. Please take a concise history and summarise your findings as you would when referring to the ENT registrar on-call.

After 6 minutes the examiner will stop you and ask you to summarise back your findings, suggest your management plan and answer some direct questions.

Case 4

You are the Foundation doctor working at a GP practice. Your next patient complaints of a lump by his left ear. Please examine this lump and present your findings and differentials to the examiner.

After 6 minutes the examiner will stop you and ask you to summarise back your findings, suggest your management plan and answer some direct questions.

Case 5

You are the Foundation doctor working in a GP practice. Your next patient complaints of a poor sense of smell. Take a full **history** from this patient.

After 6 minutes the examiner will stop you and ask you to summarise back your findings, suggest your management plan and answer some direct questions.

Case 6

You are the Foundation doctor on a GP placement. Your next patient is a 54 year old woman who has noticed the skin around her nose has changed and become red over the last few weeks. Take a short history and examine this patient presenting with nasal erythema.

After 6 minutes the examiner will stop you and ask you to summarise back your findings, suggest your management plan and answer some direct questions.

Case 7

You are the Foundation doctor working at a GP practice. Your next patient complaints of noisy breathing and his nostrils feeling blocked. **Examine** this patient's nose

After 6 minutes the examiner will stop you and ask you to summarise back your findings, suggest your management plan and answer some direct questions.

Case 8

You are the Foundation doctor working at a GP practice. Your next patient complains of a lump in her nose. **Examine** this patient presenting with a nasal lump.

After 6 minutes the examiner will stop you and ask you to summarise back your findings, suggest your management plan and answer some direct questions.

Case 9
A 12-year old boy presents to the Emergency Department (ED) minor injuries unit with complications of nasal trauma he sustained recently. You are the Foundation year doctor in ED and you are asked by your consultant to take a short history from the patient and carry out the relevant clinical examination, and offer a management plan.

After 6 minutes the examiner will stop you and ask you to summarise back your findings, suggest your management plan and answer some direct questions.

Case 10
You are the Foundation doctor in the ED and are asked to **examine** the nose of a 19-year-old male patient who presents with a bleeding nose after being assaulted outside a night club.

After 6 minutes the examiner will stop you and ask you to summarise back your findings, suggest your management plan and answer some direct questions.

Case 11
You are a Foundation doctor on a GP placement. Take a history from this 58 year old patient presenting with dysphagia.

After 6 minutes the examiner will stop you and ask you to summarise back your findings, suggest your management plan and answer some direct questions.

Case 12
You are a Foundation doctor on a rotation at a GP practice. Take a comprehensive history from a 20-year old lady presenting with odynophagia

After 6 minutes the examiner will stop you and ask you to summarise back your findings, suggest your management plan and answer some direct questions.

Case 13
You are a Foundation doctor on a rotation at a GP practice. Take a **history** from this 29-year old who complains of voice hoarseness.

After 6 minutes the examiner will stop you and ask you to summarise back your findings, suggest your management plan and answer some direct questions.

Case 14
You are the Foundation doctor in ENT, and have been asked to take a brief history and examine this 71-year old who presents with acute stridor.

After 6 minutes the examiner will stop you and ask you to summarise back your findings, suggest your management plan and answer some direct questions.

Case 15
You are a Foundation doctor working in the emergency department. You have been asked to assess a 36 year man in the emergency department with difficulty in breathing. He has been brought in with significant facial injury following a motorbike accident. He now has increasing tongue swelling and is becoming drowsy.

Discuss the immediate and escalatory management of acute airway compromise.

You have 8 minutes for this station, but will get a warning bell 2 minutes prior to the end. Please use this remaining time to collect your thoughts and discuss any other important points you will like to cover.

Case 16

You are a Foundation doctor on a GP placement. Take a history from this 79 year old lady who presents with a lump in the throat

After 6 minutes the examiner will stop you and ask you to summarise back your findings, suggest your management plan and answer some direct questions.

Case 17

You are an ED Foundation doctor. A 22-year old woman anxiously attends the emergency department (ED) with sudden palpitations and a progressively growing neck lump. The patient called her GP yesterday to book an appointment because of her neck swelling that has been increasingly growing over the past month. However, tonight she started having palpitations, shortness of breath and lightheadedness. The ED Nurse Practitioner who triaged the patient documented the following vitals (BP 140/90, HR 115, temp 37.5, SaO2 96% on air). Take a full history from this patient

After 6 minutes the examiner will stop you and ask you to summarise back your findings, suggest your management plan and answer some direct questions.

Case 18

You are the Foundation doctor in ENT outpatients and you are sitting in the head and neck consultant-led clinic. You are asked by your consultant to carry out a clinical examination of a 45 years old male patient who has a history of a progressively enlarging, but otherwise asymptomatic, right sided neck lump.

After 6 minutes the examiner will stop you and ask you to summarise back your findings, suggest your management plan and answer some direct questions.

Case 19

You are a Foundation doctor in the emergency department. You have been asked to see Agnes, an 85 year old lady who has been brought into the department complaining of loss of vision. She has no referral letter and hasn't been to the hospital before. Take a history, present your findings, suggest potentially useful investigations and a differential diagnosis.

After 6 minutes the examiner will stop you and ask you to summarise back your findings, suggest your management plan and answer some direct questions.

Case 20

A 24-year old lady has presented with right sided blurry vision. You are the Ophthalmology Foundation doctor in eye casualty and have been asked to take a focused **history and perform ishihara charts, pupillary response and fundoscopy.** Present your findings to the registrar following the examination.

After 6 minutes the examiner will stop you and ask you to summarise back your findings, suggest your management plan and answer some direct questions.

Anaesthetics & Critical Care

Case 1

Martin Williams is a 52-year-old man who has presented for elective laparoscopic inguinal hernia repair under general anaesthetic.

You are a Foundation Year doctor on your Anaesthetic rotation and you have been asked to take a short history and perform an anaesthetic pre-assessment.
After 6 minutes the examiner will stop you and ask you to summarise back your findings and suggest your management plan.

Case 2

John is a 78-year-old man who has presented for elective inguinal hernia repair under general anaesthetic.
You are a Foundation Year1 doctor on your anaesthetics rotation and you have been asked to perform an Anaesthetic pre-assessment, including answering any questions he may have.
After 6 minutes the examiner will stop you and ask you to summarise back your findings and suggest your management plan and answer some brief questions.

Case 3

Rachel is a 44-year-old woman presenting for an elective excision of a benign breast lump under general anaesthetic. You are a Foundation Year1 doctor on your anaesthetics rotation and you have been asked to perform an Anaesthetic pre-assessment.
After 6 minutes the examiner will stop you and ask you to summarise back your findings and suggest your management plan.

Case 4

You are a Foundation Year 1 doctor doing an anaesthetics rotation. A student Operating Department Practitioner (ODP) asks you for some help understanding Waveform Capnography.

Please explain to them why Waveform Capnography is used, then examine five diagrams from their textbook and explain the clinical significance of the various waveforms. Suggest what measures may need to be taken in clinical practice to identify or correct the problems leading to any abnormalities in each trace.

Case 5

Richard, patient ID 1234567D, is a 36-year-old man with a history of heroin and crack cocaine use who has presented to the Emergency Department with difficulty breathing and a productive cough. He has been triaged and 60% oxygen is being administered via a Venturi mask.
You are a Foundation Year 1 doctor working in the Emergency Department and you have been asked to review his arterial blood gas. This is shown below;

ID: 1234567D, Richard, arterial, 01/01/2016, 10:20am		
pH	7.30	
pO_2	10.1	kPa
pCO_2	3.5	kPa
HCO_3	20	mmol/L
Lactate	3.5	mmol/L
BE	-5	
Na+	137	mmol/L
Cl-	101	mmol/L
Hb	157	g/L

Review the information and when then summarise your findings and plan of action to the ED registrar.

Case 6

A 22-year-old man, Tom, has been brought in to the emergency department after having been found drowsy and unwell at home by his friend. She says he has been ill for a few days with severe vomiting and abdominal pain.

You are the Foundation year doctor in the department and have been asked by a senior colleague to analyse and comment on the following arterial blood gas result from the patient, to aid management of his condition.

After evaluating the blood gas you should present it to the examiner and answer any questions they may have.

Results

Arterial blood gas: 3/8/16 16:45
Mr Tom, DOB 15/5/95
fiO2 0.21

pH	6.94
P_aO_2	13.8kPa
P_aCO_2	2.5kPa
HCO_3^-	8mmol/L
Base excess	-19.5mmol/L
Glucose	27mmol/L

Case 7

You are the Foundation Year 1 covering the Acute Medical Unit. You are asked to see Samuel, a 53-year-old patient whose GP has referred him for investigation of ascites. The nurse admitting him is concerned that his blood pressure is low.
After 6 minutes the examiner will stop you and ask you to summarise back your findings, suggest your management plan and answer some direct questions.

Case 8

A 72-year-old man was admitted under the medical take earlier in the day for treatment of pneumonia, but has now been found unconscious by a staff nurse.

You are the Foundation Year 1 doctor on call and have been asked to assess and treat the patient appropriately.

After 6 minutes the examiner will stop you and ask you to summarise back your findings and suggest your management plan.

Case 9

You are a Foundation Year 1 doing your Emergency Department rotation. You are asked to urgently assess Lena, a 19-year-old woman brought to resus by ambulance. She is unconscious and hypotensive. Her mother called the ambulance having found her collapsed in her bedroom – she has been worried about her mood and behavior since Lena failed her first-year university exams.

You have been asked to assess and stabilise the patient and start initial management.
After 6 minutes the examiner will stop you and ask you to summarise back your findings and suggest your management plan from here on.

Case 10

You are a Foundation Year 1 on your anaesthetics placement. You are on the medical ward to pre-assess a patient for surgery on behalf of your consultant (who is in theatre). As you enter the bay the nursing staff call you over to a different patient who is having seizures.

Jonny is a 24-year-old patient with a history of epilepsy who is undergoing treatment with IV antibiotics for a community acquired pneumonia. His seizures are usually well controlled with oral sodium valproate.

After 6 minutes the examiner will stop you and ask you to summarise back your findings, suggest your management plan and ask you some direct questions.

Case 11

You are a Foundation Year 1 on your ICU placement. You are attending a patient in the Emergency Department ahead of your registrar who is due to join you imminently.

Tim is a 78-year-old gentleman with a history of benign prostatic hypertrophy, who has been moved to the Resus area after becoming hypotensive and drowsy. He was admitted with pyrexia, vomiting and loin pain.

The charge nurse in ED looking after the patient is able to provide you with much of the salient history and is fully aware of what investigations and treatment have been initiated.

After 6 minutes the examiner will stop you and ask you to summarise back your findings, suggest your management plan and ask you some direct questions.

Case 12

You are a Foundation Year 1 on the orthopaedic ward.

A staff nurse asks you to see Dan, a 28 year old awaiting wash-out of an infected elbow effusion. He complained of feeling unwell as the nurse was completing her drug rounds. Please assess him, state your diagnosis and initiate appropriate management.

After 6 minutes the examiner will stop you and ask you to summarise back your findings, suggest your management plan and answer some direct questions.

Case 13

Jeanie is a 76-year-old female who has been admitted to the Emergency Department (ED) after being found slumped in her chair by her daughter. She has lung cancer and had a lobectomy over a year ago. Her last course of chemotherapy was over a month ago.

You are the Foundation Year doctor in the ED and have been asked to perform the initial assessment. Jeanie's daughter is present and can answer any questions and an ED nurse is available to help you. Assess the patient with a view to making a diagnosis and formulate an initial management plan.

After 6 minutes the examiner will stop you and ask you to summarise back your findings, suggest your management plan and answer some direct questions.

Case 14

You are a foundation doctor working in Emergency Department and a staff nurse has asked you to urgently assist with a man who appears to be choking in the waiting room.

After 6 minutes the examiner will stop you and ask you to summarise back your findings, suggest your management plan and answer some direct questions.

Case 15

A 65 year old man admitted with SOB and pleuritic chest pain has collapsed and become unresponsive on the cardiology ward. The nurse at the bedside has shouted for help.

You are the foundation doctor on ward cover and you are the first to attend. Please assess the patient and manage accordingly.

After 6 minutes the examiner will stop you and ask you to summarise back your findings, suggest your management plan and answer some direct questions

Case 16

Daniel is a 25-year-old man who was knocked off his bike and landed on his back. He has been brought to the emergency department and is complaining that he can't move his legs.

You are a Foundation Year doctor and have been asked to finish the primary survey. Your senior colleague has already assessed Daniel's airway and breathing. He appears to have a diaphragmatic breathing pattern and respiratory rate of 25. Continue the primary survey from 'C' .
After 6 minutes the examiner will stop you and ask you to summarise back your findings, suggest your management plan and answer some direct questions.

Case 17

You are a Foundation Year doctor on your Anaesthetics rotation. You are spending the day in the labour ward and have been asked to talk to a pregnant woman about the options available for pain relief during labour.
She is a 25 year old primigravida who is 36 weeks pregnant. She has been well during her pregnancy and has no past medical history of note. She is planning to have a normal delivery in the hospital birthing suite.
After 6 minutes the examiner will stop you and ask you to summarise back your findings, suggest your management plan and answer some direct questions.

Case 18

You are a Foundation Year doctor on your Anaesthetics rotation. Today there is a year 4 medical student attending your list who has just started the first week of their Anaesthetics rotation. They are interested to talk to you about the different drugs used in Anaesthesia.
Using the labelled syringes/drugs list as an aide memoire, talk the student through the different drugs, giving as much information about each as you can, then answer any questions they may have.

Case 19

A 62-year-old man has been admitted under the Gastroenterology team. He is to undergo an elective OGD to investigate his worsening epigastric pain. He vaguely understands the procedure after reading about it on the Internet.

As the Foundation year doctor on the team, you have been asked by a nurse to speak to the patient who has some questions regarding the procedure. He seems to be most worried about being fully awake during it, and would like you to explain how he would be sedated to avoid this.
After 6 minutes the examiner will stop you and ask you to summarise back your findings, suggest your management plan and answer some direct questions.

Case 20

You are a Foundation Year doctor on your anaesthetics placement. On the labour ward a new midwifery student asks you to explain spinal anaesthesia to her.
With 2 minutes remaining the examiner will stop you and ask you some direct questions in regards to spinal anaesthesia.

Case 21

You are the Foundation Year1 on your anaesthetics placement. You have a third year medical student with you on a clinical attachment. Your consultant has asked you to provide some brief teaching to the student regarding the provision of oxygen to patients.

Review the following diagrams of oxygen delivery devices. These can be used as a reference point for your teaching.
After 6 minutes the examiner will stop you and ask you questions regarding the delivery of oxygen.

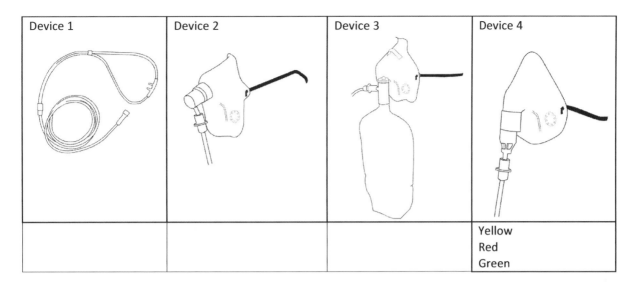

Device 1	Device 2	Device 3	Device 4
			Yellow Red Green

Case 22

You are the foundation year doctor in anaesthetics and you have been called to recovery to review Betty.

Betty is an 80 year old female who had a left total hip replacement under general anaesthetic 2 hour ago and is now reporting pain. According to the Anaesthetic record, she received 8mg of morphine IV intra-operatively, but no other analgesia.
In addition, the recovery nurse points out that the patient's drug chart has not been completed.
Please review the patient's pain and prescribe appropriate treatment.

Case 23

Clarice is a 60-year-old woman who was admitted for mastectomy for breast cancer. Her postoperative pain has been managed with IV morphine PCA, with a bolus dose of 1mg. She has used a total of 20mg in the last 24 hours. Her postoperative biochemistry is normal.
You are a Foundation Year doctor on your anaesthetics rotation and you have been asked to prescribe an appropriate dose of modified release morphine tablets, with some additional opioid for breakthrough pain. You may ask the patient questions you feel are relevant.

After 6 minutes the examiner will stop you and ask you to summarise back your drug chart and ask you to answer some direct questions.

A summary of Clarice's drug chart is shown below:

MANOR PARK NHS FOUNDATION TRUST WARD DRUG CHART	Mrs. Clarice 6579-091A 3-4-1956		Allergy status:			
				23/9/16	24/9/16	25/9/16
REGUALAR MEDICATIONS	Paracetamol 1g qds	6	*			
		12	*			
		18	*			
		22	*			
PRN MEDICATIONS	Morphine PCA 1mg bolus 5 minute lockout No background infusion	6	*			
		12	*			
		18	*			
		22	*			

Case 24

You are the Foundation Year1 doctor on your Anaesthetics rotation. Your consultant has asked you to assist in recovery where a patient from your list needs a blood transfusion following their elective colorectal procedure. The patient is haemodynamically stable and has a haemoglobin level of 75g/L.

Your consultant has prescribed 1 unit of packed red cells to be transfused. You are required to check and administer the blood with a member of staff in recovery.

After 6 minutes the examiner will stop you and ask you to summarise back your case, and ask you to answer some direct questions.

Case 25

Michelle is a 26-year-old woman who has returned to the Gastroenterology ward following a colonoscopy under sedation.

You are a Foundation Year doctor on the ward and you have been called over by the nurse, who is unhappy that Michelle seems very drowsy and is snoring. Her respiratory rate is 6 breaths/minute.

Please use the mannequin to demonstrate the manoeuvers you would perform and equipment you would use to support her airway.

Orthopaedics & Rheumatology

Case 1
A 40-year-old rugby player comes to orthopaedic clinic with a troublesome shoulder. He has experienced multiple episodes of dislocation always during rugby matches. Most of these episodes have been treated with reduction on the field however the most recent episode last week required sedation in the emergency department. He is concerned about ongoing feelings of instability.

Please take and a focused history and present your findings to the examiner along with a management plan.

You have 6 minutes to take the history before being asked to summarise your findings to the examiner.

Case 2
A 70-year-old male, retired builder has presented to orthopaedic clinics with bilateral hip and groin pain for months – now worsening in the past few weeks. He complains that he is struggling to get in and out of his car to go to the shops. Recently he has had difficulty talking his grandchildren to the park.

You are the foundation year doctor. Please take and a focused history and present your findings to the examiner along with a management plan.

You have 6 minutes to take the history before being asked to summarise your findings to the examiner.

Case 3
A 47-year old female has been referred by her GP to the orthopaedic hand clinic with a 3-month history of right hand and wrist pain which has failed to settle with activity modification and splinting.

You are the foundation year doctor. Please take and a focused history and present your findings to the examiner along with a management plan.

You have 6 minutes to take the history before being asked to summarise your findings to the examiner.

Case 4
A 25-year-old male has been referred by her GP to rheumatology clinic with a 9-month history of lower back pain. He has been using regular painkillers and sought his GP's attention due to a failure of his symptoms to resolve.

You are the foundation year doctor in the clinic. Please take and a focused history and present your findings to the examiner along with a management plan.

You have 6 minutes to take the history before being asked to summarise your findings to the examiner.

Case 5
A 75-year-old female has self-presented to the emergency department with a 2-month history of thoraco-lumbar spine pain. She has been using regular over-the-counter pain-killers but hasn't sought her GP's attention for her complaint.

You are the foundation year doctor in the clinic. Please take and a focused history and present your findings to the examiner along with a management plan.

You have 6 minutes to take the history before being asked to summarise your findings to the examiner.

Case 6
A patient has been referred by her GP to rheumatology with a 6-month history of lower back pain. They have been prescribed naproxen by their GP which hasn't settled their symptoms.

You are the foundation year doctor in the clinic and have been asked to examine the patient's gait, arms, legs and spine (GALS) and then summarize your examination findings back to the team.

After 6 minutes the examiner will stop you and ask you to summarise back your findings, suggest your differential diagnoses and your initial management plan.

Case 7

A 60-year-old male patient presents to see you in an Orthopaedic elective clinic appointment complaining of restricted range of movement in the shoulder for 6 months. He reports previous shoulder dislocations as a young rugby player which were reduced in the emergency department but no surgery required. He denies neck pain or weakness and sensory disturbance distal to the shoulder.

You are the foundation year doctor in the Orthopaedic clinic and have been asked to examine his shoulder.

After 6 minutes the examiner will stop you and ask you to summarise back your findings, suggest your differential diagnoses and your initial management plan.

Case 8

A 60-year-old female patient presents to see you in a GP clinic appointment complaining of left hip and groin pain which is restricting her gardening. She has been troubled by the pain for 2 years.

You are the foundation year doctor in the GP practice and have been asked to examine her hip.

After 6 minutes the examiner will stop you and ask you to summarise back your findings, suggest your differential diagnoses and your initial management plan.

Case 9

A 30-year-old female patient presents to see you in a GP clinic appointment complaining of knee pain and locking following a twisting injury during football.

You are the foundation year doctor in the GP practice and have been asked to examine her knee then summarize your examination findings back to the team.

After 6 minutes the examiner will stop you and ask you to summarise back your findings, suggest your differential diagnoses and your initial management plan.

Case 10

A 40-year-old female patient presents to the Emergency Department with severe lower back pain or acute onset when diving into a swimming pool. She has had back pain for 6 months and previously been seen by physiotherapists with some benefit. This acute pain presents with a central lower back pain and pain radiating down her right leg. She is able to weight bear but describes pins and needles in her right foot.

You are the foundation year doctor in the Emergency Department and have been asked to examine her back.

After 6 minutes the examiner will stop you and ask you to summarise back your findings, suggest your differential diagnoses and your initial management plan.

Case 11

A 70-year-old female patient presents to see you in a GP clinic appointment complaining of bilateral pain around the big toe and difficulty with some footwear. This pain has been a problem for a long time but worsened over 6 months.

You are the foundation year doctor in the GP practice and have been asked to examine her hand then summarize your examination findings back to the examiner.

After 6 minutes the examiner will stop you and ask you to summarise back your findings, suggest your differential diagnoses and your initial management plan.

Case 12

A 40-year-old female patient presents to the emergency department with severe neck pain of acute onset after a low energy collision as the driver of a car. Her neck pain is constant, severe and radiates down her right arm. On and off she reports tingling sensation in the arm.

You are the foundation year doctor in the emergency department and have been asked to perform a neurological examination of her upper limbs then summarize your examination findings back to the examiner.

After 6 minutes the examiner will stop you and ask you to summarise back your findings, suggest your differential diagnoses and your initial management plan

Case 13

An 85-year-old female has been brought into the Emergency Department having been found on the floor by her residential home warden. She has been unable to walk and is complaining of pain in the left hip.

You are the emergency department doctor working in the majors area and have been asked to review the radiographs. Review the radiographs and present your findings to the examiner along with an appropriate management plan.

There will be questions from the examiner following your presentation.

Case 14

You are a foundation year doctor currently working in rheumatology and help with the weekly metabolic bone clinic. A new clinical nurse specialist has just started working with the team. She has seen a complicated patient in clinic and would like to discuss the blood results. The consultant is not around and she has asked for your advice. Please discuss the results with her and help come up with an appropriate management plan.

Mr David West
DW987654
DOB; 17/7/40

The results are below with reference ranges in brackets:

Sodium (Na+)	136mmol/L (135-145mmol/L)
Potassium (K+)	4.6mmol/L (3.5-5.0mmol/L)
Creatinine(Creat)	670µmol/L (71-115 µmol/L)
Calcium (Ca++)	2.21mmol/L (2.15-2.6mmol/L)
Albumin	40g/L (35-50g/L)
Alkaline phosphatase (ALP)	293 IU/L (30-130 IU/L)
Phosphate	2.06mmol/L (0.8-1.4mmol/L)
PTH	1050 ng/L (10-70ng/L)

Case 15

You are the foundation year doctor on the orthopaedic team. You have been called to theatre to assist in a total hip replacement surgery.

Scrub up and put on a gown and surgical gloves.

Following this there will be some questions from the examiner.

Case 16

A 25-year-old walks into the Emergency Department shortly after being involved in a road traffic accident resulting in him being thrown from his motorcycle. He is complaining of neck pain.

The patient has been taken to the resuscitation area of the ED and a trauma call declared. You are the orthopaedic foundation year doctor and have been asked to immobilise the patient's cervical spine.

Another member of the trauma team is available to assist you if require.

Case 17

You are the SHO on call overnight in a busy DGH. You are called to see a young male patient who has undergone tibial nailing today for a closed NV intact tibial shaft fracture. The nurses are concerned that they can't keep him comfortable and have asked you for more analgesia.

Your brief assessment can include a short focused history, examinations for key signs and will include radiograph interpretation.

There will be some questions from the examiner following this.

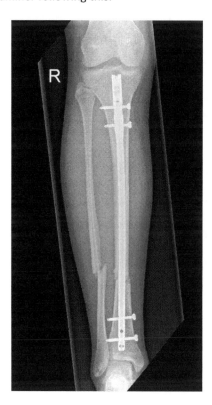

Case 18

You are on the trauma team at the major trauma centre for the area. A young adult male, not yet identified, has been brought in by HEMS following RTA. He has multiple injuries including a tibial shaft fracture with a large contaminated open wound. There is considerable skin loss and fat, muscle and bone is visible.

Your brief assessment can include a short focused history, examinations for key signs and will include radiograph interpretation.

There will be some questions from the examiner following this.

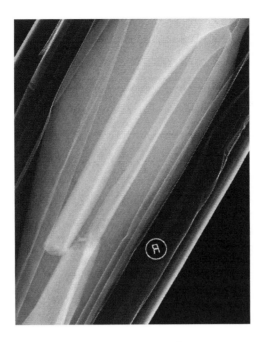

Case 19

A 19-year-old man is brought into the emergency department by the police. You have been informed he has been stabbed in his arm approximately 2 hours ago. He is complaining his hand feels cold and numb.

You are the foundation year 2 doctor in accident and emergency who has been asked to assess him and report your findings and management plan to your consultant. Your brief assessment can include a short focused history, examinations for key signs.

Once you approach the patient you see that he has sustained a deep laceration to the antecubital fossa.

There will be some questions from the examiner following this.

Case 20

A 95-year-old lady has been brought up to the orthopaedic ward from the emergency department. She is normally a nursing home resident and was found by her carers on the floor. She is complaining of pain and is disorientated in time and place.

The patient has had a hip x-ray in accident and emergency. An AMTS has been done which is 6/10. The nurses have done a set of observations.

You are the foundation year doctor on call for trauma and orthopaedics and have been asked to clerk her in. Your brief assessment can include a short focused history, examinations for key signs and will include radiograph interpretation.

Observations
BP 110/70 HR 105   RR 18   Sats 90%

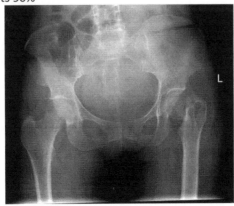

Case 21

A 56-year-old man has been brought by ambulance to the Emergency Department following falling from a ladder at a height of 3m.

You are the orthopaedic doctor in the trauma team and have been asked to perform a primary survey. Your brief assessment can include a short focused history, examinations for key signs and will include data interpretation.

There will be some questions from the examiner following this.

Case 22

A fit and healthy 21-year-old woman was admitted late last night with a broken ankle. She was placed in a temporary backslab and is on the trauma operating list today for "open reduction and internal fixation of the right ankle" where the fracture will be fixed with a small metal plate a series of screws.

You are the foundation year doctor in the orthopaedic team. Having seen this operation several times before your Consultant has asked you to go through the consent process with the patient. You will also need to answer any questions that patient may have.

You have 6 minutes to complete the task before being asked to summarise your consultation to the examiner.

Case 23

A fit and healthy 21-year-old woman was admitted 2 days ago with broken ankle she underwent surgery to fix the broken ankle (open reduction and internal fixation) yesterday and is due to be discharged home non-weight bearing in a plaster cast (below her knee).

You are the foundation year doctor in the orthopaedic team and have been asked to discharge the patient. The patient would like to know more information about preventing deep vein thrombosis (DVT) prior to going home.

You have 6 minutes to complete the task before being asked to summarise your consultation to the examiner.

Case 24

A 78-year-old woman recently fell on an outstretched hand and suffered from a distal radius fracture. She was seen in fracture clinic where they opted for conservative management. Given that the fracture occurred without significant trauma, the orthopaedic team have advised that she starts on a bisphosphonate. They have advised her to see her GP to start the medication.

You are the foundation year doctor working in general practice. Please discuss the medication with the patient and address any concerns.

You have 6 minutes to complete the task before being asked to summarise your consultation to the examiner.

Case 25

A 30-year-old woman was referred to the rheumatology clinic with an 8-week history of joint pain and swelling affecting the hands, wrists and knees bilaterally. The history and examination was suggestive of inflammatory arthritis and she was sent for further investigations. Blood tests showed a strongly positive anti-CCP antibody and ultrasound confirmed active synovitis at the wrists and MCP joints bilaterally. She has returned to clinic today to get the results and discuss the next steps.

You are the foundation year doctor in clinic and have been asked to explain the diagnosis and discuss the next steps with the patient.

You have 6 minutes to complete the task before being asked to summarise your consultation to the examiner.

Psychiatry

Case 1

You are a foundation year doctor in a GP practice. A 45-year-old supermarket cashier called Annabel attends with bleeding gums from excessive tooth brushing. She is not previously known to the practice.

Please take a history from this patient. You have 7 minutes, after which you will be asked to summarise and provide a management plan.

Case 2

You are a foundation year doctor working on a secure psychiatric ward, you have been asked by the nursing staff to come and speak with Rafael. He is the son of one of your patients and you have been warned that he appears angry.

Please meet with Rafael to explore his concerns. You have 8 minutes.

Case 3

A 25-year-old lady called Phoebe attends the emergency department (ED) following an episode of deliberate self-harm (DSH).

She has been medically cleared by the ED registrar who informs you that she has a known history of Emotionally unstable personality disorder (EUPD).

You are the foundation doctor on the liaison psychiatry team and have been asked by your registrar to take a history from the patient, with a view to forming a differential diagnosis and management plan.

You have seven minutes to take the history followed by one minute of questions.

Case 4

A 23-year-old lady called Ling has presented to the emergency department accompanied with her friend, who is concerned that she has been 'out of sorts'.

You are a foundation doctor working in the emergency department and have been asked by your consultant to take a brief history and Mental state examination (MSE) from the patient.

You have 6 minutes to take your history after which you will be asked to summarise the MSE and provide an initial management plan.

Case 5

A 27-year-old man called Kryz has been brought into the emergency department by the police on Section 136. He was found agitated in the city centre. Police say that he has been talking 'nonsense' and was found climbing onto private property.

You are a foundation doctor in the emergency department and have been asked to perform a Mental State Examination (MSE). You do not need to take a detailed history of the symptoms.

You will be stopped after 5 minutes to summarise the findings of your MSE, provide a differential diagnosis and management plan.

Case 6

You are a foundation doctor in a suburban GP practice where Annie, a 32-year-old lady has come to see you. You can see from the GP records that she has not seen a GP in quite a few years and has no significant past medical history. She did not attend her scheduled GP appointment last week due to 'anxiety'.

You have 7 minutes to take a focused history from this patient and make a primary diagnosis.

Case 7

You have been asked to speak to a 43-year-old male called Liam diagnosed with paranoid schizophrenia 5 years ago. He has already been trialled on 2 different anti-psychotics with little effect. Your consultant reviewed him earlier in the psychiatry outpatient clinic and has advised starting clozapine.

Your colleague has already performed a physical examination, ECG and bloods all of which were normal. Liam has no past medical history and no known drug allergies.

You are the foundation doctor on your psychiatry placement and your consultant has asked you to discuss clozapine treatment with this patient. You have 8 minutes.

Case 8

A 20-year-old lady called Summer has been admitted to the inpatient psychiatric unit following some unusual and reckless behaviour.

You are the foundation doctor based on the ward and have been asked by your consultant to take a history from the patient.

You have 7 minutes to take a history, after which you will be stopped and asked to present your findings and suggest an initial management plan.

Case 9

A 30-year-old lady called Charmaine has been admitted to the inpatient psychiatry ward following her first episode of mania. The consultant wants to start her on lithium to help stabilise her mood.

You are the foundation doctor based on the acute psychiatry ward. Your colleagues have taken a thorough history and Mental State Examination (MSE) and you have been asked to counsel the patient about initiating lithium therapy.

She is an informal patient and has been judged by the consultant to have capacity to consent to medication. You have 7 minutes for your discussion.

Case 10

You are the foundation doctor working on the Endocrine ward. Over the past few weeks, you have noticed that Paul, one of the senior nurses you work with has become more withdrawn and has been behaving strangely. Today, when asking him about a patient's discharge plans, he becomes tearful. You have taken him aside to talk about his feelings.

You have 7 minutes to take a psychiatric history from Paul, after which you will be asked to summarise the case and evaluate his risk

Case 11

A 17-year-old boy called Taylor has been brought into your GP surgery by his mother who is concerned that he is behaving oddly as he has become antisocial and irritable. His mother has decided not to be present during the consultation as she feels her son will be more open without her there.

You are a foundation doctor based at the GP practice and you have been asked to take a history from the patient.

You have 7 minutes to take the history, followed by 1 minute to summarise your findings and initial management plan back to the patient.

Case 12

You are a foundation doctor in the emergency department and you have been asked to examine a 48-year-old lady called Violet who came in via ambulance from the psychiatric inpatient unit.

You have been handed over by the paramedics that she has a diagnosis of schizoaffective disorder and she has recently been started on daily haloperidol injections.
She is unwell and is in Resus. You do not need to take a history. Please talk out loud during your examination.

You will be stopped after 6 minutes to give a diagnosis, initial investigations and a management plan.

Case 13
You are a foundation year doctor on your GP placement. You are seeing your own patients this morning. The first patient is 52-year-old Roya.

Please take a history. You will be stopped after 7 minutes to summarise, and provide a differential diagnosis.

Case 14
You are a foundation year doctor in the emergency department. Your next patient is a 21-year-old male called Ahmed who has been brought to the emergency department by the police after being found acting bizarrely in the middle of a busy street.

Please take a history from Ahmed. You will be stopped by the examiner after 7 minutes to summarise and provide a differential diagnosis.

Case 15
You are a foundation year doctor based at a GP surgery. A 78-year-old man called Albert has attended the practice. His daughter has recommended that he attends as he is becoming more forgetful.

Please take a history. You have 6 minutes to do so, after which you will be asked to summarise the findings and make an initial plan.
Case 16
You are a foundation year doctor working on the acute medical unit (AMU). A 92-year-old man called Reggie has been admitted following a fall at home. His wife has felt that over the past few days he has becoming increasingly confused.

You have 5 minutes to take a collateral history from Mr Hammond's wife after which the examiner will ask you a series of questions.

Case 17
A 78-year-old man called Clifford has presented to the GP accompanied by his 45-year-old daughter. She is concerned that he has been 'out of sorts' recently.

You are the foundation doctor working at the GP surgery and have been asked to take a history from the patient. You have five minutes to take your history followed by two minutes to perform an Abbreviated Mental Test Score (AMTS).

After 7 minutes you will have one minute to present your findings and formulate an initial management plan.

Case 18
You are a foundation doctor working in a busy emergency department. 15-year-old Grace has been brought to see you by her mother. Grace's mother found her crying next to an empty packet of paracetamol and an empty bottle of wine half an hour ago, so took her immediately to the emergency department. She has now admitted to taking the tablets.

Grace's mother has left to answer an urgent phone call and will not be present during the consultation.

Please take a history from the patient. You will be stopped after 7 minutes and asked to summarise and suggest a management plan.

Case 19

You are a foundation year doctor working in the emergency department. A 15-year-old girl called Natalia has attended with a deep laceration on her forearm. The ED nurse practitioner has sutured the wound. The patient has revealed that it is self-inflicted, and the nurse asks you to speak to her.

Please take a history from the patient about her history of self-harm and current risk status. You have 5 minutes to complete the history, after which the examiner will stop you to ask some further questions.

Case 20
You are a foundation year doctor currently on your CAMHS placement. You are asked by your consultant to see your own patients this morning. The first patient is a 16-year-old girl called Sam.

Please take a focused history. You will be stopped after 6 minutes to provide a diagnosis.

Surgery

Case 1

A 72-year-old man has presented to the Emergency department acutely unwell with severe abdominal pain.

You are the foundation year doctor on the surgical team and have been asked to take the initial history and then summarise your findings back to the surgical registrar on-call.

After 6 minutes the examiner will stop you and ask you to summarise back your findings, suggest your differential diagnoses and your initial management plan.

Case 2

A 22-year-old female has been brought into Emergency Department by ambulance with right iliac fossa pain for the last 12 hours.

You are the foundation year doctor on the surgical team and have been asked to take the initial history and then summarise your findings back to the surgical registrar on-call.

After 6 minutes the examiner will stop you and ask you to summarise back your findings, suggest your differential diagnoses and your initial management plan.

Case 3

A 70-year-old man has been referred directly to the on-call surgical registrar by his GP with abdominal pain and vomiting.

You are the foundation year doctor on the surgical team and have been asked to take the initial history and then summarise your findings back to the surgical registrar on-call.

After 6 minutes the examiner will stop you and ask you to summarise back your findings, suggest your differential diagnoses and your initial management plan.

Case 4

A 62-year-old male has presented to the general surgical clinic with difficulty opening his bowels.

You are the foundation year doctor the surgical team and have been asked to take the initial history and then summarise your findings back to your consultant.

After 6 minutes the examiner will stop you and ask you to summarise back your findings, suggest your differential diagnoses and your initial management plan.

Case 5

A 68-year-old female has been brought into Emergency Department by ambulance with haematemesis.

You are the foundation year doctor the surgical team and have been asked to take the initial history and then summarise your findings back to the surgical registrar on-call.

After 6 minutes the examiner will stop you and ask you to summarise back your findings, suggest your differential diagnoses and your initial management plan.

Case 6

A 41-year-old lady with right upper quadrant pain is the next patient to be seen on the surgical take list.

You are the foundation year doctor on the surgical team and have been asked to take the initial history and then summarise your findings back to the surgical registrar on-call.

After 6 minutes the examiner will stop you and ask you to summarise back your findings, suggest your differential diagnoses and your initial management plan.

Case 7

A 68-year-old male has presented to hospital unable to move his left leg.

You are the foundation year doctor on the general surgical team and have been asked to take the initial history and then summarise your findings back to the team.

After 6 minutes the examiner will stop you and ask you to summarise back your findings, suggest your differential diagnoses and your initial management plan.

Case 8

You are the foundation year doctor attached to the GP practice and have been asked to see a 75 year old male who is complaining of intermittent haematuria. You have been asked to take the initial history and then summarise your findings back to your GP Consultant.

After 6 minutes the examiner will stop you and ask you to summarise back your findings, suggest your differential diagnoses and your initial management plan.

Case 9

You have been asked to see a 27-year-old male who is complaining of a dull ache in his left testicle.

You are the foundation year doctor on the urology team and have been asked to take the initial history and then summarise your findings back to the surgical registrar on-call.
After 6 minutes the examiner will stop you and ask you to summarise back your findings, suggest your differential diagnoses and your initial management plan.

Case 10

A 49-year-old female has attended her General Practice clinic with a lump in her right breast. You are the foundation year doctor and have been asked to take the initial history and then summarise your findings back to the GP Consultant.

After 6 minutes the examiner will stop you and ask you to summarise back your findings, suggest your differential diagnoses and your initial management plan.

Case 11

You are the foundation year doctor in the in general surgery. Jack is an 80-year-old man who underwent an emergency repair of an incarcerated inguinal hernia 2 days ago. Prior to surgery he lived independently with his wife with no medical history apart from hypertension. The ward nursing staff has contacted your team because he is allegedly confused. Your registrar has asked you to obtain a history to the best of your abilities in order to assess their mental status.

After 6 minutes the examiner will stop you and ask you to summarise back your findings, suggest your differential diagnoses and your initial management plan.

Case 12

You are the foundation year doctor in the surgical assessment unit. John is a 60-year-old man who has been reviewed with intermittent rectal bleeding. He is to be invited back to the endoscopy unit for a flexible sigmoidoscopy to investigate this. This will occur in the next two weeks.

You have been asked by your registrar to explain the procedure 'flexible sigmoidoscopy 'to the patient.

Case 13

You are the foundation year doctor in the surgical assessment unit. Samantha is the 35-year-old mother of Tom a 9-year-old child who is currently being operated on for an emergency splenic rupture. He was with his father when he apparently fell from off his bicycle.

She is very upset and the nursing staff has asked you to speak with her and address her concerns.

Case 14

You are the foundation year doctor on the general surgical team. David has been admitted under your consultant's care. He is a 57 year old gentleman who has presented with severe gallstone pancreatitis. He has severe epigastric pain radiating to his back, which is not being controlled by regular oral analgesics and PRN IV morphine.
Latest observations are:

Temperature   38.2
Heart Rate   120bpm
Blood pressure   105/65
Respiratory Rate   26 per minute

You have performed an arterial blood gas as he appeared to be becoming more breathless on air

pH 7.33   PO2 7.9
PCO2 3.5   Lac 4.3
HCO3 24

His recent blood results are:

WCC 18.6   Urea 13.2
ALT 253   LDH 420
Ca 1.9   Alb 28
Glu 7.8

After discussing the case with your senior who is in theatre, you have have been asked to contact the ITU registrar for advice and review.
The ITU on-call registrar is on the phone.

Case 15
You are a foundation doctor working in the Emergency Department. A 71-year-old man was brought in an hour ago as a trauma call. He was a restrained driver of a car who crashed into a tree at 45 mph. He has had a full primary and secondary survey and has just come back from a CT scan to the resuscitation department. The CT shows the only injury sustained is a right-sided pneumothorax and you have just reviewed these images yourself. The Emergency Department consultant has said he'll supervise and assist you putting in your first surgical chest drain.
Before starting the procedure tell the consultant what equipment you will need, and how you wish to prepare the patient. Then turn to the patient and insert the chest drain.

Case 16

You are the foundation year doctor in general surgery. A 72-year-old female patient with a background of relapsing remitting multiple sclerosis presents to the acute surgical take. She describes severe generalised abdominal pain. You request an abdominal radiograph to investigate for an underlying cause. You are now asked by the consultant on the post take ward round to describe the abdominal radiograph in a systematic manner, assemble a differential diagnosis and management plan for this patient.

Abdominal plain radiograph examples for Interpretation:

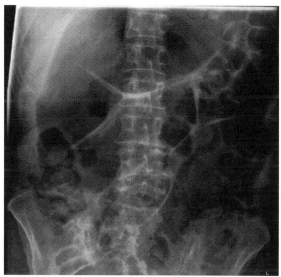

Example one

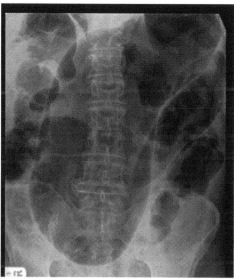

Example two

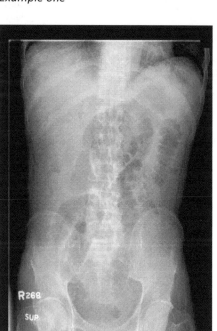

Example three

Case 17

You are the foundation year doctor in general surgery. A 72-year-old presents with severe generalised abdominal pain with shortness of breath on exertion. You request an erect chest radiograph to investigate for an underlying cause.

You are now asked by the consultant on the post take ward round to describe the chest radiograph in a systematic manner, assemble a differential diagnosis and management plan for this patient.

Chest plain radiograph examples for Interpretation

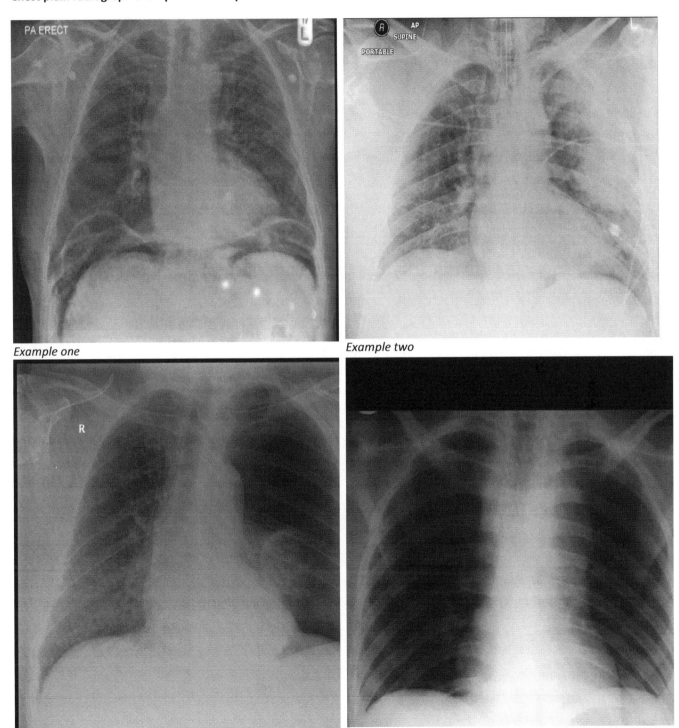

Example one

Example two

Example 3

Example four

Case 18

You are the foundation year doctor on the surgical team. A 25-year-old man named James presents with a laceration to the dorsum of his hand after cutting it against a can.

Perform an appropriate examination of the injury and close the wound using three interrupted sutures. Explain any further management.

After 6 minutes the examiner will stop you and ask you to summarise back what you have done and ask you a direct question.

Case 19

You are an foundation year doctor working in General Surgery. You receive a call from your Registrar, who is in theatre, asking you to examine the abdomen of Reuben who is a 50 year old man in the Surgical Admissions Unit. The patient was seen earlier in the day by their GP and referred directly to the surgical team with an acute abdomen. He has central severe pain, which started suddenly four hours ago.

Explain to the examiner what you are doing as you conduct your abdominal examination. The examiner will provide you with the clinical findings that you request.

Case 20

A 78-year-old man is referred to clinic with a large mass in his left groin. He does not describe any associated pain, nausea or vomiting. The patient is usually in good health, and is keen to be discharged from hospital.

You are the foundation year doctor on the surgical team and have been asked to examine the hernia, and present your findings to the examiner.

Case 21

You are the foundation year doctor attending a Breast Surgical Clinic. Your consultant has asked you to perform a breast examination on Clarissa, a 49-year-old who has a lump in her right breast. Explain to the examiner what you are doing as you conduct your examination.

Please note that in the exam it is possible that you are given a model to perform the breast examination. But you will need to speak to the actor as though you are performing the examination on her.

Case 22

A 35-year-old woman has attended her GP practice complaining of anxiety and fatigue. You are the foundation year doctor on rotation and your GP supervisor asks you to do a full thyroid examination and present your findings.

You have 6 minutes after which you will be asked to summarise your findings and asked two questions about the examination.

Case 23

You have been asked to see a 54-year-old male who is complaining of an abnormal lump and an uncomfortable dragging sensation in his left testis. You are the foundation doctor on the General Surgical Team and have been asked by your consultant to examine this patient. Please report your findings to the examiner.

Case 24

You are a foundation doctor working in the emergency department. A man is brought into resuscitation department, following a traumatic road traffic accident. You assess the patient along with an ED registrar, and an experienced ED nurse who will assist with tasks.

Your registrar requests you conduct the primary survey. Talk the examiner through how you would perform this and they will provide you with the clinical findings/observations/investigation results.

Case 25

You have been asked to see a 72-year-old woman, who has presented to the vascular clinic complaining of pain in her calves on walking.

You are the foundation doctor on vascular team and have been asked by your consultant to conduct an examination of the peripheral vasculature. Please report your findings back to the examiner.

Emergency medicine

Case 1
You are a foundation doctor working in the Emergency Department of a district general hospital. An ambulance is on its way with a 27-year-old male cyclist who was hit by a car. His C-spine has been immobilised by the ambulance team.
Please assess this patient, stating any interventions you would like to perform as you go along.

Case 2
You are a foundation doctor working in the Emergency Department when you discover a 60-year-old unresponsive male in a cubicle. Assess and manage this patient according to the principles of Advanced Life Support.
After 6 minutes the examiner will stop you and ask you to summarise back your findings and your management plan.

Case 3
You are the foundation doctor on call for general medicine. The crash bleep goes off and tells you that there is an arrest on the ward next to yours. You are the first of the crash team to arrive on the ward.

Case 4
You are the foundation doctor in the Emergency Department in the resus area overnight. A 19-year-old man gets brought in by ambulance after being picked up outside a kebab shop where they have reported difficulty in breathing. They have also been noted to have developed a widespread rash and prominent lip swelling.

The ambulance crew hand over that they don't think there is any Past medical history.
Please assess and manage this patient.

Case 5
You are a foundation doctor in the Emergency Department who has been asked to see this 35-year-old asthmatic who has been brought around by the triage nurse. The nurse informs you he is an office worker who had just walked in and was found to have oxygen saturations of 93% and is struggling to complete sentences.
Please take a short history and examine the patient. Start treatment as appropriate.

Case 6
You are the foundation doctor working in the Emergency Department. A 24-year-old university student has just been brought into the ED with profuse vomiting for the past 12 hours. He had been at a barbeque with friends yesterday enjoying a few beers and some food. He had gone to bed early after 'not feeling quite right'. He thought he might have had a few too many drinks but he awoke at 2am with abdominal pain and perfuse vomiting. You have a nurse with you to help.

An arterial blood gas has been done:
pH 7.22
PCO2 3.2
PO2 17
Bicarbonate 5.8
Base excess -25
Na 147
K 6.2
Glucose 32
Lactate 6

Take a focused history from the patient and perform an initial assessment. Decide on a likely diagnosis, discuss this with the nurse and give a plan for any urgent investigations and treatment required, along with treatment goals. Ensure you complete the fluid prescription chart if any fluids are required.

Case 7

A 25-year-old man is brought into the Emergency Department having a generalised tonic-clonic seizure, which started 15 minutes ago. The paramedic team have been unable to secure IV access but have administered one dose of rectal diazepam 10 minutes ago. The patient has no past medical history and does not take any regular medication.

You are the foundation doctor on the acute medical take and have been called to the Emergency Department to manage this patient. You have an experienced staff nurse with you to help.

After 6 minutes the examiner will stop you and ask you to summarise back your findings, suggest your differential diagnoses and your management plan from here on.

Case 8

You are a foundation doctor working in the resuscitation area of the emergency department when a new patient arrives. A 62-year-old lady has been referred in by the GP with 'abnormal blood results'.

Her past medical history includes congestive cardiac failure, chronic kidney disease, hypertension and gout.
Perform an initial assessment A through E assessment correcting any abnormalities as you go.

Case 9

You are the foundation doctor in the Emergency Department. You have been asked to see this 24-year-old lady who has presented with shortness of breath. Please take a full history.

After 6 minutes the examiner will stop you and ask you to summarise back your findings, suggest your differential diagnoses and your initial management plan.

Case 10

You are the foundation doctor working in the emergency department. You pick up the notes for the next patient to be seen and the presenting complaint states 'headache'. The patient is a 24-year-old female called Gaby Howard with no previous ED attendances. Take a full history from the patient and address any concerns she has.

After 6 minutes the examiner will stop you and ask you to summarise back your findings, suggest your differential diagnoses and your initial management plan.

Case 11

You are a foundation year doctor working in the Emergency Department and have been asked to see this patient by your consultant. A 45-year-old male patient has attended the following an innocuous head injury at home. He currently has a GCS of 15 and walked into the department.

Please take a focused history and advise the patient about your management plan.

After 6 minutes the examiner will stop you and ask you to summarise back your findings, suggest your differential diagnoses and your initial management plan.

Case 12

You are the foundation doctor in the Emergency Department. Your next patient, 25-year-old James, has been brought in by his friends. They tell the triage nurse they found him unconscious at home with empty bottles of vodka and paracetamol packets around him. He is now alert but refusing to talk to the triage nurse. Please take a full history.

After 6 minutes the examiner will stop you and ask you to summarise back your findings, suggest your differential diagnoses and your initial management plan.

Case 13

You are the foundation doctor in the Emergency Department in the majors area. You have been asked by your consultant to see a 54-year-old man has been brought to the ED with a PR bleed. Currently the man is haemodynamically stable but reports feeling nauseous and seeing fresh red blood coming from the back passage. Please take a full history.

After 6 minutes the examiner will stop you and ask you to summarise back your findings, suggest your differential diagnoses and your initial management plan.

Case 14

You are the foundation doctor in the Emergency Department in the majors area and have been asked to see a 25-year-old man who has collapsed today. Please take a full history.

After 6 minutes the examiner will stop you and ask you to summarise back your findings, suggest your differential diagnoses and your initial management plan.

Case 15

You are the foundation doctor in the Emergency Department in the majors area.

A 66-year-old lady has presented to the ED because she has been feeling unwell since getting back from holiday in Australia a week ago. She has had a chesty cough for a few days and awoke this morning shaking and unable to get warm, she is also feeling a bit breathless. She has no history of lung disease or smoking. She is normally fit and well and was swimming daily in the hot springs in Australia while away.

Perform a respiratory examination on this patient and present your findings to the examiner. Outline any bedside investigations that should be performed and how you will manage this patient in the ED.

Case 16

You are the foundation doctor in the Emergency Department in the majors area.

A 69-year-old female patient has been brought into the Emergency Department by ambulance after collapsing outside a shopping centre.

Please examine her cardiovascular system. After 6 minutes the examiner will stop you and ask you to summarise back your findings.

Case 17

You are the foundation doctor in the Emergency Department resus area and have been asked to see a 65-year-old man who has been brought in by ambulance complaining of left sided chest pain and shortness of breath.

The senior registrar in ED asks you to undertake the initial structured assessment. You are asked to report your findings and management plan at each stage to the team. You have 6 minutes to complete your assessment.

After 6 minutes the examiner will stop you and ask for a diagnosis. A competent nurse is assisting you.

Case 18

You are the foundation doctor in the Emergency Department in the majors area. A 30-year-old man self-presents to ED with severe right sided loin pain.

Please take a full history.

After 6 minutes the examiner will stop you and ask you to summarise back your findings, suggest your differential diagnoses and your initial management plan.

Case 19

You are the foundation doctor in the Emergency Department in the minors area.

A 39-year-old gentleman presents to ED after developing severe lower lumbar back pain with associated left sided lower limb numbness and feels he is having difficulties mobilising over the last 5 days. He has had ongoing back issues since having lumbar spinal surgery when he was 25 after a rugby accident.

After 6 minutes the examiner will stop you and ask you to summarise back your findings, suggest your differential diagnoses and your initial management plan

Case 20

You are the foundation doctor in the Emergency Department in the majors area.

You have been asked to perform a cerebellar examination on a 48-year-old male who presents with severe dizziness, sickness, and instability on his feet. You need to ascertain whether this is a cerebellar or labyrinthine disorder as this will affect the management.

After 6 minutes the examiner will stop you and ask you to summarise back your findings, suggest your differential diagnoses and your initial management plan.

Case 21

You are the foundation doctor working in the Emergency Department. A colleague has already taken a history from this patient but is called away so asks you to examine his knee.

He is a 24-year-old man has been brought to the Emergency department with a painful swollen knee sustained after being tackled by another player whilst playing football yesterday - the other's player's boot went into his left knee. Since then he has had pain on the inside of his left knee and is finding it difficult to walk. Today he woke up and his knee was more swollen so he has come to the ED.

Case 22

You are the foundation doctor in the Emergency Department and you are asked to see a 50-year-old woman has self-presented to ED with left shoulder pain after falling from her bicycle onto her left shoulder earlier that day. She is complaining of pain and restricted movements. Please perform a full shoulder examination, you do not need to take a history.

After 6 minutes the examiner will ask you to present your findings and provide the most likely diagnosis.

Case 23

You are the foundation doctor in the resuscitation room of the ED and have been asked if a final year medical student can shadow you for the day.

The team has received a priority call informing them that a female patient with a reduced GCS is expected to arrive in the department shortly. She is reported to be heavily intoxicated with no evidence of any injuries.
Using the equipment provided explain to the student the basics of airway management. Include in your teaching, basic airway manoeuvres, as well as the selection and insertion of airway adjuncts and devices. You should demonstrate how you would escalate your control of an airway if your initial techniques were unsuccessful.

For the purpose of this station the attachment of oxygen and demonstration of intubation is not required.

Case 24

You are the foundation year doctor in the Emergency Department working in the majors area and the nurse asks you to see a 67-year-old man with significant abdominal pain who has not passed urine for 12 hours.

Perform a quick history and examination, and explain your next steps in the management. The patient will need a catheter so you will have to prepare for this and insert one using the provided model.

Case 25

You are the foundation year doctor in the Emergency Department working in the resus area.

You have just assessed John, a 66-year-old man with 2 days history of worsening shortness of breath on a background history of COPD who has been brought in by ambulance. He is breathing oxygen at 15L per minute via non re-breathe bag.

Please analyse the following arterial blood gas and explain your findings to a medical student who is shadowing you today.

ABG
Name: John
Date of birth: 10/04/1950
Date: 15/09/2016, Time 10:26 am

PH –   7.150
PO2 –   12.9
PCO2 –   9.7
HCO3 –   39
Base excess : +10.5

Obstetrics & Gynaecology

Case 1

You are the Foundation Year Doctor in the Gynaecology outpatient clinic. Huda is a 26-year-old woman presenting with a history of painful periods. Please take a history but you do not need to examine the patient.

After 6 minutes the examiner will stop you and ask you to summarise back your findings, suggest your management plan and answer some direct questions.

Case 2

You are the Foundation Year Doctor in the Gynaecology outpatient clinic. Celeste is a 34-year-old woman presenting with a history of heavy menstrual bleeding. Please take a history but you do not need to examine the patient.

After 6 minutes the examiner will stop you and ask you to summarise back your findings, suggest your management plan and answer some direct questions.

Case 3

You are the Foundation Year Doctor in the Emergency Department. Martha is a 24-year-old woman who has presented with lower abdominal pain and discharge. Please take a focused gynaecological and sexual history. You do not need to examine the patient.

After 6 minutes the examiner will stop you and ask you to summarise back your findings, suggest your management plan and answer some direct questions.

Case 4

You are the Foundation Year Doctor in the Gynaecology outpatient clinic. Ellie is a 34-year-old woman who has been referred by her GP for difficulty conceiving. Please take a history but you do not need to examine the patient.

After 6 minutes the examiner will stop you and ask you to summarise back your findings, suggest your management plan and answer some direct questions.

Case 5

You are the Foundation Year Doctor in the General Obstetrics Clinic. Natalie is a 27-year-old woman who is 30 weeks pregnant and has been referred by her GP due to ongoing pruritus. Please take a history but you do not need to examine the patient.

After 6 minutes the examiner will stop you and ask you to summarise back your findings, suggest your management plan and answer some direct questions.

Case 6

You are the Foundation Year Doctor in the Maternity Triage Unit. Kiran is a 27-year-old woman who is 32 weeks pregnant and has presented with vaginal bleeding. Please take a history but you do not need to examine the patient.

After 6 minutes the examiner will stop you and ask you to summarise back your findings, suggest your management plan and answer some direct questions.

Case 7

You are the Foundation Year Doctor in a GP practice. Winona is a 32-year-old woman who has presented feeling generally unwell 5 days after giving birth. Please take a history but you do not need to examine the patient.

After 6 minutes the examiner will stop you and ask you to summarise back your findings, suggest your management plan and answer some direct questions.

Case 8

You are the Foundation Year Doctor in a GP practice. Yee is a 29-year-old woman who has come in for her 6 weeks after giving birth. Please complete her 6-week postnatal check.

You do not need to examine the patient, although please describe to the examiner what you wish to assess. You do not need to assess the baby.

After 6 minutes the examiner will stop you and ask you to summarise back your findings, suggest your management plan and answer some direct questions.

Case 9

You are the Foundation Year Doctor in a GP practice. Kyra is a 25-year-old woman who is due to have her first cervical smear and has booked a double appointment. Please explain the procedure in order to take verbal consent and discuss any concerns she may have.

You do not need to examine the patient or demonstrate the procedure.
You have eight minutes.

Case 10

You are the Foundation Year Doctor in the Gynaecology Clinic. Frances is a 58-year-old woman who has been experiencing postmenopausal bleeding. A transvaginal ultrasound showed a slightly thickened endometrium. She is to have an urgent hysteroscopy and you have been asked by your consultant to explain this procedure to her and discuss her concerns.

You do not need to examine the patient.
You have eight minutes.

Case 11

You are the Foundation Year Doctor in a GP surgery. Megan is a first year student midwife who has just started her community placement today. The practice midwife has just called in sick and your trainer has asked if you could talk to Megan about the mechanisms and stages of birth.
You may use the model pelvis and doll available to you.
You have eight minutes.

Case 12

You are the Foundation Year Doctor in a GP surgery. Sia is 25-year-old woman who has presented with PV discharge and intermittent bleeding. You have been asked to perform a cervical smear and bimanual examination. She has already been consented for the procedure.

Please use the model provided.
You have eight minutes.

Case 13

You are the Foundation Year Doctor in the General Obstetrics clinic. Lucy is 28-year-old woman who is currently 28 weeks pregnant. She has come in for a routine check. You have been asked to perform an examination of her pregnant abdomen. Please present your findings to the examiner and discuss.

Please use the mannequin provided.
You have eight minutes.

Case 14

You are the Foundation Year Doctor in a GP surgery. Gina is a 35-year-old woman who has been sent a letter asking to attend a routine appointment at her GP surgery due to abnormal smear results. You have the results that states:

Mild dyskaryosis, HPV positive.

Please counsel the patient regarding investigation and follow up in view of these findings and answer any questions she may have.

You do not need to examine the patient.
You have eight minutes.

Case 15

You are the Foundation Year Doctor in a GP surgery. Celia is an 18-year-old woman who has asked to speak to you about starting the oral contraceptive pill. Please counsel the patient regarding the oral contraceptive pill and answer any questions she may have. Please also ask a focused history to elicit suitability for the chosen method of contraception.

You do not need to examine the patient.
You have eight minutes.

Case 16

You are the Foundation Year Doctor in the Genitourinary Medicine (GUM) clinic. Marc is a 19-year-old man who has come in for a routine STI screen after having had unprotected sexual intercourse with a casual partner. Please take a focused history and counsel this patient for a HIV test. You do not need to examine the patient.
You have ten minutes.

Case 17

You are the Foundation Year Doctor in the Genitourinary Medicine (GUM) clinic. David is a 27-year-old man who was diagnosed with HIV in a routine STI check and informed last week at the clinic. He has come back today for follow up. Please answer any questions he may have, but you do not need to examine the patient.
You have ten minutes.

Case 18

You are the Foundation Year Doctor in a GP surgery. Avanti is a 24-year-old woman who has requested an urgent appointment as she has recently discovered she is pregnant. Please discuss the patient's concerns and how she wishes to proceed with the pregnancy.
You do not need to examine the patient.
You have eight minutes.

Case 19

You are the Foundation Year Doctor at a GP surgery. You have been asked to see Gloria, a 25-year-old Nigerian woman who is intending on starting a family. She is a known carrier of sickle cell disease and would like to discuss how this will impact her pregnancy. Please counsel her and discuss her concerns.

You do not need to examine the patient.
You have eight minutes.

Case 20

You are the Foundation Year Doctor at a GP surgery. Heidi is a 30-year-old pregnant woman who has made an appointment to discuss the whooping cough vaccination. Please counsel her about the vaccination and discuss any concerns she may have.

You do not need to examine the patient.
You have eight minutes.

Medicine

Case 1
You are the foundation year doctor on call for medicine. You have been called urgently to the acute medical unit to assess a patient who has suddenly become short of breath, wheezy and developed a rash.
With 2 minutes remaining the examiner will stop you and ask you to summarise your findings and ask you some direct questions.

Case 2
You are the foundation year doctor on the admitting medical team. You have been asked to assess a gentleman in the emergency department that the triage nurse is concerned about. The patient is an elderly gentleman who has been admitted generally unwell, confused and pyrexial. The district nurse changed his long-term catheter yesterday. His family say that he was well yesterday and the confusion is new.
With 2 minutes remaining the examiner will stop you and ask you to summarise your findings and ask you some direct questions.

Case 3
You are the foundation year doctor on the liver ward. You have been called urgently to assess a patient who is having haematemesis and melena. The nurse tells you that the patient is known to have cirrhosis with portal hypertension and varices.
With 2 minutes remaining the examiner will stop you and ask you to summarise your findings and ask you some direct questions.

Case 4
You are the foundation year doctor in respiratory clinic. Your consultant has asked you to examine a patient and report back your findings. Jim is a 75-year-old gentleman who worked in a shipyard his whole life before retiring 15 years ago. He has noticed that he has become increasingly short of breath on exertion and has a dry tickly cough.
With 2 minutes remaining the examiner will stop you and ask you to summarise your findings and ask you some direct questions.

Case 5
You are the foundation year doctor in renal clinic. Sarah is a 42-year-old female with type 1-diabetes who has attended for review.
Your consultant has asked you to examine Sarah and report back your findings.
With 2 minutes remaining the examiner will stop you and ask you to summarise your findings and ask you some direct questions.

Case 6
You are the foundation year doctor in cardiology clinic. Your consultant has asked you to examine a patient and report back your findings. Mable is a 80-year-old female who has come for her annual check up. Her past medical history includes rheumatic fever as a child.
With 2 minutes remaining the examiner will stop you and ask you to summarise your findings and ask you some direct questions.

Case 7
A 45-year-old lady comes into the emergency department with a 3 day history of worsening balance and falls. You see from her previous clinic letters that she was diagnosed with multiple sclerosis 10 years ago.
Your consultant has asked you to do a thorough cerebellar examination and present your findings.
With 2 minutes remaining the examiner will stop you and ask you to summarise your findings and ask you some direct questions

Case 8

A 45-year-old lady has been admitted to the Acute Medical Unit with a chest infection. This morning on the ward round, she mentioned that she has had pain in her hands for a few months, but has not yet seen her GP about this.

You are the foundation doctor and have been asked to perform a hand examination then present your findings back to your team.

Case 9

You are the foundation year doctor in a General Practice surgery. A 78-year-old gentleman has presented with a tremor in his hands. Your trainer has asked you to examine the patient and present your findings.

With 2 minutes remaining the examiner will stop you and ask you to summarise your findings and ask you some direct questions.

Case 10

You are a foundation year doctor in the emergency department. A 65-year-old gentleman has been brought in with a 2 hour history of crushing central chest pain. An ECG has been done as well as routine bloods.

You have been asked to interpret the ECG and explain to the patient what you have found. Please talk through your interpretation of the ECG out loud.

At 6 minutes you will be asked how you would like to assess and manage this patient.

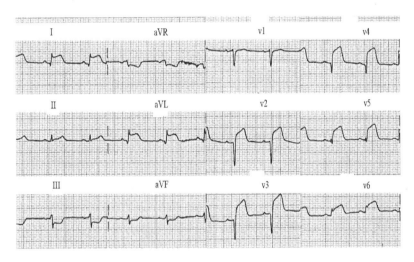

Case 11

You are the foundation year doctor in the emergency department. A 42-year old gentleman has been referred to you from his GP with a week's history of cough and worsening shortness of breath.

He has been adequately resuscitated and started on appropriate initial treatment based on clinical findings. You have been asked to chase his chest x-ray and interpret the results.

Interpret the chest x-ray and briefly explain the findings to the patient.

With 2 minutes remaining the examiner will stop you and ask you to summarise your findings and ask you some direct questions.

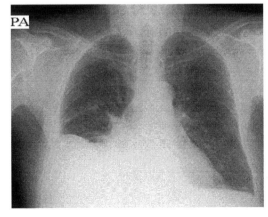

Case 12

You are the foundation year doctor on call for the medical wards. You are bleeped to see Joe a 60-year-old man with COPD who has become increasingly drowsy and breathless.

As part of your initial ABC assessment, you perform an arterial blood gas. Interpret the ABG result given to you and present your findings to the examiner.

ABG Print out

Patient:	Joe					
FiO_2:	21%					
Sample:	Arterial					
Blood Gas Values						
pH	7.293		[	7.350	-	7.450	]
pCO_2	9.00	kPa	[	4.00	-	6.50	]
pO_2	7.2	kPa	[	12.0	-	15.0	]
Acid Base Status						
HCO_3^-	32	mmol/L	[	22	-	28	]
BE	8.9	mmol/L	[	-3.0	-	3.0	]
Oximetry Values						
Hb	135	g/L	[	135	-	175	]
SaO_2	84.0	%	[	95.0	-	100.0	]
Electrolyte Values						
K^+	4.2	mmol/L	[	3.5	-	5.0	]
Na^+	137	mmol/L	[	135	-	145	]
ion Ca^{2+}	1.15	mmol/L	[	1.10	-	1.35	]
Cl^-	102	mmol/L	[	96	-	106	]
Anion Gap	3.0	mmol/L	[	8.0	-	16.0	]
Metabolic Values						
Lact	1.0	mmol/L	[	0.5	-	2.0	]
Bili	6	µmol/L	[		-		]

Case 13

You are the medical foundation year doctor on call. You have been asked to see James a 32-year-old gentleman, with generalised abdominal pain and vomiting. On examination, he appears sweaty and has a tremor. James would like to know the results of his blood tests taken earlier today. Please interpret the following results, summarising and discuss your findings with the patient. Discuss the likely causes and suggest further management.

BLOOD RESULTS

Patient Name: James
DOB: 15/05/1984
Hospital No: M1234567

Hb	131
MCV	106
PLT	118
WCC	4.7
Na	132 mmol/l
K	3.2 mmol/l
Urea	2.5 mmol/l

Creatinine	58 µmol/l
Albumin	30 g/l
AST	34 IU/l
ALT	33 IU/l
GGT	139 IU/l
Bilirubin	11 µmol/l
ALP	65U/l

Case 14

You have been asked to set up a syringe driver for a palliative patient on your ward who is struggling with pain and can no longer to take medications by mouth. The patient already has a subcutaneous butterfly needle in situ.

On the advice of the palliative care team your colleague has prescribed;
5mg diamorphine over 24 hours
10mls water for injection

Please set up and start the syringe driver. Paper and a calculator are provided for you if needed for workings out. There is a nurse available to help you.

Case 15

You are the foundation year doctor working in geriatrics outpatients. Winston, an 85 year old gentleman, has been experiencing calf pain on the left side whilst mobilising.

Please measure an ABPI, on the left hand side only, and document this procedure on the paper provided.

With 2 minutes remaining the examiner will stop you and ask you to summarise your findings and ask you some direct questions.

Case 16

You are the foundation year doctor on the gastroenterology ward. One of your patients has just returned from endoscopy, where they found a bleeding duodenal ulcer, which was clipped and injected. The patient is no longer bleeding, is haemodynamically stable and has a haemoglobin level of 69g/L. 2 units of packed red cells have been prescribed by your senior colleague.

Please check and administer the first unit. A nurse is available to help you. The cannula has a working cannula.

Case 17

You are the foundation year doctor on a medical ward. You have been informed by the nursing staff that a patient has spiked a temperature of 38.1°C. You decide to take blood cultures as part of the septic screen.

Demonstrate how you would do so using the equipment provided.

Case 18

You are the foundation year doctor working on the acute medical take. Frank is a 75 year old man who has presented with shortness of breath. Please take a focused history from her.

At 6 minutes you will be asked to present your history, give a differential diagnosis and provide a management plan.

Case 19

You are a foundation doctor on attachment to a general practice surgery. A 23-year-old man has come to his GP with a history of diarrhoea. He is normally well with no other medical conditions. Please take a focussed history from him.

At 6 minutes you will be asked to present your history, give a differential diagnosis and provide a management plan.

Case 20

You are a foundation year doctor in the emergency department. Brenda is a 71-year-old lady who has presented to the emergency department with collapse. Please take a focussed history.

At 6 minutes you will be asked to present your history, give a differential diagnosis and provide a management plan.

Case 21

You are a foundation year doctor attached to a general medical ward. Brenda is a 65-year old lady who has presented with weight loss. Please take a focussed history.

At 6 minutes you will be asked to present your history, give a differential diagnosis and provide a management plan.

Case 22

You are a foundation year doctor attached to a General Practice. Edward is a 43-year-old gentleman who has recently had some routine blood tests. These blood tests show that he has Type 2 Diabetes. The diabetic nurse at the practice has asked you to inform the patient of his diagnosis and explain the condition.

Case 23

Patricia is a 52-year old lady attending outpatient's gastroenterology clinic for troublesome, persistent reflux. She is scheduled for a gastroscopy in two weeks' time.

You are the gastroenterology foundation doctor and your consultant has asked you to explain the procedure to the patient. You are not required to consent Patricia for the procedure, or discuss the risks associated with the procedure.

Case 24

An elderly patient had a fall on the ward overnight. This was not witnessed by the nursing staff and he was found by a healthcare assistant sat on the floor. He appears to have sustained no injuries. This morning his family phoned the ward to check on his progress and were shocked to hear that he had fallen. They are very upset and demanding to speak to a doctor on the ward. They would like an explanation as to why this happened and what will be done next.

You are the junior doctor on the ward. The nursing staff have approached you and asked if you could speak with the family. Please explore the relative's concerns and offer a plan of action.

Case 25

You are a foundation year doctor working on a general medical ward. Cara is a 72-year-old woman who presented with a five day history of worsening shortness of breath and productive cough of green sputum. She has been admitted to the ward for treatment for a Community Acquired Pneumonia.

Unfortunately Cara has been administered a dose of IV Co-Amoxiclav despite a documented penicillin allergy and went on to develop anaphylaxis. She received all the appropriate emergency medical management and is now stable and being monitored on HDU.

You have been asked by the nursing staff to speak with Cara's family, explaining the medication error and eliciting any concerns that they may have.

Paediatrics

Case 1

A 10 year old boy called Paul has come into ED via ambulance with his father after witnessing him having a fit. Paul is currently sitting on a trolley with a GCS of 15.

You are the FY1 doctor in the paediatric team and have been asked to take a history.

With 2 minutes remaining the examiner will stop you, ask you to summarise back your findings and will ask you some direct questions.

Case 2

An 8 month old boy has been brought in by his parents with a 3 day history of cough reduced feeding and some difficulty in breathing.

You are the FY1 doctor in the paediatric team and have been asked to take a history and then summarise your findings back to the team.

With 2 minutes remaining the examiner will stop you, ask you to summarise back your findings and will ask you some direct questions.

Case 3

A 3 year old girl is brought in by her mother via ambulance after an episode of shaking all over. The toddler is alert and active but miserable with a fever in triage.

You are the FY1 doctor in the Emergency Department and have been asked to take a history and then summarise your findings your findings back to the team.

With 2 minutes remaining the examiner will stop you, ask you to summarise back your findings and will ask you some direct questions.

Case 4

A mother has brought her 14 month old baby girl to the Paediatric Outpatient Department. She was referred by her GP, who was concerned that her growth has been poor.

You are the FY1 doctor in the paediatrics team and have been asked to take the history, and then to summarise your findings to the team.

With 2 minutes remaining the examiner will stop you, ask you to summarise back your findings and will ask you some direct questions.

Case 5

A mother brings her four month old baby to the local Emergency Department. He burned his arm.

You are the FY1 in the Emergency Department, and have been asked to see the child immediately as the nurse has concerns about the burn. You have been asked to take the history, and to summarise back to your team. You will need to discuss your next steps and management plan.

With 2 minutes remaining the examiner will stop you, ask you to summarise back your findings and will ask you some direct questions.

Case 6

A 5 day old baby is referred into the Emergency Department by the community midwife, who is worried because the baby has lost 12% of his birth weight.

You are the FY1 doctor in the Paediatric team and have been asked to take the history, and then to summarise your findings to the team. You will need to explain your management plan to the mother.

With 2 minutes remaining the examiner will stop you, ask you to summarise back your findings and will ask you some direct questions.

Case 7

Alice is a twelve-year old girl who has been bought in to ED by her mother, after school noticed numerous cut marks on her forearms.

You are the FY1 doctor in Paediatric ED. The team have seen Alice with her mother and have dressed her forearm injuries, which are superficial and not of medical significance.

They ask you to speak to Alice without her mother present in order to assess her suicide risk. Both Alice and her mother have agreed to this.

With 2 minutes remaining the examiner will stop you, ask you to summarise back your findings and will ask you some direct questions.

Case 8

Oscar is a three week old baby boy who has been brought to ED by his parents, after he had a floppy episode whilst feeding. You are the FY1 doctor in Paediatric ED. The team ask you to take a history of the event from Oscar's mother. Oscar has normal observations, and the Paediatric nurse tells you he looks alert and active at triage.

With 2 minutes remaining the examiner will stop you, ask you to summarise back your findings and will ask you some direct questions.

Case 9

You are the FY1 doctor for Paediatrics and you have been asked to perform a routine newborn examination on a baby and present your findings back to your registrar. All the equipment that you need will be available on request.

With 2 minutes remaining the examiner will stop you, ask you to summarise back your findings and will ask you some direct questions.

Case 10

You are an FY1 doctor in the Paediatric Outpatient Clinic. You have just seen a 9 year old child with recurrent abdominal pain and the consultant asks you to perform a focused abdominal examination and present your findings.

With 2 minutes remaining the examiner will stop you, ask you to summarise back your findings and will ask you some direct questions.

Case 11

You are an FY1 doctor in Paediatrics. A 12 year old girl has been referred in by her GP for review as he noted a raised blood pressure (130/75) on examination in the surgery today. Your registrar asks you to examine her cardiovascular system and present your findings.

With 2 minutes remaining the examiner will stop you, ask you to summarise back your findings and will ask you some direct questions.

Case 12

You are an FY1 doctor in Paediatrics. You have just seen a 15 year old boy with a chronic chest condition on the ward round and you have been asked to perform a respiratory examination and present your findings.

With 2 minutes remaining the examiner will stop you, ask you to summarise back your findings and will ask you some direct questions.

Case 13

You are an FY1 doctor in Paediatrics Paediatric Outpatient Department. A 9 year old girl presents with weakness in her arms. Your registrar has asked you to assess the motor neurology in the upper limbs of this patient and present your findings.

Case 14
An 8 year old boy who was born at 28 weeks gestation, who has a history of grade 3 IVH has been brought to clinic for his routine follow up.
You are an FY1 doctor in the Paediatric Outpatient clinic. You have been asked to examine the child's lower limb neurology and gait and then summarise your findings to your senior.
With 2 minutes remaining the examiner will stop you, ask you to summarise back your findings and will ask you some direct questions.

Case 15
Sarah is 14 and she has recently been diagnosed with asthma. You are the FY1 on the ward and your Consultant has asked you to explain to Sarah what asthma is and why she needs to take inhalers. They had a brief chat about asthma on the ward round this morning, but a more detailed explanation is required before Sarah goes home. You should explain to Sarah what asthma is and that she will need preventer and reliever inhalers after discharge from hospital. As part of your explanation, you should ensure that Sarah knows when to seek advice from an adult.
You see Sarah on the ward with her Mum before she goes home.

With 2 minutes remaining the examiner will stop you, ask you to summarise back your findings and will ask you some direct questions.

Case 16
Ben is 18 months old. He was admitted to the children's ward following a febrile convulsion. He had a runny nose and temperature for 3 days before the convulsion. His fever was 39.2C at the time. It lasted 3 minutes and his mother described shaking of both his arms and his legs and Ben was not responding to her. It stopped by itself before the ambulance arrived and Ben has been very well since admission to the ward. You are the FY1 doctor on the ward and have been asked to explain to Ben's mother exactly what a febrile convulsion is.

With 2 minutes remaining the examiner will stop you, ask you to summarise back your findings and will ask you some direct questions.

Case 17
Jack is 18 months old and has been diagnosed with a viral upper respiratory tract infection. He attended the Emergency Department with a 24-hour history of a runny nose, dry cough and a fever. He is generally well in himself, eating and drinking as usual and playing in the waiting room. His mother wants him to have antibiotics for his infection but these have not been prescribed. You are the FY1 doctor in ED and have been asked to talk to Jack's mother.

Case 18
A woman who is 25 weeks pregnant has been admitted to Labour ward with contractions. On examination her cervix is found to be 5cm dilated and the obstetric team expect her to deliver in the next few hours. This is her first pregnancy and except for being treated for a UTI 1 week ago there has been nothing else untoward during the antenatal period.
You are a junior doctor in the paediatric team and have been asked to speak to the mother about her impending premature delivery.
With 2 minutes remaining the examiner will stop you, ask you to summarise back your findings and will ask you some direct questions.

Case 19
A newborn baby boy was born in poor condition following shoulder dystocia. He has been intubated and ventilated due to low Apgar scores. Blood gases have been borderline and for the first two hours the baby was doing well but then was noted to be having focal seizures. The baby was given phenobarbitone and the seizures stopped. However, in view of this it is decided to transfer the baby to a tertiary centre for therapeutic hypothermia and further investigations.
You are the junior doctor in the paediatric team and have been asked to speak to the family to explain the change in his condition and need to transfer the baby to a tertiary centre for ongoing care.
With 2 minutes remaining the examiner will, ask you to summarise back your findings and will ask you some direct questions.

Case 20

A 7 month old boy has attended the Emergency Department with coughing, coryza, wheezing and poor feeding. On examination he is active and alert but is wheezing a lot and has some subcostal recessions. His oxygen saturations are 89% in air but go up to 98% on nasal cannula oxygen. His older brother has similar symptoms. He was examined by the Registrar who diagnosed him with bronchiolitis and asks for the child to be admitted to the short stay ward.

You are the FY1 doctor in the paediatric team and have been asked to explain to the family that the child will need to be admitted and talk to them about his diagnosis.

With 2 minutes remaining the examiner will stop you, ask you to summarise back your findings and will ask you some direct questions.

Case 21

You are an FY1 doctor on the General Paediatric ward. Iris, a 2 year old girl, was admitted two days ago with acute viral wheeze requiring nebulised salbutamol. Iris is being discharged home today. You have been asked by your team to explain and demonstrate how to use a metered dose inhaler (MDI) with a mask and spacer to the parent who is anxious about going home.

Iris is not by the bedside. You can use a nearby doll or teddy bear to demonstrate inhaler + spacer + mask technique to the parent.

Case 22

You are an FY1 doctor working on the postnatal ward with the Paediatric team. You are carrying out routine newborn baby checks when the senior midwife on the ward approaches you and asks if you would kindly speak to a mother who was yesterday informed her new baby son Simon is likely to have Down's Syndrome. She is anxious and has some questions she would like to ask.

Case 23

You are the FY1 doctor on the Special Care Baby Unit. Benjy, an ex 32 week premature baby is now 8 weeks old and due his first set of routine immunisations.

Please obtain verbal consent from his mother and perform the task using the equipment provided.

Case 24

A parent on the ward has rushed out of their cubicle shouting that their child "is not waking up".

You are the Paediatric FY1 covering the ward and have been fast-bleeped by the nurse to urgently assess this child and start treatment.

Case 25

You are an FY1 doctor in the Emergency Department and have clerked a 9 year old boy who presented after falling onto his left hand whilst ice-skating.

He has returned from X-ray and your consultant would like you to interpret the radiograph and then present your findings to the medical student on your team in order to teach them about basic radiograph interpretation.

Please then discuss your differential causes followed by your management plan.

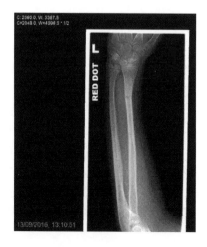

General Practice

Case 1
You are the foundation year doctor working in General Practice. The practice nurse has asked this 60 year old gentleman Peter to see you as his blood pressure was 150/95 mmHg on three separate occasions last week.

After 6 minutes the examiner will stop you and ask you to summarise back your findings, suggest your differential diagnoses and your initial management plan.

Case 2
You are the foundation year doctor working in General Practice and have been asked to see Amanda a 50 year old lady who presents to your practice after experiencing palpitations.

After 6 minutes the examiner will stop you and ask you to summarise back your findings, suggest your differential diagnoses and your initial management plan.

Case 3
You are the foundation year doctor working in General Practice and have been asked to see a 70 year old woman Diana, who has presented to the GP surgery complaining of increased breathlessness and cough.

After 6 minutes the examiner will stop you and ask you to summarise back your findings, suggest your differential diagnoses and your initial management plan.

Case 4
You are the foundation year doctor working in General Practice and have been asked to see Jack a 60 year old man who has presented to the GP surgery complaining of a chronic cough.

After 6 minutes the examiner will stop you and ask you to summarise back your findings, suggest your investigations and your initial management plan.

Case 5
You are the foundation year doctor working in General Practice and have been asked to see a 33 year old woman, Bekah who attends your GP practice with a headache.
After 6 minutes the examiner will stop you and ask you to summarise back your findings, suggest your differential diagnoses and your initial management plan.

Case 6
You are the foundation year doctor working in General Practice and have been asked to Colleen who has presented to the GP surgery as she is worried about her husband's progressing confusion. Please take a collateral history from the relative.

After 6 minutes the examiner will stop you and ask you to summarise back your findings, suggest your differential diagnoses and your initial management plan.

Case 7
You are the foundation year doctor working in General Practice and have been asked to see a 38 year old lady Philippa who has presented to the GP surgery complaining of feeling unwell. You note from recent letters that she has recently been diagnosed with multiple sclerosis following two admissions to hospital under the Neurology team but has not seen her GP since her diagnosis.

Please take a history and address the patient's ideas, concerns and expectations. After 6 minutes the examiner will stop you and ask you to summarise back your findings, suggest your differential diagnoses and your initial management plan.
Case 8

You are the foundation year doctor working in General Practice and have been asked to see a 45 year old gentleman Harry who has presented to the GP surgery as he would like to cut down on his alcohol intake. Please take a full history.

After 6 minutes the examiner will stop you and ask you to summarise back your findings, suggest your differential diagnoses and your initial management plan.

Case 9

You are the foundation year doctor working in General Practice and have been asked to see a 37 year old gentleman Sam who has presented to the GP surgery complaining of rectal bleeding. Please take a full history.

After 6 minutes the examiner will stop you and ask you to summarise back your findings, suggest your differential diagnoses and your initial management plan.

Case 10

You are the foundation year doctor working in General Practice and have been asked to see a 50 year old woman Sarah has presented to the GP surgery after having found a lump in her breast. Please take a full history.

After 6 minutes the examiner will stop you and ask you to summarise back your findings, suggest your differential diagnoses and your initial management plan.

Case 11

You are the foundation year doctor working in General Practice and have been asked to see a 64 year old gentleman Winston who has presented to the GP surgery complaining of blood in his urine. Please take a full history.

After 6 minutes the examiner will stop you and ask you to summarise back your findings, suggest your differential diagnoses and your initial management plan.

Case 12

You are the foundation year doctor working in General Practice and have been asked to see a 55 year old woman Geeta who has presented to the GP surgery complaining of feeling unwell. Take a full history and address their ideas, concerns and expectations.

After 6 minutes the examiner will stop you and ask you to summarise back your findings, suggest your differential diagnoses and your initial management plan.

Case 13

You are the foundation year doctor working in General Practice and have been asked to see a 42 year old gentleman Praveen who has attended the GP surgery for a routine diabetic follow up but he is complaining of feeling funny in the last few weeks. Please take a full history.

After 6 minutes the examiner will stop you and ask you to summarise back your findings, suggest your differential diagnoses and your initial management plan.

Case 14

You are the foundation year doctor working in General Practice and have been asked to see a 38 year old gentleman Spencer who has presented to the GP surgery with a rash. The rash is seen on both elbows on the flexors surfaces and is raised with dry scaly plaques. Please take a full history and perform a brief examination.

After 6 minutes the examiner will stop you and ask you to summarise back your findings, suggest your differential diagnoses and your initial management plan.

Case 15

You are the foundation year doctor working in General Practice and have been asked to see a 59 year old gentleman Hugo who has presented to the GP surgery with a small mole.
Please take a full history.

After 6 minutes the examiner will stop you and ask you to summarise back your findings, suggest your differential diagnoses and your initial management plan.

Case 16

You are the foundation year doctor working in General Practice and have been asked to see a 30 year old gentleman Robert who has presented to the GP surgery complaining of back pain. Please take a full history.

After 6 minutes the examiner will stop you and ask you to summarise back your findings, suggest your differential diagnoses and your initial management plan.

Case 17

You are the foundation year doctor working in General Practice and have been asked to see a 30 week pregnant lady, Debbie, aged 29, who has presented to the GP surgery for a routine antenatal appointment. Please take a focused history and perform a routine antenatal examination.

After 6 minutes the examiner will stop you and ask you to summarise back your findings, suggest your differential diagnoses and your initial management plan

Case 18

You are the foundation year doctor working in General Practice and have been asked to see a 24 yr old lady Keely, who has had a baby 6 weeks ago, has presented to the GP surgery for her routine postnatal check. Please take a fully history.

After 6 minutes the examiner will stop you and ask you to summarise back your findings, suggest your differential diagnoses and your initial management plan.

Case 19

You are the foundation year doctor working in General Practice and have been asked to see a A 28 year old Claire who has presented to the GP to discuss her periods as she is very concerned about them becoming heavier than usual.

After 6 minutes the examiner will stop you and ask you to summarise back your findings, suggest your differential diagnoses and your initial management plan.

Case 20

You are the foundation year doctor in the GP and have been asked to see Tessa a 28 year old woman, has been asked to come to the GP surgery to discuss the results of a recent cervical smear. The result shows mild dyskaryosis and HPV Type 16 (high risk) positive.

Take a focused history and discuss the results with the patient and then suggest an appropriate management plan and address their ideas, concerns and expectations.

Examiner's instructions

ENT	**47**
Anaesthetics & Critical Care	**53**
Orthopaedics & Rheumatology	**62**
Psychiatry	**69**
Surgery	**74**
Emergency medicine	**79**
Obstetrics & Gynaecology	**88**
Medicine	**91**
Paediatrics	**97**
General Practice	**103**

ENT

Case 1

This is a scenario of a child complaining of left sided hearing impairment. He is otherwise well, up to date with his vaccinations, and cooperative throughout the entire history, though the candidate should demonstrate an ability to ask specific questions in order to get the full history from the child.

The main focus of this station is for the candidate to focus his history taking around the 2 most common causes of paediatric ear presentations; foreign body and infection

After 6 minutes, please stop the candidate and ask:

"Please summarise your findings and discuss how you would like to investigate and manage this patient."

Case 2

This is a scenario of a 35 year old man presenting with a 5 day history of discharge from the left ear. Please assess the candidate specifically on how concise the history is. The candidate should appreciate that unilateral otorrhoea in an adult should be taken seriously as it can indicate an infection, or more rarely, head and neck malignancies.
The candidate should very clearly ascertain if the symptoms are acute, chronic, or associated with signs/symptoms of malignancy.

After 6 minutes, please stop the candidate and ask:

"Please summarise your findings and discuss how you would like to investigate and manage this patient."

Case 3

This is a scenario of a 6 year old boy presenting acutely with blood from the left ear.

Asses the candidate specifically on how concise the history is. The candidate should appreciate that unilateral bloody-otorrhoea in a child is most likely to be trauma or foreign body related, and as such, the questions asked whilst the candidate takes the history should be along these lines.

Ensure the candidate understands the range of differentials with this particular presentation in a paediatric setting, in order of how common they are, i.e. trauma and foreign body being most common in a child at school, followed by infection (acute or chronic) and less commonly, malignancies. If the candidate describes malignancy as a top differential, challenge them on this and emphasize the importance of mentioning the commoner differentials first.

The candidate should suggest an ear (with a comprehensive ENT) examination + +/- toileting as the first line management in an emergency department setting.

After 6 minutes, please stop the candidate and ask:

"Please summarise your findings and discuss how you would like to investigate and manage this patient.

Case 4

This is a scenario of a 30 year old man presenting with a 1 year history of a lump behind the left ear.

Please assess the candidate specifically on how fluent the lump examination is. The candidate should very clearly assess for tenderness prior to touching the lump

After 6 minutes, please stop the candidate and ask:

"Please summarise your findings and discuss how you would like to investigate and manage this patient."

Examination findings:
The lump is behind the left ear, it is fixed to the skin but not to any underlying structures
There is no pain
There is no mastoid tenderness
There is no erythema
Examination of the canal is NORMAL

Case 5

The station is directed towards history taking only and therefore the candidate should be reminded of that should he/she try to carry out a clinical examination.
After 6 minutes, please stop the candidate and ask:

"Please summarise your findings and discuss how you would like to investigate and manage this patient."

Case 6

This is a station where the candidate has to elicit a history of the presenting complaint. The candidate is then to perform a focused examination of a patient with facial erythema.
When the patient is being examined give the appropriate clinical findings if the candidate performs the correct examination technique or describes what they would like to do to elicit a clinical sign.
Ask the candidate to summarize their findings and offer a differential diagnosis with a management plan.
After 6 minutes, please stop the candidate and ask:

"Please summarise your findings and discuss how you would like to investigate and manage this patient."

Examination findings:

Observations
Comfortable at rest on room air
Respiratory rate 16, SpO2 100% on room air
Pulse 80, BP 150/95 Capillary refill time 3 seconds, Warm peripheries
36.5°

Inspection
Rash in a malar distribution
Nasolabial folds are spared

Palpation
Area not tender
Not warmth compared to other skin
Not raised

Case 7

When the patient is being examined give the appropriate clinical findings if the candidate performs the correct examination technique or describes what they would like to do to elicit a clinical sign.
Ask the candidate to summarize their findings and offer a differential diagnosis with a management plan.
After 6 minutes, please stop the candidate and ask:

"Please summarise your findings and discuss how you would like to investigate and manage this patient."

Examination findings:
There is no pain. There is no discharge. There is no erythema. Examination of the nose reveals a deviated septum towards the right with narrowing of the air passages.

Case 8

When the patient is being examined give the appropriate clinical findings if the candidate performs the correct examination technique or describes what they would like to do to elicit a clinical sign.

Ask the candidate to summarize their findings and offer a differential diagnosis with a management plan.

After 6 minutes, please stop the candidate and ask:

"Please summarise your findings and discuss how you would like to investigate and manage this patient."

Examination findings:

There is no pain. There is no current discharge. Examination of the nose reveals an irregular raised lump on the inside of the left nostril fixed to skin and extending into the nasal cavity.

Case 9

This is a scenario of complicated nasal trauma in a 15 years old boy. The candidate is asked to take a history and carry out a comprehensive examination of the patient.

After 6 minutes, please stop the candidate and ask:

"Please summarise your findings and discuss how you would like to investigate and manage this patient."

Examination findings:
The physical examination should reveal:

An infected septum bilateral haematoma
A bony deformity of the nasal bones towards the left
No other neurological, orbital or maxillo-facial abnormalities
A temperature of 38.7 degrees
No neurological signs, your limbs and vision are normal
You have some mucky mucus in your nostrils but no blood and no watery discharge
The partition inside your nose is boggy and swollen filling your nostrils on both sides, and your nose skin is red and tender to touch
Your bony nose bridge is tender, mildly swollen and is deviated towards the left
You have no other facial deformities, bruising or tenderness

The candidate should suggest the following plan of action:

Admitting the patient and prepare him for a possible GA
Secure an IV access and take bloods for FBC, U&Es, CRP and clotting
Inform senior and discuss the need for IV antibiotics and for a manipulation of nasal bones and incision and drainage of nasal septum infected haematoma under GA
Counselling the patient and relatives regarding the diagnosis of nasal bones fracture and the need for manipulation under anaesthesia after 7-14 days from the trauma
Counselling patient and relatives regarding the diagnosis of an infected nasal septum haematoma and the need for an incision and drainage under GA to prevent the dissemination of sepsis

Case 10

This is a scenario of complicated nasal trauma in a 19 years old man. The candidate is asked to carry out a comprehensive examination of the patient's nose.

After 6 minutes, please stop the candidate and ask:

"Please summarise your findings and discuss how you would like to investigate and manage this patient."

Examination findings:
The bridge of the nose is deviated to the left and is tender.
There is a small laceration to the skin and a red eye.
No eye signs/andormailities.
There is obvious epistaixs, but no other nasal (CSF, catarhh etc) discharge.

Case 11

The station is directed towards history taking only and therefore the candidate should be reminded of that should they try to carry out a clinical examination.
After 6 minutes, please stop the candidate and ask:

"Please summarise your findings and discuss how you would like to investigate and manage this patient."

Case 12

The station is directed towards history taking only and therefore the candidate should be reminded of that should he/she try to carry out a clinical examination.
After 6 minutes, please stop the candidate and ask:

"Please summarise your findings and discuss how you would like to investigate and manage this patient."

Case 13

The station is directed towards history taking only and therefore the candidate should be reminded of that should they try to carry out a clinical examination.
After 6 minutes, please stop the candidate and ask:

"Please summarise your findings and discuss how you would like to investigate and manage this patient."

Case 14

When the patient is being examined give the appropriate clinical findings if the candidate performs the correct examination technique or describes what they would like to do to elicit a clinical sign.
After 6 minutes, please stop the candidate and ask:

"Please summarise your findings and discuss how you would like to investigate and manage this patient."

Examination findings:

Patient appears panicked, sat upright and is using accessory muscles to breath
She can only give very short answers to questions, is in severe pain and is pointing to her neck

She appears in distress and is constantly spitting saliva into a bowl
A: Audible stridor from the foot of the bed
B: Appears peripherally cyanosed, but centrally well perfused
      Respiratory rate is 40, Oxygen Sats on air 80%, on high flow oxygen 98%
      Trachea is central, equal chest expansion and air entry bilaterally, chest percussion sounds normal >> no signs of a pneumothorax
C: Heart rate is 125 beats/minute, BP 170/88mmHg
D: She is fully alert but distressed

Case 15

At each stage press the candidate as to what the next step would be if that intervention failed. The patient suffered facial trauma and has a swollen tongue.

It is unknown whether he has a skull base fracture but he has no evidence of a cervical spine injury. He had morphine from the ambulance crew and has been given a dose of intravenous Co-Amoxiclav.

The tongue may be swollen due to haematoma or possibly allergic reaction to the antibiotic

The candidate has 8 minutes for this station, but please give them a warning with 2 minutes to go.

Case 16

The station is directed towards history taking only and therefore the candidate should be reminded of that should he/she try to carry out a clinical examination.

After 6 minutes, please stop the candidate and ask:

"Please summarise your findings and discuss how you would like to investigate and manage this patient."

Case 17

This is a scenario of a 22 year old woman who attends the emergency department (ED) with sudden palpitations and a progressively growing neck mass. The patient's presentation suggests thyrotoxicosis with a thyroid goitre and atrial fibrillation; the candidate should be able to elicit that through the information he/she gathers from the patient.

The station is directed towards history taking only and therefore the candidate should be reminded of that should he/she try to carry out a clinical examination.

After 6 minutes, please stop the candidate and ask:
"Please summarise your findings and discuss how you would like to investigate and manage this patient."

Case 18

The candidate is tasked to carry out a comprehensive clinical examination of a 45 years old man who presents to the head and neck clinic with a right sided neck mass that has been gradually enlarging over two months. The patient is concerned that this mass is malignant due to a family history of cancer.

The session is aimed towards a clinical examination only, and the candidate should be reminded of that should he/she attempt to take any history.
After 6 minutes, please stop the candidate and ask:

"Please summarise your findings and discuss how you would like to investigate and manage this patient."

After summarising their findings, the candidate should conclude that the patient requires an urgent workup of the potentially neoplastic presentation. Within the outpatient setting the candidate should request (or perform if capable) an FNE, and a fine needle aspiration for cytology of the mass (FNAC).

The most prudent first line investigations of the neck node should include imaging (MRI neck) and blood testing (blood film, FBC, LFT's, U&Es, LDH, Viral serology [EBV/CMV/HIV], other serology [Bartonella / Toxoplasmosis], ESR / CRP, autoimmune profile [ANCA / RF]). Pending the results, second line investigations could include further imaging studies (USS / CT), TB testing, and a pan-endoscopy +/- node biopsy under GA.

Examination findings:
The examination reveals no upper airway noises and a normal.

The patient is well hydrated, has a normal weight, and his basic observations are (temperature 36.3, BP 140/85, HR 90, RR 14, SaO2 97% on air).

The inspection and palpation of the neck reveal a 5X5cm right sided firm neck mass at the upper half of the sternocleidomastoid muscle (levels 2&3). The lump is mobile, non-tender, not associated with skin changes and does not move on swallowing.

The examination of the oral cavity and oropharynx shows no abnormalities.

Facial inspection and anterior nasal examinations are unremarkable, and the patient has no other palpable masses.

If fibre-optic Naso-endoscopy (FNE) is available (even if only by an illustration that is provided to the candidate), it will be normal.

Case 19

This is a station where the candidate has to elicit a history from a patient with monocular vision loss.

After 6 minutes, please stop the candidate and ask:

"Please summarise your findings and discuss how you would like to investigate and manage this patient."

Case 20

A 24-year old lady has presented with right sided blurry vision. The candidate has been asked to take a focused history and examination.

After 6 minutes, please stop the candidate and ask:

"Please summarise your findings and discuss how you would like to investigate and manage this patient."

Examination findings:

Right			Left
6/36	Visual Acuity	(unaided)	6/6
6/36	Visual Acuity	(pinhole)	6/6
3/17	Colour Vision		17/17
Equal	Pupil inspection		Equal
Reacts slowly	Pupillary reaction		Normal reaction
Normal	Red reflex		Normal
Normal	Retina		Normal
Pale, swollen	Optic disc		Normal

Normal accommodation bilaterally

Right relative afferent pupillary defect (RAPD) - on shining light into right eye the pupil dilates. Light shone into the left eye causes pupillary constriction.

Anaesthetics & Critical Care

Case 1

Martin is a 52-year-old man who has presented for elective laparoscopic inguinal hernia repair under general anaesthetic.

He is an obese gentleman, body weight 115kg, height 182cm (BMI 34), who takes Ramipril 5mg for hypertension.

He had an anaesthetic 5 years ago for a cholecystectomy, and was told after the operation that there had been a problem putting a tube into his airway. He doesn't remember much more detail, but says his throat was very sore afterwards.

After six minutes, ask the candidate to summarise the case and suggest what they would do next. Can they suggest a safe plan for providing anaesthesia?

Case 2

John is a 78-year-old male who has presented for elective inguinal hernia repair under general anaesthetic.

He has a history of cardiac disease and suffered a myocardial infarction 2 years ago. He has two coronary stents and is currently asymptomatic. He can climb two flights of stairs, walks 2 miles every day and lives independently at home. He has no signs or symptoms of cardiac failure. His baseline blood pressure is 145/70 and his oxygen saturations are normal.

After six minutes ask the candidate to summarise the case and the important issues. Ask them to comment on his risk and fitness for general anaesthesia and what further investigations they would like to review before his operation. Ask them then how the situation would be different if the patient had recently started to complain of worsening chest pain and shortness of breath.

Case 3

Rachel is a 44-year-old patient who has presented for an excision of a benign breast lump under general anaesthetic.

She has had a previous general anaesthetic for an appendicectomy twenty years ago, which was uneventful.

Significantly, she suffers from asthma. She has had multiple Emergency Department admissions with acute asthma attacks, and three years ago had an admission to ICU after use of diclofenac led to a life-threatening exacerbation of her asthma. She was intubated and ventilated for 48 hours on that occasion.

Currently her asthma is well controlled using inhalers and oral montelukast. Otherwise she has no long-term medical problems, and is a lifelong non-smoker.

After six minutes ask the candidate to summarise the case and say how they would proceed. Ask them if there are any further investigations they would request prior to general anaesthetic.

Case 4

The candidate is to take the role of a Foundation Year doctor in Anaesthetics, teaching a student ODP about Waveform Capnography.
Present them with six Capnography waveforms.
Ask them to outline the reason capnography is used in clinical practice, and then explain each of the capnography traces to the student ODP, including any abnormalities, the clinical significance of these abnormalities, and what steps should be taken to further identify or treat the problem.

Waveform 1: Normal capnography trace.
Waveform 2: Trace suggesting obstruction to expiration.
Waveform 3: Trace suggesting sudden loss of cardiac output.
Waveform 4: Trace suggesting patient making respiratory effort against ventilator.
Waveform 5: Trace suggesting disconnection from breathing circuit.

Case 5

Richard is a 28-year-old man who has presented to the ED acutely short of breath and with a productive cough.
He has a history of heroin and crack cocaine use. As part of his work up today he has had an arterial blood gas taken.
The candidate should interpret the results and summarise their findings. The SpR will then ask them the following questions.

What they would like to do next?
What tests they would like (if any)?
What their treatment would be if the CXR showed consolidation of the Right Middle Lobe?
What changes may they see on the arterial blood gas if the patient was tiring?
How they would treat the lactic acidosis?
What arterial PO2 they would expect with an inspired oxygen concentration of 60% in a healthy subject?

Case 6

A 22-year-old man is brought to the emergency department semi conscious with a prior history of severe vomiting and abdominal pain.

The patient is being resuscitated and assessed by an ED doctor, who has asked the F1 doctor to analyse and interpret an arterial blood gas sample in order to manage the patient.

Allow 6 minutes for the candidate to present the data in a structured manner, and then summarise their analysis. When they have presented their findings, ask the following questions:

What is the likely diagnosis?
What further investigations would you order in this patient?
What management would you institute?
What other causes of a metabolic acidosis do you know?

Results

> Arterial blood gas: 3/8/16 16:45
> Mr Tom, DOB 15/5/95
> fiO2 0.21
>
> | | |
> |---|---|
> | pH | 6.94 |
> | P_aO_2 | 13.8kPa |
> | P_aCO_2 | 2.5kPa |
> | HCO_3^- | 8mmol/L |
> | Base excess | -19.5mmol/L |
> | Glucose | 27mmol/L |

Case 7

Samuel is a 53-year-old patient with alcohol dependence whose GP has referred him for investigation of ascites. The nurse admitting him is concerned that his blood pressure is low.

The admitting nurse has noticed that he has a tachycardia of 120 and blood pressure of 75/40. The candidate should perform an ABCDE assessment which will reveal signs of hypovolaemia and presence of malaena.

They should concurrently take a basic history which should reveal the patient's excessive alcohol consumption, and a 2-day history of copious amounts of black offensive stools. The patient will deteriorate during the station with signs of worsening haemorrhagic shock. The candidate will be expected to administer fluids and request flying squad/O -ve blood in addition to calling for appropriate help.

In the final two minutes, ask them to provide a differential diagnosis, outline what abnormalities they will be looking for in laboratory investigations, and state that the patient will require an urgent OGD. Establish if they understand the rationale for antibiotic therapy and terlipressin.

Case 8

A 72-year-old man, admitted to a medical ward for treatment of pneumonia, is found unconscious by a staff nurse.

The Foundation Year 1 doctor has been asked to assess and treat the patient appropriately. The candidate is to use an A-E approach and may ask for relevant history and investigations, results of which would be provided.

Stop the candidates after 6 minutes and ask them to summarise the case. Then ask them:
what other medications would you prescribe on the drug chart to be used in the event of recurrent hypoglycaemia?
what is the target capillary blood glucose level for a patient with critical illness?

Case 9

Lena is a 19-year-old woman who has been brought to the Emergency Department by ambulance. She was found unconscious by her mother, who has been concerned about Lena's low mood and erratic behaviour since she failed her first-year exams.

The candidate should perform an A to E assessment, where they will discover signs of tricyclic overdose.

If they probe for further history, the paramedic is able to report that Lena's mother takes Amitriptyline for back pain, and several empty packets of the drug were found hidden in a bin in the bathroom.

The candidate should begin appropriate resuscitation while requesting senior help and support from ICU/Anaesthetics. In the final two minutes ask them to summarise the case and list the clinical features of Tricyclic overdose. If not clear from the scenario, clarify whether they know how to obtain information on treating a potential poisoning or drug overdose, and if they know of a specific intervention for tricyclic poisoning.

Case 10

Jonny is a 24-year-old patient with a history of epilepsy (generalised seizures). His epilepsy is normally well controlled with twice daily oral sodium valproate (300mg). He has been an in-patient on the medical ward since yesterday, requiring treatment with IV antibiotics for community-acquired pneumonia. He is penicillin allergic, so is being treated with IV levofloxacin.

The patient has been having generalised seizures on the ward for 7 minutes now, and has not responded to initial buccal midazolam by the nursing staff. He has jaw clenching, but with high flow oxygen through a reservoir mask has maintained saturations of 96%. He is tachycardic (105 beats per minute), has normal blood pressure (134/69), and is apyrexial (temperature 37.4).

The candidate has been asked to assist in the immediate management by nursing staff, and should assess the patient with an ABCDE approach. The scenario requires knowledge of the step-wise approach to the management of status epilepticus.

With 2 minutes remaining ask the candidate for possible causes of the onset of seizures – relevant to this scenario these would include acute infection and pharmacological interaction (with a quinolone antibiotic). If it has not been volunteered enquire about escalation of care for refractory status epilepticus.

Case 11

Tim is a 78-year-old patient with a history of benign prostatic hypertrophy who is being assessed in the Emergency Department (ED) Resus area. He has no significant past medical history, and is generally active and well, with no allergies.

For the last 18 hours he has developed left loin pain, vomiting and rigors. He had a temperature of 38.9°C on arrival to the ED 20 minutes ago and was normotensive with a tachycardia of 108 beats/minute. He now has a blood pressure of 85/37mmHg, and tachycardia at a rate of 113/min. He is drowsy and much less responsive than when he arrived.

The ED staff have inserted a large bore IV cannula, and are administering a bolus of 250ml crystalloid. They sent routine bloods (FBC, UE, CRP), but no serum lactate measurement or blood cultures when the cannula was inserted. He has received no antibiotics.

The experienced nurse with the patient is able to provide all of the relevant history points, and can provide the candidate with details of the investigations and treatment so far.

With 2 minutes remaining the examiner should ask the candidate to present back their finding and should be asked directly to summarise the approach to treating a septic patient.

Case 12

Dan is a 28 year old awaiting wash-out of an infected elbow effusion. He began feeling unwell shortly after an infusion of Flucloxacillin commenced.

The candidate should perform an A to E assessment of a mannequin, where they should initially note lip swelling, mild wheeze, a modest tachycardia and hypotension

The patient will go on to show signs of deterioration - worsening airway oedema, worsening wheeze, shock and rash as a late sign.

They should declare an emergency, summon appropriate help, and administer IM adrenaline at the correct dose.

With 2 minutes remaining ask the candidate to summarise the case, the management so far, and next steps, including the need for ICU admission.

Case 13

Jeanie is a 76-year-old female who has been brought into the ED having been found slumped in her chair at home. She has lung cancer and has been treated with a lobectomy and chemotherapy. She currently takes paracetamol and furosemide only. Jeanie's daughter is present and can answer any questions. There is no history of diabetes, stroke or epilepsy and Jeanie no longer smokes or drinks any alcohol.

The Foundation Year doctor in the ED team has been asked to take perform the initial assessment and formulate a management plan. The relevant findings are as follows:

A: The airway is patent and the patient responds to a question with a confused answer
B: The patient's oxygen saturations are 94% on air
The respiratory rate is 20/min
Respiratory examination is normal
C: Pulse is 100/min. Blood pressure is 110/80.
D: The patient is V on the AVPU scale
There is no external sign of head trauma
Pupils are equal and reactive to light

There is no meningism
All 4 limbs appear to be moving and reflexes are normal
Glucose is 7.0 mmol/L

Temperature is 35.5 C
Sodium is 110 mmol/L on a venous gas. Other parameters are normal.

With 2 minutes remaining ask the candidate to summarise their findings, the management so far, and ask directly about the hyponatraemia.

Case 14

The foundation doctor has been called to assist with a man that is choking in the waiting room of the Emergency Department.

The scenario should be conducted using a mannequin. The candidate is required to progress through the ALS choking algorithm with assistance from a helper who will play the role of the nurse in the scenario.

With 2 minutes remaining ask the candidate to summarise their management and ask how the foreign body could be removed after the patient has arrested. As a follow up question, ask the candidate what other means are available for oxygenation should attempts to relive the upper airway obstruction be unsuccessful.

Case 15

A 65 year old man admitted with SOB and pleuritic chest pain has collapsed on the cardiology ward. The nurse at the bedside has shouted for help. The candidate is the foundation doctor on the ward and is the first to attend.

They are expected to confirm cardiac arrest and put out a cardiac arrest call. They should identify and initial rhythm of VF on the defibrillator and deliver a shock appropriately. Following one shock and 2mins of CPR the rhythm will switch to PEA. Following administration of adrenaline and further 2mins of CPR there is return of spontaneous circulation (ROSC).

Ask the candidate to identify the reversible causes of cardiac arrest (4 Hs & 4 Ts) and which is the most likely in this case.

Case 16

Daniel is a 25-year-old man who was knocked off his bike and landed on his back. He has been brought to the emergency department and is complaining that he can't move his legs. His airway and breathing have already been assessed. He has a diaphragmatic breathing pattern and respiratory rate of 25. A C-spine collar is already in situ.

The candidate should continue the primary survey.

The clinical findings are as follows:
Heart rate of 40/min
Blood pressure of 80/50
GCS 15
Pupils equal and reactive to light
No external signs of head trauma
Flaccid paralysis of the lower limbs
Absent patellar reflexes, intact upper limb reflexes
Sensory level at T4
Soft abdomen
No obvious long bone or pelvic injuries
Normal temperature and blood glucose

Ask the candidate to summarise the case and answer the following questions

What would you like to do now?
What imaging is required?
What is the pathophysiology of neurogenic shock?

Case 17

Lisa is a 25 year old primigravida who has attended the hospital for a midwifery appointment and has asked to speak to a doctor about pain relief during labour.

She is very anxious about the pain of childbirth, but has heard some very worrying stories from friends about the risks of having an epidural. She doesn't know what to do and is getting increasingly worried about having her baby.

The candidate is a Foundation Year doctor who will be expected to explore the patient's concerns and offer simple advice about the options for pain relief during labour in a reassuring and understandable way.

With 2 minutes remaining ask the candidate to summarise the discussion and suggest a plan for this woman.

Case 18

The candidate has been asked to talk to a year 4 medical student about the drugs that are commonly used in Anaesthetics. To help them they should be provided with labelled syringes to use as an aide memoire (or alternatively a list of drugs can be used). The candidate has been instructed to give as much information as they can - the most salient facts are included in the mark scheme.

They will be expected to identify each class of drug and give a brief summary of their clinical usage. They should also field any questions the student may pose
The list of drugs is as follows:

Hypnotics/induction agents Propofol Thiopental	Opiates Fentanyl Morphine	Muscle Relaxants Suxamethonium Rocuronium	Anti-emetics Ondansatron Cyclizine
Sympathomemetics Ephedrine Metaraminol	Vagolytics Atropine Glycopyrollate	Local Anaesthetics Lidocaine Laevobupivicaine	

Case 19

A 62-year-old man is to undergo an elective OGD to investigate his worsening epigastric pain.

The Foundation year doctor has been asked to explain the process of conscious sedation to the patient who is worried about being awake during the procedure. The patient has some prior knowledge about the process as his friend has previously undergone one with a bad experience.
The candidate is to focus on sedation and not necessarily the indication for the OGD.

With 2 minutes remaining ask the candidate to summarise the case, the management so far, and next steps, including the as instructions to be given to the patient after the procedure.

Case 20

The candidate has been instructed to explain spinal anaesthesia to a midwifery student.

They should to be able to approach this task by using language and terminology that a junior member of the labour ward team would be expected to understand. The actor has been instructed to seek clarification on a number of points, and may not immediately grasp some concepts. The mark scheme reflects the necessity for a patient approach!

One aspect of this station is to consider the safe conduct of anaesthesia. With 2 minutes remaining ask the candidate directly regarding checks prior to commencing a spinal anaesthetic, patient monitoring during regional anaesthesia, and the emergency management of potential complications after spinal anaesthesia (hypotension and high spinal block). Specific management is not crucial, rather the application of a systematic ABC approach and calling for senior help.

Case 21

The candidate should review the diagrams of 4 oxygen delivery devices. They should then provide brief teaching to the medical student, including some of the advantages and disadvantages of each oxygen delivery device. Some points in the accompanying mark scheme will be covered during the teaching.

With 2 minutes remaining in the station directly ask the candidate any of the following questions that have not already been explained /answered. These form two parts; the first part relates to the achievable oxygen concentrations offered by each device, the second part consists of 4 clinical scenarios.

The answers regarding oxygen concentrations are provided as absolute figures. In reality there is a wide degree of variation in oxygen concentrations, so these values (apart from atmospheric oxygen) can be considered as estimates. Answers within 2% are acceptable.

The text in italics after each clinical scenario is for information purposes and can be reviewed with the candidate after the station has been completed if time allows.

Questions:

1) As a percentage, what is the atmospheric concentration of oxygen (i.e., that found in room air)?
21%.

2) Identify Device 1: Nasal cannulae / speculae

3) What percentage of oxygen will the patient receive if this device is attached to oxygen at 2 L/min?
~28%

4) And at 6 L/min?
~38%

5) Identify Device 2: Hudson mask / face mask

6) What percentage of oxygen will the patient receive if this device is attached to oxygen at 6 L/min?
~50%

7) Identify Device 3: Reservoir mask / non-rebreathe mask

8) What percentage of oxygen will the patient receive if this device is attached to oxygen at 15 L/min?
90%

9) How do you inflate the reservoir bag after the mask is attached to an oxygen supply before applying the mask to the patient?
Occlude the valve inside the mask.

10) Identify Device 4: Venturi mask

11) These devices have colour-coded adapters to control the inspired concentration of oxygen. For each of the colours listed in the table can you indicate the oxygen percentage each should supply?
Yellow 35%   Red 40%   Green 60%

12) What else relating to oxygen supply allows the device to administer the specified oxygen percentage?
Oxygen flow rate.

13) Where can the appropriate flow rate for each adapter be found?
It is printed on the collar of the Venturi attachment.

14) Which of the above devices are 'fixed performance devices'?
Venturi mask only.

Clinical scenarios
For each of the following scenarios choose the most appropriate device.

Scenario 1: 24-hours post-operatively, a patient on the surgical ward has an SpO_2 of 93%. They are comfortable and have a normal respiratory rate.
Answer: Nasal cannulae.

The incidence of atelectasis post operatively leads to a short-term additional FiO2 requirement. In this instance the most practical choice best tolerated by the patient would be nasal cannulae.

Scenario 2: A patient with severe COPD has presented with an exacerbation of his disease. He is responding to nebulised treatment, and requires an arterial blood gas sample.
Answer: Venturi face mask.

Controlled oxygen therapy is important for patients with severe COPD. As the disease progresses, there may be chronic hypercapnoea which can affect the sensitivity of the brainstem's respiratory centres to changes in PaCO2. A small proportion of these patients may rely on relative hypoxia to maintain their respiratory effort - the 'hypoxic drive'. Venturi masks play an important role in providing supplemental oxygen in these situations especially.

Scenario 3: A patient admitted into the Emergency Department resuscitation area as a trauma call after a road traffic collision, with chest wall bruising and an obvious femoral fracture.
Answer: Reservoir / non-rebreathe mask.

This patient may have significant chest wall and pulmonary injuries, with blood loss from the femoral injury. Until the injury pattern is fully elucidated the patient should receive maximal oxygen therapy.

Scenario 4: A normally fit and well patient recovering in the endoscopy department after a colonoscopy under light sedation.
Answer: Hudson face mask.

Procedural sedation can result in a temporarily reduced respiratory drive. The most practical device to administer supplemental oxygen in the short term for a drowsy patient is the face mask.

Case 22
The candidate is the foundation year doctor in anaesthetic and has been called to recovery to review Betty an 80 year old lady who is 2 hours post left total hip replacement.

She is currently reporting pain in her left hip and has been given no medication since leaving theatre. She received 8mg IV morphine on the table, but no other analgesia.

The candidate is expected to review her pain and prescribe appropriate treatment.

Case 23
Clarice is a 60-year-old woman who was admitted for mastectomy for breast cancer. Her postoperative pain has been managed with IV morphine patient controlled analgesia system (PCA), with a bolus dose of 1mg. She has used a total of 20mg in the last 24 hours.
The candidate should take a pain history (including allergies) and formulate a pain management plan that should include a prescription for an appropriate dose of oral morphine.

Ask the candidate the following questions:

What other medications may be useful to administer in this scenario?
What emergency drug should also be prescribed?
What advice would you give the patient?

Case 24
The candidate is a Foundation Year doctor on their Anaesthetics rotation. They have been asked to check and administer a blood transfusion to a patient who is in recovery after his elective colorectal procedure this morning.

The candidate must safely check and prepare the unit of blood for administration, assisted by the recovery nurse.

With 2 minutes remaining at the end of the station the candidate may require direct questioning regarding frequency of observations during transfusion and time limits for product administration after removal from temperature controlled storage.

Case 25

Michelle is a 26-year-old woman who has returned to the GI ward following a colonoscopy under sedation.

The nurse on the ward is unhappy that Michelle seems very drowsy and is snoring. Her respiratory rate is 6 breaths/minute. Ask the candidate to address the partial airway obstruction by demonstrating on the mannequin some simple airway manoeuvers, correctly sizing and inserting airway adjuncts, and demonstrating they can use the bag-valve mask to support ventilation.

Any requests to know what sedation the patient has received (100mcg of fentanyl, 4mg of midazolam) or obtain antagonists such as naloxone or flumazenil should be acknowledged, but keep them focused on the practical aspects of the station.

They should ask for help, and should be assured that whatever assistance they request is on its way, but they need to continue to manage the patient until that help arrives.

Orthopaedics & Rheumatology

Case 1

A 40-year-old rugby player comes to orthopaedic clinic with a troublesome shoulder. He has experienced multiple episodes of dislocation always during rugby matches. Most of these episodes have been treated with reduction on the field however the most recent episode last week required sedation in the emergency department. He is concerned about ongoing feelings of instability.

The foundation year doctor in clinic has been asked to take the initial history and then summarise their findings back to the team.

After 6 minutes stop the candidate whatever stage they are at and ask them to 'please summarize your findings and your management plan from here'.

Ask the candidate what the likely diagnosis is and what further investigations they would like to organize.

Case 2

A 70-year-old male, retired builder has presented to orthopaedic clinics with bilateral hip and groin pain for months – now worsening in the past few weeks.

The foundation year doctor in clinic has been asked to take the initial history and then summarize their findings back to the team.

After 6 minutes stop the candidate whatever stage they are at and ask them to 'please summarize your findings and your management plan from here'.

Ask the candidate what the likely diagnosis is and what further investigations they would like to organize.

Case 3

A 47-year old female has been referred by her GP to the orthopaedic hand clinic with a 3-month history of right hand and wrist pain which has failed to settle with activity modification and splinting. The GP believe this could be carpal tunnel syndrome requiring surgery.

The foundation year doctor in clinic has been asked to take the initial history and then summarize their findings back to the team. The doctor should consider and directly ask about exacerbating factors.

After 6 minutes stop the candidate whatever stage they are at and ask them to 'please summarize your findings and your management plan from here'.

Ask the candidate what the likely diagnosis is and what further investigations they would like to organize.

Case 4

A 25-year-old male has been referred by her GP to rheumatology clinic with a 9-month history of lower back pain. He has taken over-the-counter Ibuprofen 400mg TDS for over 4 weeks and was recently prescribed Co-Codamol 30/500mg QDS by his GP which hasn't settled her symptoms. The GP is concerned about the possibility of an inflammatory aetiology to his pain. His symptoms are highly suggestive of an ankylosing spondylitis and include early morning stiffness, a history of bilateral Achilles tendonitis and an episode of uveitis 3 years previously which resolved with topical steroids. He has no peripheral articular symptoms.

The foundation year doctor in the clinic has been asked to take the initial history and then summarize their findings back to the team. The patient will disclose a family history of inflammatory bowel disease and psoriasis affecting two close relatives.

After 6 minutes stop the candidate whatever stage they are at and ask them to 'please summarize your findings and your investigation and management plan from here'. Ask the candidate what the likely diagnosis is and what further investigations they would like to organize.

Case 5

A 75-year-old female has self-presented to the emergency department with a 2-month history of thoraco-lumbar spine pain. Her pain suddenly worsened over the last 48 hours. She has taken over-the-counter Ibuprofen 200mg TDS for over 4 weeks but this hasn't helped. She hasn't seen her GP for this ailment. She has red flag symptoms including nocturnal pain, unintentional weight loss (approximately 10kg over the past 4 weeks) and poor appetite. Her symptoms are highly suggestive of an underlying malignancy. She has no peripheral articular symptoms. On further questioning, the patient will disclose a history of perianal sensory loss and difficulty passing urine over the past 24 hours. She has also had one episode of faecal incontinence earlier today. Of note, she is an ex-smoker with a 30 pack-year history and has had a chronic cough for 4 months which she hasn't sought medical attention for.

The foundation year doctor in the emergency department has been asked to take the initial history and then summarize their findings back to the team.

After 6 minutes stop the candidate whatever stage they are at and ask them to 'please summarize your findings and your investigation and management plan from here'. Ask the candidate what the likely diagnosis is and what further investigations they would like to organize.

Case 6

A patient has been referred by their GP rheumatology clinic with a 3-month history of muscle and joint pain. The foundation year doctor in clinic has been asked to take perform a GALS examination and then summarize their findings back to the team. If the candidate attempts to take a clinical history, please confirm this is a clinical examination station and eliciting a history is not required, aside from the three screening questions (listed below) that are routine in GALS assessment.
Do you have any pain or stiffness in your muscles, joints or back?
Can you dress yourself completely without any difficulty?
Can you walk up and down the stairs without any difficulty?

After 6 minutes stop the candidate whatever stage they are at and ask them to 'please summarize your findings and your planned investigations'.

Case 7

In this case a 60-year-old male patient has attended Orthopaedic outpatient clinic with restricted range of shoulder movement over 6 months. The patient has had previous dislocations successfully reduced in the emergency department but not required any surgery. The candidate is expected to illicit weakness in rotator cuff function and exclude frozen shoulder. The candidate is in the role of an foundation year doctor and has been asked to examine the affected shoulder.

The doctor has to examine the affected shoulder. The candidate to allowed to ask some introductory questions but the focus of the station should be examination of the shoulder. If required, prompt the candidate to examine the affected shoulder only.

After 6 minutes stop the candidate whatever stage they are at and ask them to present their findings and suggest relevant investigations and management.

Case 8

In this case a 60-year-old female patient has attended GP appointment for hip and groin pain affecting her over 2 years. The candidate is in the role of an foundation year doctor and has been asked to examine the affected hip.

The doctor has to examine the affected hip. The candidate to allowed to ask some introductory questions but the focus of the station should be examination of the knee. If required, prompt the candidate to examine the affected hip only.

After 6 minutes stop the candidate whatever stage they are at and ask them to present their findings and suggest relevant investigations and management.

Case 9

In this case a 30-year-old female patient has attended GP appointment for knee pain and locking following a sports injury. The candidate is in the role of an foundation year doctor and has been asked to examine the affected knee.

The doctor has to examine the affected knee. The candidate to allowed to ask some introductory questions but the focus of the station should be examination of the knee. If required, prompt the candidate to examine the affected knee only.

After 6 minutes stop the candidate whatever stage they are at and ask them to present their findings and suggest relevant investigations and management.

Case 10

In this case a 40-year-old female patient has attended the emergency department with acute onset back pain following a dive into a swimming pool. The central lower back pain radiates down her right leg and is affecting her sensation around the right foot.

The foundation year doctor has to examine the spine and should progress to focus on examination of the sciatic nerve. The candidate to allowed to ask some introductory questions but the focus of the station should be examination.

The station should provide a tendon hammer for reflexes and you are allowed to prompt the candidate to make us of this during the examination.

After 6 minutes stop the candidate whatever stage they are at and ask them to present their findings and suggest relevant investigations and management.

Case 11

A 70-year-old female patient presents to see you in a GP clinic appointment complaining of bilateral pain around the big toe and difficulty with some footwear. This pain has been a problem for a long time but worsened over 6 months.

The foundation year doctor has to examine the affected feet and is allowed to focus on a single foot to demonstrate this skill. The candidate to allowed to ask some introductory questions but the focus of the station should be examination of the foot. If required, prompt the candidate to examine one hand only.

After 6 minutes stop the candidate whatever stage they are at and ask them to present their findings and suggest relevant investigations and management.

Case 12

A 40-year-old female patient presents to the emergency department with severe neck pain of acute onset after a low energy collision as the driver of a car. Her neck pain is constant, severe and radiates down her right arm. On and off she reports tingling sensation in the arm.

The foundation year doctor has to examine the upper limb neurological status. The candidate to allowed to ask some introductory questions but the focus of the station should be examination.

The station should provide a tendon hammer for reflexes and you are allowed to prompt the candidate to make us of this during the examination.

After 6 minutes stop the candidate whatever stage they are at and ask them to present their findings and suggest relevant investigations and management.

Case 13

An 85-year-old female has been brought into the ED having been found on the floor by her residential home warden. She has been unable to walk and is complaining of pain in the right hip.

After 6 minutes, please stop the candidate and ask: "Please summarise your findings and discuss how you would like to investigate and manage this patient."

X Ray Review:

Assume the radiographs have the complete patient identifiers and date they were taken.

They are technically adequate with an AP projection of both hips including the proximal femurs and both iliac crests and a lateral projection of the left hip. There is no excessive rotation and the penetration is acceptable.

The most obvious abnormality is a left displaced intracapsular neck of femur fracture. Joint space is maintained, and all other joints are appropriately aligned. There are no soft tissue abnormalities and no other fractures identified on reviewing the cortical outline of all the bones.

Questions;

1. What is the most common cause of fragility fractures?
Osteoporosis

2. Which arteries contribute blood supply to the femoral head?
Medial circumflex femoral artery (main contributor)
Lateral circumflex femoral artery
Inferior Gluteal artery
Superior gluteal artery
Artery of Ligamentum Teres (patent in children, minimal supply in adults)

3. What is the main concern with intracapsular fractures?
Loss of blood supply to the femoral head

4. How should intracapsular fractures be treated in the older population?
Arthroplasty (hemiarthroplasty or total hip replacement)

5. How should extracapsular fractures be treated?
Fixation with dynamic hip screw or intramedullary nailing

Case 14
A patient with known kidney disease and non-specific joint pains has been referred to the metabolic bone clinic. They were seen in the clinic yesterday by the new clinical nurse specialist along with the consultant. Several investigations were requested and the results are now available. The consultant is not around and the nurse specialist would like to discuss the results with another member of the team.

The results show secondary hyperparathyroidism in a patient with known end stage renal failure. It is not primary or tertiary hyperparathyroidism because the calcium level is low.

Case 15
The candidate is required to demonstrate scrubbing up technique and appropriate donning of a gown and gloves.

A sink with appropriate taps, surgical brush and surgical scrub are provided. A packed surgical gown and towels are provided as are appropriately sized packed sterile gloves.

You will finish by asking the candidate the following questions:

1. Which patient allergy group should be identified and acted upon before theatre management?
Latex allergy, some hospitals still use latex containing surgical gloves

2. Once scrubbed up – which parts of your gown and gloves can be considered sterile?
a. Hand to elbow and nipple to mid-waist only

3. What is sterilisation?
a. A process of removal or deactivation of micro-organisms from a surface including bacteria, fungi and viruses

4. What types of sterilisation do you know?
a. Heat sterilisation, Chemical sterilisation, Radiation sterilization

5. What steps would you take in you sustained a needlestick injury?
a. Expose the wound and thoroughly irrigate encouraging bleeding. Document injury and inform line manager/ theatre manager. Attend Occupational Health or ED for further management according to local Trust policies.

Case 16

A 25-year-old motorcyclist has attended the ED shortly after being involved in a road traffic accident resulting in him coming off his motorcycle. He has removed his own helmet and walked at the scene. He has self-presented to the ED complaining of neck pain. He has been transferred to the resuscitation area and is standing up next to the bed.

The orthopaedic foundation year doctor on call has been asked to immobilise the patient's cervical spine.

A stiff cervical spine collar, blocks and a Velcro strap/tape is provided. A third person is available to assist in providing in line immobilisation if requested by the candidate.

Case 17

This is a case of postoperative compartment syndrome of the leg following tibial nailing earlier today.

Ask the candidate to assess the patient including brief history, examination and management.

Once the assessment shows that the patient has had high levels of opioid analgesia without relief the candidate should state that they are considering compartment syndrome. Candidate should recognise the need for urgent surgical decompression. During the assessment the candidate will examine the limb and when performing appropriate tests you will offer the positive findings of tense compartments, severe tenderness and worsening pain on passive stretch. The limb remain perfused with a palpable pulse but reduced sensation in the foot.

You should allow the candidate 6 minute for assessment and then a further 2 minutes to present their findings and management plan and answer your questions.

You should ask the following questions;

What is the definition of compartment syndrome?
What are the signs of a compartment syndrome?
Describe the underlying pathology of compartment syndrome?
Outline the main management points in the BOAST guideline for compartment syndrome?

Case 18

The candidate is on the trauma team at the major trauma centre for the area. A young adult male, not yet identified, has been brought in by HEMS following RTA. He has multiple injuries including a tibial shaft fracture with a large contaminated open wound. There is considerable skin loss and fat, muscle and bone is visible.

Ask the candidate to describe their initial management approach to this scenario which should be guided by ATLS protocol.

Following a satisfactory answer please ask the candidate to now focus on the open fracture management. Candidate should recognise the need for antibiotics, tetanus and urgent surgical debridement.

You should allow the candidate 6 minute for assessment and then a further 2 minutes to present their findings and management plan and answer your questions.

Describe a classification system for open fractures?
Describe the key points of the BOAST guidelines for management of open fractures?
What is the indication for immediate out of hours debridement?

Case 19

A 19-year-old man is brought into the emergency department by the police. You have been informed he has been stabbed in his arm approximately 2 hours ago. He is complaining his hand feels cold and numb.

The candidate is a foundation year 2 doctor in ED who has been asked to assess him and report their findings and management plan to their consultant. When they go to see the patient, you are presented with a deep laceration to the antecubital fossa.

The patient has no median nerve function, no radial pulse and a cold hand.

You should allow the candidate 6 minute for assessment and then a further 2 minutes to present their findings and management plan and answer your questions.

What are the signs of a vascular injury?
What are the signs of a radial nerve injury?
What are the signs of a median nerve injury?
What are the signs of an ulnar nerve injury?
When should a neurovascular injury be treated?

Case 20

A 95-year-old lady has been brought up to the orthopaedic ward from the emergency department. She is screaming out in pain and trying to get out of her bed. The patient has had a hip x-ray and a chest x-ray in accident and emergency. The nurses have done a set of observations.

The candidate is the foundation year doctor on call for trauma and orthopaedics and has been asked to clerk her in. They have been presented with the following x-rays and observations.

You should allow the candidate 6 minute for assessment and then a further 2 minutes to present their findings and management plan.

Case 21

A 56-year-old man has been brought by ambulance to the Emergency Department following falling from a ladder at a height of 3m.
The orthopaedic doctor in the trauma team has been asked to perform a primary survey.

If asked by the candidate for the patient's examination findings:

Airway is clear, no abnormal sounds.

Chest expands equally, central trachea, normal percussion note, equal normal breath sounds, no chest wall tenderness.

Palpable radial pulse. No obvious haemorrhage sites. Soft, non-tender abdomen, no stigmata of pelvic injury. No pain in upper limbs, no pain in thighs, pain in both ankles and feet.

Observations:- HR 120   BP 95/65   RR 22   Sats 90% on 2l

Case 22

A fit and healthy 21-year-old woman was admitted late last night with a broken ankle. She was placed in a temporary backslab and is on the trauma operating list today for "open reduction and internal fixation of the right ankle" where the fracture will be fixed with a small metal plate a series of screws.

The foundation year doctor has been asked to answer the patient's questions and go through the consent process. They have seen this operation before several times and are therefore able to explain it to the patient. They need to obtain informed consent and documented proof of this by signing the consent form with the patient.

After 6 minutes stop the candidate whatever stage they are at and ask them to 'please summarize your consultation'.

Case 23

A fit and healthy 21-year-old woman was admitted 2 days ago with broken ankle she underwent surgery to fix the broken ankle (open reduction and internal fixation) yesterday and is due to be discharged home non-weight bearing in a plaster cast (below her knee).

The foundation year doctor has been asked to answer the patient's questions about preventing deep vein thrombosis (DVT) as part of the discharge process. The patient will voice concern about getting a DVT whilst in a plaster cast the candidate is expected to perform a Venous thrombo-embolism (VTE) assessment on the patient and explain the role of Enoxaparin injections and compression stockings.

After 6 minutes stop the candidate whatever stage they are at and ask them to 'please summarize your consultation'.

Case 24

A 78-year-old woman with a recent history of fragility fracture has been asked to attend her GP to start a bisphosphonate. She has done some reading online about bisphosphonates and is very concerned about starting on the medication. She will be particularly concerned about the risk of osteonecrosis of the jaw and atypical femoral fractures.

The candidate should be aware that the risk of osteoporotic fragility fracture far outweighs the risk of atypical fragility fractures and osteonecrosis of the jaw in this instance.

The candidate should give adequate advice on how the medication should be taken. Alendronic acid is the first line biologic in the UK. It is given as a once weekly preparation. The BNF advises "Tablets should be swallowed whole with plenty of water while sitting or standing; to be taken on an empty stomach at least 30 minutes before breakfast (or another oral medicine); patient should stand or sit upright for at least 30 minutes after taking tablet"

After 6 minutes stop the candidate whatever stage they are at and ask them to 'please summarize your consultation'.

Case 25

A 30-year-old woman with an 8-week history of joint pain and swelling in a distribution that is typical for rheumatoid arthritis (RA) has attended clinic today. She has been seen once before and investigations were requested. These have confirmed a diagnosis of RA. She has returned to clinic today to get the results and discuss the treatment options.

The candidate should explain the diagnosis in simple terms minimising the use of jargon or where medical terms are used give a lay explanation for them.

The candidate should be aware that modern treatment strategies advocate starting treatment with disease modifying anti-rheumatic drugs (DMARDs) early to prevent permanent damage. The most commonly used first line drug is methotrexate and this should at least be discussed. However, methotrexate is potentially teratogenic and the candidate should explain that alternatives are available without having to give specific examples.

The candidate should appropriately re-assure the patient that the risk of her future children being affected by the disease is low.

After 6 minutes stop the candidate whatever stage they are at and ask them to 'please summarize your consultation

Psychiatry

Case 1

A 45-year-old supermarket cashier called Annabel has attended their GP surgery with bleeding gums from excessive tooth brushing. She is not previously known to the practice.

The foundation year doctor based at the practice has been asked to take a history from this patient, with a view to summarise the findings.

At 7 minutes, ask the candidate for a summary and ask the following questions:

What do you think the most likely diagnosis is for this patient? (Obsessive Compulsive Disorder)

What differential diagnosis would you consider?

What would you like to include in your initial management plan?

Case 2

The foundation year doctor working on a secure psychiatric ward has been asked to speak to the son of one of the patients, Rafael, who is angry. The candidate should meet with Rafael and speak with him in a way that de escalates his anger, remains non-confrontational but also tries to address his concerns and provide some reassurance.

The candidate should remain calm in the face of threats by the relative and should not make derogatory comments about colleagues in order to win the relatives favour.

Pay close attention of the candidate's body language and voice, they should aim to lower the tone and volume of their voice and appear attentive to the angry relative.

Case 3

A 25-year-old lady called Phoebe attends the emergency department following an episode of deliberate self-harm. She has been medically cleared by the emergency department registrar.

The foundation doctor on the liaison psychiatry team has been asked to take a detailed history from the patient with a view to forming a differential diagnosis and initial management plan.

Pay particular attention to the candidate's interaction with this young lady who is prone to becoming irritable and defensive. If the candidate fails to establish a good rapport, the actor may threaten to end the discussion.

At 7 minutes, please ask the candidate to summarise the case, and then ask the following two questions:

What differential diagnoses would you consider for this patient?

What would you like to include in your initial management plan?

Case 4

A 23-year-old lady called Ling has come into the emergency department She is 6 weeks postpartum. Her friend was concerned with her recent behaviour so has brought her in for assessment. Currently Ling looks anxious and seems to acting oddly and responding to voices.

The foundation doctor in the emergency department has been asked to take a brief history and present the Mental State Examination (MSE).

At 6 minutes stop the candidate and ask them to summarise the MSE, and what they would include in their initial management plan.

Case 5

The candidate has been asked to complete a Mental State Examination (MSE) on Kryz, a 27-year-old male brought into the emergency department by police on Section 136. He was found agitated in the city centre, talking 'nonsense' and was found climbing onto private property

The candidate should focus on performing the MSE rather than take a history.

Please stop the candidate after 5 minutes and ask them to summarise the MSE, provide a differential diagnosis and management plan.

Please look out for the following phrases when the candidate is presenting the MSE:

MSE component	Description
Appearance and behaviour	Anxious, casually dressed, dirty clothes, poor eye contact, fidgety, irritated, difficulty concentrating
Speech	Pressure of speech, normal form and content
Mood and affect	Stressed, nervous, scared, anxious, paranoid, irritable. Mood is not low or elated
Thought	Secondary delusion of a persecutory nature and normal thought form
Perception	Third person auditory hallucinations, some visual illusions e.g. cameras
Cognition	Poor concentration, orientated
Insight	No insight
Risk	Medium risk to himself – not eating, poor sleep, may get hurt whilst 'removing cameras' around the city. High risk to neighbours – has had thoughts of attacking neighbours for the good of society, only protective factor is that the police won't believe him

Case 6

The candidate is a foundation doctor working in a suburban GP surgery. They have been asked to take a history from Anne, a 32-year-old lady who has come to see her GP due to increasing anxiety and fear of leaving the house.

Pay particular attention to the candidate's communication skills and their ability to put an anxious patient at ease. You also need to assess their awareness of anxiety disorders and ability to take a focused history.

Please stop the candidate after 7 minutes and ask them to summarise their findings and give a diagnosis.

Case 7

The candidate has been asked to speak to a 43-year-old male called Liam diagnosed with paranoid schizophrenia 5 years ago. He has already been trialled on 2 different anti-psychotics with little effect. His consultant reviewed him earlier in the psychiatry outpatient clinic and has advised starting clozapine.

Their colleague has already performed a physical examination, ECG and bloods all of which were normal. Liam has no past medical history and no known drug allergies.

The candidate has been asked to counsel this patient regarding their clozapine treatment. They have 8 minutes.

Case 8

A 20-year-old lady called Summer has been admitted to the inpatient psychiatric unit following some unusual and reckless behaviour.

The foundation doctor based on the acute psychiatry ward has been asked to take a history from the patient.
At 7 minutes, please ask the candidate to summarise the case, and then ask the following three questions:

What do you think is the most likely diagnosis for this patient? (Bipolar affective disorder)
What differential diagnoses would you also consider?
What would you like to include in your initial management plan?

Case 9

A 30-year-old lady called Charmaine has been admitted on the inpatient psychiatry ward following her first episode of mania. The consultant wants to start her on lithium to help stabilise her mood.

The foundation doctor based on the acute psychiatry ward has been asked to counsel the patient about starting this drug. She is an informal patient and has been judged by the consultant to have capacity to consent to medication.

Pay particular attention to the candidates use of medical jargon

Case 10
A 29-year-old nurse called Paul has been acting more withdrawn at work and the foundation doctor has been become concerned regarding his behaviour. They have been asked to take a psychiatric history and evaluate risk.

After 7 minutes stop the candidate and ask them to summarise their findings. Once complete ask the following questions:

How would you rate this patient's suicide risk?
What aspects of his case led you to give him this risk rating?

Case 11
A 17-year-old boy called Taylor has been brought into the GP surgery by his mother who is concerned that he is behaving oddly as he has become antisocial and irritable. His mother has decided not to be present during the consultation as she feels her son will be more open without her there.

The foundation doctor based at the GP practice has been asked to take a history and formulate a management plan and explain this plan to the patient.

At 7 minutes, if the candidate has not already done so, prompt them to summarise their consultation and discuss their management plan with the patient.

Case 12
The candidate has been asked to examine a 48-year-old lady called Violet in the emergency department. The aim of the station is to test the candidate's ability to recognise neuroleptic malignant syndrome and its symptoms.

Please inform the candidate of their findings at their request, e.g. when looking at the patient from the end of the bed you can inform them that she is clammy and sweaty. Positive findings are listed below:

Danger: The patient is in the resus bed and you are safe to proceed
Response: The patient is drowsy. She is not responding to voice. But opens her eyes to her name
Airway: No snoring, swelling, stridor or evidence of airway obstruction
Breathing: Tachypneoic (respiratory rate 26), Sats 98% on 35% oxygen venturi, using accessory muscles to breathe, symmetrical chest expansion, chest clear.
Circulation: Pyrexic 39.5 degrees Celsius, Tachycardic (pulse 104), Hypotensive (blood pressure 94/50), Hot centrally and peripherally, capillary refill time <2 seconds, looks pale, sweaty and clammy. Incontinent of urine.
Disability: Confused GCS E3, V2, M5 10/15, lead pipe rigidity (increased tone) in upper and lower limbs, significant tremor in both arms
Everything Else:Abdomen soft and non tender, glucose 4.8.

Investigations include
Bloods – FBC, U&E, calcium, LFTs, CK, INR – Sent for analysis
ABG – pO2 24.4, pCO2 3.4 BE -4.5, Bicarb 16.0 Lactate 5.6
Urinary drug screen – Sent for analysis
CXR – Clear lung fields
ECG – Sinus tachycardia Rate 110

Management includes
IV Fluids
Cooling – Take clothes off whilst maintaining dignity as much as possible
Benzodiazapines if catatonic
Doperminergic agents (however the evidence is limited and use is controversial)

Stopping the offending medication is vital
ICU referral If signs of respiratory distress, temp >40 or requiring sedation/IV cooling

Case 13
A 52-year-old woman, Roya, has come into her GP surgery to discuss her mood. The foundation year doctor has been asked to take a history from her, followed by a summary and differential diagnosis based on the symptoms described.

Please stop the candidate at 7 minutes and ask them to summarise and state the differential diagnoses. Please prompt the candidate to justify the severity of the diagnosis (mild, moderate or severe) if they do not do so, and to explain why.

Case 14
The police have brought a 21-year-old male called Ahmed to the emergency department. The foundation year doctor has been asked to take a history from him.

Please stop the candidate at 7 minutes and ask them to summarise and provide a differential diagnosis. Please prompt the candidate to justify the diagnosis if they do not do so, and to explain why.

Case 15
A 78-year-old man called Albert attends his GP surgery. He lives with his daughter and she encouraged him to make an appointment with his GP as she feels he has been more forgetful lately.

The foundation year doctor has been asked to take a history from the patient. Please stop the candidate after 6 minutes and ask them to make a summary, including a brief risk assessment, differential diagnosis, and an initial plan.

Case 16
Reggie is a 92-year-old gentleman, his wife has come to visit him at the hospital and the candidate has been asked to take a collateral history.

At 5 minutes please stop the candidate and ask the following questions:

1. How would you classify Mr Hammond's confusion?

2. What might be causing his acute confusion/delirium?

3. What are some causes of chronic confusion?

4. How would you like to manage Mr Hammond's acute confusion?

Case 17
A 78-year-old man called Clifford has come into the GP practice with his daughter. She is concerned that he has been 'out of sorts' recently.

The foundation doctor at the GP surgery has been asked to take a history from the patient and present their findings.
At 5 minutes stop the candidate and ask them to perform an abbreviated mental test score (AMTS).

At 7 minutes stop the candidate and ask them to: 'please present your history and formulate an initial management plan.'
At the end ask the candidate these questions:

1. What is the Most likely diagnosis?

2. What initial investigations would you perform?

3. What is your initial management plan?

Case 18

The candidate has been asked to take a history from 15-year-old Grace who took an overdose of paracetamol this evening and has been brought to the emergency department department by her mother.

Grace's mother has gone off to answer a phone call and will not be present during the consultation. This station will test the candidate's history taking skills and their ability to evaluate suicide/self harm risk.

Please stop the candidate after 7 minutes and ask them to summarise their history, suggest a suicide risk category and formulate a management plan.

If the candidate mentions taking paracetamol levels in their management plan ask them when they should be taken.State that the "levels have come back above the treatment line" and ask them how would this affect management?

Case 19

A foundation year doctor is working in a busy eemrgency department. They are asked to see a 15-year-old called Natalia, who self-harmed. The doctor is asked to take a history of her self-harm and to establish her current risk.

Emphasis should be placed on the candidate's ability to ask potentially difficult questions sensitively and to behave professionally and compassionately towards the patient.

They should also clearly distinguish deliberate self-harm from attempted suicide in the risk assessment.

Please stop the candidate at 5 minutes, so that you can ask some further questions:

QUESTION: What do you consider the risk to be?
Prompt the candidate to describe the risk to self and to others.

QUESTION: Now that she has spoken to you she feels ready to be discharged from A&E and is planning to go home. What options would you consider in your management plan?

QUESTION: Who else would you speak to?

Case 20

A 16-old girl called Sam has been referred to CAMHS by her GP. The foundation year doctor has been asked to take a focused history from her and to formulate a diagnosis based on the symptoms described.

Please stop the candidate at 6 minutes and ask them to state the diagnoses and discuss potential triggers for this.
QUESTION: What is your diagnosis?
QUESTION: How would you grade the severity, and why? (Mild, moderate or severe)

Surgery

Case 1

A 72-year-old man has presented to the Emergency department acutely unwell with severe abdominal pain. The foundation year doctor has been asked to take the initial history and summarise their findings.

After 6 minutes stop the candidate and ask them to 'please summarise your findings, including a differential diagnosis and immediate management plan' for 2 minutes.

Please follow the mark sheet and grade appropriately.

Case 2

A 22-year-old female has been brought into Emergency Department by ambulance with right iliac fossa pain for the last 12 hours. The foundation year doctor has been asked to take the initial history and summarise their findings.

After 6 minutes stop the candidate and ask them to 'please summarise your findings, including a differential diagnosis and immediate management plan' for 2 minutes.

Please follow the mark sheet and grade appropriately.

Case 3

A 70-year-old man has been referred directly to the on-call surgical registrar by his GP with abdominal pain and vomiting. The foundation year doctor has been asked to take the initial history and summarise their findings.

After 6 minutes stop the candidate and ask them to 'please summarise your findings, including a differential diagnosis and immediate management plan' for 2 minutes.

Please follow the mark sheet and grade appropriately.

Case 4

A 62-year-old male has presented to the general surgical clinic with difficulty opening his bowels. The foundation year doctor has been asked to take the initial history and summarise their findings.

After 6 minutes stop the candidate and ask them to 'please summarise your findings, including a differential diagnosis and immediate management plan' for 2 minutes.

Case 5

A 68-year-old female has been brought into Emergency Department by ambulance with haematemsis. The foundation year doctor has been asked to take the initial history and summarise their findings.

After 6 minutes stop the candidate and ask them to 'please summarise your findings, including a differential diagnosis and immediate management plan' for 2 minutes.

Please follow the mark sheet and grade appropriately.

Case 6

A 41-year-old lady with right upper quadrant pain is the next patient to be seen on the surgical take list. The foundation year doctor has been asked to take the initial history and summarise their findings.

After 6 minutes stop the candidate and ask them to 'please summarise your findings, including a differential diagnosis and immediate management plan' for 2 minutes.

Please follow the mark sheet and grade appropriately.

Case 7

A 68 year old gentleman has come to the hospital unable to move his left leg.

The foundation year doctor has been asked to take the initial history and summarise their findings.

After 6 minutes stop the candidate and ask them to 'please summarise your findings, including a differential diagnosis and immediate management plan' for 2 minutes.

Please follow the mark sheet and grade appropriately.

Case 8

A 75-year-old man has presented to the GP practice complaining of blood in his urine. The foundation year doctor has been asked to take the initial history and summarise their findings.

After 6 minutes stop the candidate and ask them to 'please summarise your findings, including a differential diagnosis and immediate management plan' for 2 minutes.

Please follow the mark sheet and grade appropriately.

Case 9

A 27-year-old male has presented to the department complaining of a dull ache in his left testicle. The foundation year doctor has been asked to take the initial history and summarise their findings.

After 6 minutes stop the candidate and ask them to 'please summarise your findings, including a differential diagnosis and immediate management plan' for 2 minutes.

Please follow the mark sheet and grade appropriately.

Case 10

A 49-year-old female has attended her General Practice clinic with a lump in her right breast. The foundation year doctor has been asked to take the initial history and summarise their findings.

After 6 minutes stop the candidate and ask them to 'please summarise your findings, including a differential diagnosis and immediate management plan' for 2 minutes.Please follow the mark sheet and grade appropriately.

Case 11

The candidate has been asked to obtain a history/assess the mental status of Jack an 80-year-old gentleman two days after an emergency hernia repair.

The patient will maintain a confused affect throughout the scenario and is likely to cooperate minimally with the candidates questioning/assessment.

The candidate should address/introduce themselves to the patient as normal. They should go on to ask basic screening questions of the patients in terms of symptoms. It will soon become apparent that the patient is confused. The candidate should then attempt to perform an abbreviated mental test.

This is likely to be performed with limited success but all aspects should be attempted.

The candidate should persevere with the patient in order to assess them as fully as possible. This should be done reassuringly, with no element of frustration or pressure on the patient so as not to cause any agitation or confusion.

If the candidate attempts to examine the patient then prompt them that it is a history taking station.

After 6 minutes stop the candidate and ask the following questions for 2 minutes

What AMT score has been achieved?

What are the differentials for the patient's clinical state?

What are the causes of an acute delirium particularly in this patient?

How would you manage this patient?

How would you investigate this patient?

Case 12

The candidate has been asked to explain the flexible sigmoidoscopy procedure to a patient, John who is to be referred for this as an outpatient as an urgent two-week referral.

The patient knows nothing of the procedure and wishes to know all about it in terms of what to expect, how he should prepare and what risks and benefits the procedure entails. He is anxious as a friend has been recently diagnosed with colon cancer and he is worried his symptoms may be due to this.

The candidate should establish the patient's knowledge of the procedure and his concerns and expectations of the consultation. From there he should explain the procedure practically and in terms of what risks and benefits it entails. The candidate's explanation should address all concerns and expectations. This should be done in a structured manner to enable better understanding. By the end of the station the candidate should confirm the patient's understanding much like a formal consenting.

If the candidate begins to delve into the patient's symptoms and history in detail please interrupt in order to remind them that the history has been taken and that their role is to explain the investigation only.

The scenario should be handled with subtlety and sensitivity.

Please follow the mark sheet and grade appropriately.

Case 13

The candidate has been asked to hold a conversation with an upset mother who is very concerned that her 9-year-old child Tom has been rushed in for an emergency theatre for splenic rupture.

The candidate should demonstrate adequate breaking bad news skills in an empathic manner and manage patient's frustrations by listening appropriately before exploring patient concerns and addressing any expectations they are able to.

The scenario should be handled with subtlety and sensitivity.

Please follow the mark sheet and grade appropriately.

Case 14

The foundation doctor has been given a scenario of severe pancreatitis, they have been asked to make a referral to the ITU Registrar. This doctor who is under a lot of pressure today due to a lack of staffing and lots of sick patients to assess and manage. They will expect a structured SBAR handover.
After 6 minutes give a warning that there are 2 minutes remaining.

Case 15

The candidate has seen a 71-year-old man was brought in an hour ago as a trauma call. He was a restrained driver of a car who crashed into a tree at 45 mph. He had a full primary and secondary survey; a CT scan has confirmed the only injury sustained is a right-sided pneumothorax. The Emergency Department consultant has said he'll supervise and assist the foundation doctor putting in their first surgical chest drain.

The purpose of this task is to assess the knowledge required to insert a surgical chest drain:

The candidate knows the required equipment
The candidate knows how best to prepare the patient
The candidate knows the steps to safely insert a chest drain

Assist the candidate by organising their equipment and preparing the sterile field. Before the candidate makes an incision ask them what are the anatomical borders of the safe triangle.

Case 16

The candidate will be required to describe the plain abdominal radiograph presented to them (one of three examples).
The candidate will be allowed a pen and paper to scribe notations to aid in the presentation of their findings. No comments from the examiner will be provided during this assessment.

At six minutes the candidate should summarise their findings, presenting the abdominal x ray in an informed and logical and systematic manner. It must be appreciated by the examiner that there are different techniques in presenting plain radiographs, as long as the key points are reviewed, the candidate will score.

Case 17

The candidate will be required to describe the plain chest radiograph presented to them (one of four examples).
The candidate will be allowed a pen and paper to scribe notations to aid in the presentation of their findings. No comments from the examiner will be provided during this assessment.

At six minutes the candidate should summarise their findings, presenting the abdominal x ray in an informed and logical and systematic manner. It must be appreciated by the examiner that there are different techniques in presenting plain radiographs, as long as the key points are reviewed, the candidate will score. Please follow the mark sheet and grade appropriately.

Case 18

The foundation year doctor has been asked to close a wound laceration with three simple interrupted sutures.
With two minute remaining, if the candidate has not yet advised on further management, interrupt them and prompt with the question:

'Is there anything more you would like to do or advise the patient about?'

Case 19

The foundation year doctor has been asked to perform an abdominal examination on a 50 year old man who has presented with acute generalized abdominal pain

You must relay the below information to the candidate when it is appropriate. After 6 minutes, stop the candidate and ask him what further examinations he would like to perform, what investigations he would like, and ask for three possible diagnoses.

	Clinical findings
End of the bed	Looks generally unwell
Hands and nails	Cool and clammy, normal nails
Pulse	110 beats per minute
Examines the face	Dry mucus membranes Sunken eyes Normal conjunctiva Normal skin colour
Inspects abdomen	Mildly distended abdomen Open Appendicectomy Scar
Palpates abdomen for tenderness	Rigid abdomen – epigastric area most tender. Guarding in upper abdomen.
Palpates abdomen for masses	No masses and no abnormal pulsations
Palpates abdomen for Liver, Spleen and Kidneys	Normal
Percusses abdomen	Normal percussion but results in pain in the upper abdomen
Auscultates abdomen	Absent bowel sounds
Examines hernial orifices	No hernias present

The observations are:
Heat Rate – 110bpm, Respiratory Rate – 30bpm, Blood Pressure 100/70, Temperature 38.5°C, Oxygen Saturations 96% on Air

Case 20

The foundation year doctor has been asked to perform an inguinal hernia examination.
After 6 minutes stop the candidate and ask them to 'please summarise your findings, including a differential diagnosis and immediate management plan' for 2 minutes.
Please follow the mark sheet and grade appropriately.

Case 21

The foundation year doctor has been asked to perform a breast examination on a 49-year-old who has a lump in her right breast.

After 6 minutes stop the candidate and ask them to 'please summarise your findings, including a differential diagnosis and immediate management plan' for 2 minutes.

Case 22

The foundation year doctor has been asked to do a full thyroid examination and present their findings. Please ensure a glass of water is available at the station.

After 6 minutes stop the candidate and ask them to 'please summarise your findings, including a differential diagnosis and immediate management plan' for 2 minutes.

Ask the candidate the following questions:
What clinical thyroid state is the patient in? Describe 2 differences on examination between a goitre and a thyroglossal cyst.

Case 23

The candidate has been asked to see a 54-year-old male who is complaining of an abnormal lump and an uncomfortable dragging sensation in his left testis.
There will be a patient present in the station. The candidate has been instructed to initiate the consultation with the patient and undertake an appropriate examination.

After 6 minutes stop the candidate and ask them to 'please summarise your findings, including a differential diagnosis and immediate management plan' for 2 minutes.

Case 24

The candidate has been asked to conduct a primary survey on a man brought into the resuscitation department, following a traumatic road traffic accident. The candidate has been instructed to talk you through the examination.

You must relay the below information to the candidate when it is appropriate. After 6 minutes, stop the candidate and ask them what further tests they would like to perform and for an immediate management plan.

	Observations	Clinical findings	Results
Airway		Airway is patent.	
C-spine		Patient has significant pain in the neck.	
Breathing	RR-22 Sats – 92%	Diminished air-entry on right. Percussion: more resonant on right. Asymmetrical chest wall movement (left > right). Trachea shifted to the left.	CXR – Right sided large pneumothorax.
Circulation	HR – 110 BP – 105/60	HS I+II+0 CRT 4 seconds. Cool peripheries. Patient slightly pale.	ECG – sinus tachycardia.
Disability	PEARL GCS: E4/V4/M6 Temp: 37	Blood glucose: 8	

The purpose of this task is to assess the following:
An understanding of the ATLS assessment

Case 25

The candidate has been asked to see a 72-year-old woman who has presented to the vascular clinic complaining of pain in her calves on walking. There will be a patient present in the station.

The candidate has been instructed to conduct an examination of the peripheral vasculature and report their findings to you.

After 6 minutes stop the candidate and ask them to please summarise their findings.

Emergency medicine

Case 1

A 27-year-old male cyclist who was hit by a car is being brought to the Emergency Department by ambulance. His C-spine has been triple immobilised by the ambulance team.

If asked by the candidate, please provide the following information:
The trauma team are on their way to assist you but you must start your assessment immediately.

A – Patent, no obvious facial deformities, no upper airway noises

B – RR 42, oxygen saturations are 74% on room air, 86% on high flow oxygen, significantly increased work of breathing, right side of chest not moving with respiration, decreased air entry to right side of chest on auscultation, right side of chest hyper-resonant on percussion and mild tracheal deviation.

C – Pulse rate 120, blood pressure 88/50, cool peripheries, sweaty, capillary refill time 3 seconds

D – GCS 14/15, confused and agitated

E – Few superficial cuts and bruises to the lower limbs, no limb deformities.
Once candidate states/performs needle decompression, saturations improve to 99%, HR decreases to 90 and BP starts to improves to 110/80. Ask what the candidates next management would be ideally this would be to speak to ITU and to start the insertion of a chest drain.

Case 2

A 60-year-old male has become unresponsive in a cubicle in the emergency department. The doctor has discovered this patient and is willing to lead the resuscitation.

The candidate must do this according to the principles of ALS.

After 6 minutes stop the candidate whatever stage they are at and ask them to 'please summarise your findings and your management plan from here'

Case 3

This station examines the candidate's knowledge of the ALS protocol. When the candidate arrives on scene the nurse has already started performing chest compressions. They should confirm the cardiac arrest themselves.

They will need prompting with examination findings should they ask for them throughout the scenario.

When the pads are attached pause for a rhythm and pulse check. The monitor will show a VF arrest. They should identify this as a 'shockable rhythm' and instruct for CPR to be resumed.

Once they have delivered one shock and asked for CPR to be restarted, ask the candidate to tell you how long they would continue compressions for before they check the rhythm (answer 2 minutes)?

Once this has been covered tell them that their 2 minutes are up. They should recheck the rhythm. The patient has returned to normal sinus rhythm and the candidate should check the pulse to confirm that this is not PEA.

You can then end the scenario and ask the following questions:

Which drugs are used in a VF arrest situation and when are they given?

Adrenaline and Amiodarone are given after the third shock only in a VF arrest.

Can you list the 8 reversible causes of cardiac arrest?

(4 H's) - Hypoxia, Hypothermia, Hypo/hyperkalaemia and other electrolyte abnormalities and Hypovolaemia, (4 T's) – Tamponade, Tension pneumothorax, Thrombus and Toxins

Extra marks are awarded for good communication with their team.

Case 4
This 19-year-old gets brought into ED resus at 2am. They've been brought in by ambulance after being picked up outside a kebab shop where the patient said they suddenly could not breathe and was noted to have developed a rash with lip swelling.

The foundation doctor in resus overnight has been asked to assess and manage this patient.

They should follow a methodical A to E approach:

A - The girl will become increasingly short of breath and wheezy if oxygen isn't given as part of A. Lip swelling noted (Angioedema).

The candidate should also know that even though medicines usually come later in an A-E assessment, 500mcg 1:1000 adrenaline IM and 10mg chlorphenamine IV(or other antihistamine of choice) should be given in the first instance of anaphylaxis during assessment.

If the candidate asks for an anaesthetist/ICU to be bleeped, they will be enroute ASAP, but are currently delayed in theatre.

B - The patient will struggle to talk or breathe given her SOB, wheeziness and lip swelling. O2 saturations read 92-94%. Reduced air entry at lung bases but loud upper airway sounds on auscultation with inspiratory stridor. Salbutamol and Ipratropium bromide can be given at this point.

Candidate will have difficulties eliciting a history from her till later in the assessment when she's had treatment.

C - IV fluids will need to be given through 2 large bore cannulae. Bloods can be taken at this point. ABG is also appropriate

D - GCS 15 and Glucose is 5 (normal)

E - Widespread, itchy, blanching rash on chest, arms and legs.

Continually re-assess ABCDE again post intervention.

2nd stage of re-assessing:

O2 has come up to 100%. BP has dropped to 80/50.

Part two for examiner to read out:

"The nurse notifies you that the patient has fallen asleep and she sounds like she's snoring."

3rd stage of re-assessing:

Reassess again from A-E and fast bleep anaesthetists:

After 5 minutes if there is an ongoing reaction more adrenaline can be given 500mcg of 1:1000 IM or only if expert seniors are present 50mcg of 1:10000 IV

They need to attempt airway maneuvers and insert an airway adjunct. Shows how to size and insert Guedel airway appropriately.

Only after they've done airway maneuvers with an airway adjunct do the anesthetists arrive.

Case 5

The candidate should take a short history and get an idea of severity of asthma attack. The patient has acute severe asthma with a PEFR of 220. He will benefit from nebulised salbutamol and ipratropium bromide as well as steroids in an appropriate dose. The candidate should select oxygen to drive the nebuliser. He can offer intravenous magnesium sulphate. He can ask for help from others for the therapies to be administered as well as help putting in an IV cannula or getting an arterial blood gas (ABG). The candidate should have an idea of features of life threatening asthma and a low threshold to ask for senior help.

As part of the assessment, you can provide the following information if asked.

A - patent

B - Trachea central,
Wheezy chest sounds, equal air entry, symmetrical chest rise, resonant to percussion
Observations: RR 28, SpO2 93%, PEFR 220. ABG PH 7.4 PO2 8.5 PCO2 4.1 HCO3 28

C - BP 120/70, HR 115, Cool peripheries

D - GCS 15/15

E - Afebrile, some cyanosis

After initial therapy

A - patent

B - Trachea central, clear breath sounds

Observations: RR 22, SpO2 99%, PEFR 450. ABG PH 7.4 PO2 13.5 PCO2 4.0 HCO3 28

C - BP 120/70, HR 120, cool peripheries

D - GCS 15/15

E - Afebrile

Case 6

The doctor has been asked to see a 24-year-old insulin dependent diabetic patient who has just been brought into the emergency department with a 12-hour history of vomiting and abdominal pain. The patient had been out in the sun all of the previous day and had a moderate amount of alcohol. He had not eaten much all day and so he did not take his insulin. He has DKA.

The candidate has been asked to take a focused history - this should centre on the presenting complaint and the events leading up to this presentation. Salient points from his medical history should also be covered (diagnosis of diabetes) as well as his drug history.

The candidate has been asked to do an initial assessment of the patient, this should consist of an A-E approach. As the patient is examined and monitoring is placed the following is found:

A - Patent

B - Respiratory rate 24, Saturations 100% on room air, Chest is clear with bilateral air entry

C - A little cool peripherally, Heart rate 117, Blood pressure 120/67, ECG sinus. No abnormality. Normal T waves.

D - GCS 15 but very tired and only occasionally answering questions fully
Blood glucose 32

E - No obvious injuries, No rashes, Temperature 36.8, Abdomen is mildly tender to palpation. No focus. No guarding. Normal bowel sounds.

The candidate has been asked to identify a likely diagnosis and outline to the nurse any urgent investigations and management. Although they may wish to rule out other causes of the patient's presentation they should identify DKA as the most likely diagnosis and focus their answer on this.

Investigations	Management	Treatment goals (60 min)
Urine dip to confirm diagnosis	Fluids - 0.9% saline without potassium. 1L over 1-2 hours to begin replacement. Fluid bolus not required.	Restore circulating volume (reduce heart rate)
ECG	Insulin - Fixed rate IV insulin infusion at approximately 0.1 units/Kg/ hour.	Reduce blood ketone concentration by 0.5 mmol/L/hour
CXR	Treatment of hyperkalaemia	Reduce blood glucose by 3-5 mmol/L/hour
Blood tests - FBC, renal profile, serum osmolarity, lab glucose, serum ketones. Allow others if well justified.	Critical care referral	Maintain K+ between 4-5mmol/L

Do not award marks for:
Venous/ arterial gas as this has been made available in the question.
Sodium bicarbonate as it is not considered mainstay treatment.

One minute before the end of the station: Stop the candidate and ask them to confirm what they think the likely diagnosis is (if not already stated) and to name two potentially life-threatening complications of DKA.

Case 7

A 25-year-old man is brought into the Emergency Department having a generalised tonic-clonic seizure that started 15 minutes ago. The paramedic team have been unable to secure IV access but have administered one dose of rectal diazepam 10 minutes ago.

The foundation doctor has been called to manage this patient. If asked by the candidate please provide the following information:

The medical emergency team/senior help is on their way to assist you.
On initial assessment:

Patient is having a tonic-clonic seizure

A – jaw clenched, foaming at the mouth, gurgling noises from upper airway.
Once airway suctioned and nasopharyngeal airway inserted, noises from upper airway improve.
B – shallow breathing, RR 30, oxygen saturations 88% in room air, increased to 100% on high flow oxygen, clear lung fields on auscultation
C – pulse rate 120, blood pressure 140/88, warm peripheries, capillary refill time <2sec
D – GCS 3/15, blood sugar 3.5
E – no rashes, temperature 37.0

You may speed up intervals between drugs being administered and ask the candidate what they would like to do next during the scenario however no other prompts please.

After 6 minutes, if not done so, please prompt the candidate for a diagnosis and ask the candidate to summarise a handover of the case to an ICU colleague.

Case 8

This 62-year-old lady had a set of blood tests at the GP this morning. The GP has requested she attend the emergency department immediately as the plasma potassium came back at 7.1mmol/l.

The student should perform a systematic A to E assessment.

A - Patent

B – Equal air entry, Clear chest, RR 18, Sats 98% on Air

C – HR-84, BP 118/75, Cap refill < 2. The venous gas results show a potassium of 7.1mmol/l and a PH 7.35 with all other results within normal limits. The student should request an ECG. They must be handed a good example of the changes seen in hyperkalaemia.

Allow the student to interpret the ECG, without prompting. They must identify that this is a medical emergency and treat appropriately. Tall tented T waves, with loss of P waves and widening of the QRS are common features to look out for,

D - GCS 15, BM 5.1

E – General muscle ache, No signs of haemorrhage

Case 9

This 28-year-old woman has presented to the ED with shortness of breath. The foundation doctor has been asked to take a history with a view to discussing the differential diagnosis and further management plan.

She has a PE with a history consistent with a DVT as well. She has returned from New Zealand two days ago and takes the oral contraceptive pill.

This station allows the candidate to demonstrate their ability to take a history of shortness of breath and chest pain.

They should specifically ask for VTE risk factors. There is a cardiac family history which should be elicited both as part of this history and to establish that she is most worried about having a heart attack. There is a personal history of anxiety, which should be touched on, but not explored too deeply. While a panic attack is part of the differential, a PE should be excluded.

Stop the candidate at 6 minutes to discuss their further management plan. This should include as a minimum examination, observations, blood tests and a chest x-ray.

If they are able to identify PE as the most likely diagnosis on the basis of the history, tell them that this is correct and continue the discussion. If not tell them that the patient has a PE and continue from there.

The candidate should be able to discuss scoring systems for a PE. They should be aware of the Well's score and how to apply the score in clinical practice. Without further observations the Well's score cannot be calculated but from the history alone she is sufficiently high risk to warrant further imaging. The candidate should be aware that a d-dimer is only of use in low risk patients and that a negative d-dimer in the context of a high risk patient is insufficient to exclude a PE.

Tell them that the patient does have a PE. Ask them what their treatment plan would be? They should know that the patient needs a low molecular weight heparin followed by warfarin or a novel oral anti-coagulant. Ask whether the candidate knows of another treatment in the context of a life-threatening PE. They should be aware that thrombolysis is an option but the criteria for thrombolysis is not required information.

Case 10

The candidate is a foundation doctor in the emergency department. They have been asked to see Gaby, a 24-year-old professional dancer who has attended because of a headache. She has undiagnosed migraines, which have been ongoing for a few months and are related to her menstrual cycle. She has several risk factors for migraine including: female, smoking and use of the combined oral contraceptive pill.

She has also been taking codeine on a near daily basis for an ankle injury. She had become a little dependent on it because she cannot take time off work with the injury. Her ankle has improved and she stopped taking codeine a few days ago, putting her at risk of medication overuse headache.

The candidate is expected to take a full history from the patient, decide upon their top three differential diagnoses and formulate a management plan with the patient. Migraine should be identified as a potential diagnosis, but it does not need to be the candidate's primary diagnosis to obtain full marks. They should formulate a clear and safe management plan that involves a neurological examination including fundoscopy.

The patient is worried because her mother had a stroke, which was preceded by some similar features to her current headache. The candidate should identify the patient's concern and address it directly. There is no indication for a head CT and they need to be able to explain this to the concerned patient.

Stop the candidate with two minutes remaining of the station and ask for their differential diagnoses.

Case 11
A 45-year-old male patient has attended the Emergency Department following a head injury at home. He currently has a GCS of 15 and walked into the department.

A foundation doctor working in the ED has been asked to take the history and explain the management plan to the patient. If the candidate states that they would like to perform a full neurological examination, state that this is normal, and move them on to explaining a management plan for the patient.

The patient is concerned that there is bleeding in his brain and will request a scan. He becomes annoyed with the junior doctor if told there is no indication for a scan however if relevant guidelines are explained to him then he will be reassured.

Case 12
This station examines the candidate's knowledge of the management of a paracetamol overdose as well as their risk assessment of a patient with self harm and their psychiatric history skills. Establishing a rapport with the patient in the time available is obviously challenging. So, as long as the candidate illustrates that they are making an attempt to put the patient at ease, the patient should open up and give the required information. If the candidate does not demonstrate an empathetic attitude, the patient will shut down and this will become a very difficult station. They can however pick up marks during the discussion at the end with their basic knowledge about a paracetamol overdose.

After 6 minutes stop the candidate and ask them to summarise their findings. They should be able to present in an efficient and succinct manner, establishing that this patient took a paracetamol overdose 6 hours ago, at a possibly toxic level, in what was a high-risk suicide attempt! Their initial management should include baseline blood tests (as outlined in the mark scheme) with a paracetamol level (as it has been more than 4 hours since the overdose). They should be able to explain the need to calculate how much was ingested in mg/kg. Toxicity is unlikely to occur under a dose of 75mg/kg. Knowledge of the mg/kg dose is not expected.

There is normally no need to start NAC without a paracetamol level as long as the result can be obtained and acted on within 8 hours. However treatment should not be delayed if more than 150mg/kg has been ingested. Again, the mg/kg dose is not required, but candidates should be aware that it is reasonable to wait for a paracetamol level (unless a very high dose has been ingested).

Ask them what resources they can use to establish whether or not treatment is required. They should be aware of the paracetamol overdose nomogram and suggest consulting toxbase to guide management. They should know that N-Acetylcysteine (NAC) would be the treatment of choice.

Case 13

A 54-year-old man has been brought to the Emergency department with a PR bleed. Currently the man is haemodynamically stable but reports feeling nauseated and seeing fresh red blood coming from the back passage.

The foundation doctor in the emergency medicine team has been asked to take the initial history and also ascertain if there are any red flags present in this patient in relation to the PR bleed. Allow the candidate to take a history in the time provided and carefully elicit if they ask about red flag symptoms and signs.

After 6 minutes stop the candidate and ask them to present back their findings, the differential diagnoses and list the signs and symptoms of red flags in a patient with a PR bleed.

Case 14

The candidate is a foundation doctor in the Emergency Department in the majors area who has been asked to see a 25-year-old man who has presented after a collapse and take a full history and decide upon the likely differential diagnoses and the initial management plan.

Case 15

The candidate has been asked to perform a respiratory examination on the patient who has presented with symptoms of pneumonia shortly after returning from a holiday in Australia. The candidate should perform a full respiratory examination and present their findings. The examination should be conducted in a methodical manner and with minimal discomfort to the patient, it is therefore preferable to examine the anterior chest all at once and the back all at once, the custom of inspection, palpation, percussion and auscultation should be followed each time.

To extend their initial assessment the candidate should be able to identify at least three bedside tests, accept pulse oximetry, arterial blood gas, sputum sample, blood (specifically inflammatory markers or cultures) and urinary antigen tests. Also award marks for chest x-ray. This lady has symptoms of moderate severity and it would be appropriate to prescribe antibiotics, supportive treatment, symptom control and admit her to hospital.

Stop the candidate 6 minutes into the station and ask, if not already stated, what their primary diagnosis would be at this stage. Ask them to state three findings on examination of the chest that they could expect to find in a patient with pneumonia. Ask if there is an objective scoring system, which can be used to determine the severity of the pneumonia. CRB-65 (accept CURB-65).

Case 16

A 69-year-old female patient has been brought into the Emergency Department by ambulance after collapsing outside a shopping centre. The candidate has been instructed to examine the patient's cardiovascular system.

With two minutes remaining stop them and ask them to describe their examination findings. Do not prompt the candidate in any other way.

Case 17

A 65-year-old man has been brought into the ED resus via ambulance complaining of left sided chest pain and shortness of breath.

The foundation doctor has been asked to undertake the initial structured assessment of the patient and feed back his findings and management plan at each stage. Please provide the candidate with the following values as requested

A   Patent

B   On auscultation-fine creps and fine wheeze bi-basally
     RR 26, sats 91% RA, sats 98% on 15L via non-rebreathe mask

ABG results- on their way
CXR- upper lobe diversion, fine patchy shadowing both bases, Kerley B lines

C   HR 90, BP 100/60, CRT 2s, T36.8

The patient appears clammy, grey and sweaty
ECG- widespread ST depression, sinus rhythm, HS- regular, no added sounds

D   BM 12.3

E   No abnormalities

As the candidate reaches E, the nurse informs them that the patient is no longer breathing. Ask the candidate their immediate escalation plan.

At 6 minutes stop the scenario and ask the candidate to give his impression of the diagnosis.

Case 18

A 30-year-old man self-presents to ED with severe right sided loin pain.
The candidate has been asked to take a history and formulate a management plan.
After 6 minutes please bring the consultation to a close and ask the candidate to present their history and management plan.

If not offered ask the candidate directly about:
Initial treatment
Investigations required to confirm diagnosis and exclude complications
Follow up plans

Case 19

The candidate is a foundation year doctor in the minors area of ED. A 39-year-old gentleman presents to minors after developing severe lower lumbar back pain with associated left sided lower limb numbness and feels he is having difficulties mobilizing over the last 5 days. He has had ongoing back issues since having lumbar spinal surgery when he was 25 after a rugby accident.

The candidate should assess the lower limbs only in 6 minutes and should examine for:

Tone
Power
Sensation
Coordination
Reflexes
The candidate should mention that they would assess for perianal tone and saddle anaesthesia.

With 2 minutes remaining ask the candidate to summarize their findings and to give your their differential diagnoses.

Case 20

The candidate is a foundation doctor in the Emergency Department in the majors area who has been asked to see a 48-year-old man with unsteadiness and to perform a cerebellar examination and decide upon the likely differential diagnoses and the initial management plan.

Case 21

A 24-year-old man has been brought to the Emergency department with a painful swollen knee. He has an MCL sprain
He reports being tackled by another player whilst playing football yesterday - the other player's boot went into his left knee. Since then he has had pain on the inside of his left knee and is finding it difficult to walk. Today he woke up and his knee was more swollen so he has come to the emergency department.

The foundation doctor in the emergency medicine team has been asked to examine the knee to assess what investigations and treatment are required.
On examining the knee, when the candidate specifies the part of the examination they are doing, you can tell them:

Look- the left knee is generally swollen with bruising over the medial area of the left knee. There is no deformity.
Feel- The joint is not red or hot. It is tender to palpation over the medial joint line and origin/insertion of the MCL
Move- On active movement the knee cannot fully straighten. On passive movement, there is full ROM in the knee.
Ligaments: all ligaments are intact but there is pain on ligamentous testing of the MCL
Neurovascular: Sensation in the lower limb dermatomes are normal. Motor power in the left lower limb is normal except for knee flexion, which has reduced power due to pain.
Femoral, popliteal, posterior tibial and dorsalis pedis pulses are present.
Other joints: The left hip and left ankle examination is normal.
Gait- The patient is limping on the left and partially weight bearing.

Case 22

The candidate is a foundation doctor in the Emergency Department in the minors area who has been asked to see a 50-year-old woman has self-presented to ED with left shoulder pain after falling from her bicycle onto her left shoulder earlier that day. She is complaining of pain and restricted movements.

The candidate must perform a full shoulder examination but is not required to take a history. After 6 minutes stop the candidate and ask them to summarise back their findings and the likely diagnosis

Case 23

The foundation doctor is working in the resuscitation area of the emergency department. They have been asked to supervise a final year medical student for the day. A priority call is received pre-warning the department of the arrival of an intoxicated female with reduced consciousness. She is likely to require interventions to protect her airway. She has not been involved in a traumatic incident and there is no clinical suspicion of a head injury. The doctor has been asked to demonstrate to the medical student the basic principles of airway management and escalation.

The doctor should demonstrate basic airway manoeuvres, bag valve mask ventilation, the selection and use of airway adjuncts and the use of a supraglottic airway device. They are not expected to demonstrate endotracheal intubation, although they should be aware of this as an advanced method of gaining airway control. They should be aware of the need to urgently seek senior/anaesthetic help when a patient has a compromised airway. They have been asked to focus on the escalation of airway management.

They should establish and address the medical student's learning needs, be supportive and demonstrate an ability to facilitate learning.

Case 24

The candidate is a foundation doctor in the Emergency Department in the majors area who has been see a 67-year-old man with significant abdominal pain who has not passed urine for 12 hours.

They will take a brief history and examination then insert a catheter. After they have inserted the catheter ask which investigations they would like to request and what steps they would take if the procedure had failed.

Case 25

The candidate is a foundation year doctor in the Emergency Department working in the resus area. They have a medical student shadowing them today who is keen to be taught about data interpretation.
They have just assessed John, a 66-year-old man with 2 days history of worsening shortness of breath on a background history of COPD who has been brought in by ambulance. He is breathing oxygen at 15L per minute via non re-breathe bag.

They have performed an arterial blood gas and should now explain the findings to the medical student in a structured and succinct manner.

Appropriate management plan includes, but not limited to; blood tests, chest x-ray, trial of oxygen therapy to keep Sats 88-92 %, or NIV/BiPAP and critical care referral, nebulisers/steroids and repeat ABG after intervention.

Starting NIV prior to obtaining a chest x-ray is not an appropriate management plan.
The examiner's role is to observe only and not to ask any direct questions.

Obstetrics & Gynaecology

Case 1

The candidate is a Foundation Year Doctor in the Gynaecology outpatient clinic. They have been asked to speak to Huda, a 26-year-old woman presenting with a history of painful periods. The candidate should take a history and present their findings.

After 6 minutes, please stop the candidate and ask:

"Please summarise your findings and discuss how you would like to investigate and manage this patient."

Case 2

The candidate is a Foundation Year Doctor in the Gynaecology outpatient clinic. They have been asked to speak to Celeste, a 34-year-old woman presenting with a history of heavy periods. The candidate should take a history and present their findings.

After 6 minutes, please stop the candidate and ask:

"Please summarise your findings and discuss how you would like to investigate and manage this patient."

Case 3

The candidate is a Foundation Year Doctor in the Emergency Department. They have been asked to speak to Martha, a 24-year-old woman who has presented with lower abdominal pain and discharge. The candidate should take a focused gynaecological and sexual history and present their findings.

After 6 minutes, please stop the candidate and ask:

"Please summarise your findings and discuss how you would like to investigate and manage this patient."

Case 4

The candidate is a Foundation Year Doctor in the Gynaecology clinic. They have been asked to speak to Ellie, a 34-year-old woman who has been referred by her GP for difficulty conceiving. The candidate should take a history and present their findings.

After 6 minutes, please stop the candidate and ask:

"Please summarise your findings and discuss how you would like to investigate and manage this patient."

Case 5

The candidate is a Foundation Year Doctor in the General Obstetrics Clinic. They have been asked to speak to Natalie, a 27-year-old woman who has been referred by her GP due to ongoing pruritus. The candidate should take a history and present their findings.

After 6 minutes, please stop the candidate and ask:

"Please summarise your findings and discuss how you would like to investigate and manage this patient."

Case 6

The candidate is a Foundation Year Doctor in the Maternity Triage Unit. They have been asked to speak to Kiran, a 27-year-old woman who has presented with vaginal bleeding and is 32 weeks pregnant. The candidate should take a history and present their findings.

After 6 minutes, please stop the candidate and ask:

"Please summarise your findings and discuss how you would like to investigate and manage this patient."

Case 7

The candidate is a Foundation Year Doctor in a GP practice. They have been asked to speak to Winona, a 32-year-old woman who has presented feeling generally unwell 5 days after giving birth. The candidate should take a focused history and present their findings.

After 6 minutes, please stop the candidate and ask:

"Please summarise your findings and discuss how you would like to investigate and manage this patient."

Case 8

The candidate is a Foundation Year Doctor in a GP practice. They have been asked to speak to Yee, a 29-year-old woman who has attended the practice for her 6-week postnatal check. The candidate should complete the postnatal check and report to the examiner what they would like to examine and assess. They do not need to assess the baby.

After 6 minutes, please stop the candidate and ask them to present their findings and detail what they would like to assess to complete the postnatal check if they have not covered this already.

Case 9

The candidate is a Foundation Year Doctor in a GP surgery. They have been asked to speak to Kyra, a 25-year-old woman who is due to have her first cervical smear and has booked a double appointment. The candidate should explain the procedure in order to take verbal consent and discuss any concerns she may have.

The candidate has been informed they do not need to examine the patient or demonstrate the procedure.

Case 10

The candidate is a Foundation Year Doctor in the Gynaecology Clinic. They have been asked to speak to Frances, a 58-year-old woman who has been having postmenopausal bleeding. A transvaginal ultrasound showed a slightly thickened endometrium and she is to have an urgent hysteroscopy. They have been asked by your consultant to explain this procedure to her and discuss her concerns.

The candidate has been informed that they do not need to examine the patient.

Case 11

The candidate is a Foundation Year Doctor in a GP practice. They have been asked to speak to Megan, a first year student midwife who has just started her community placement today. The practice midwife has just called in sick and the candidate has been asked to talk to Megan about the mechanisms and stages of birth.

Case 12

The candidate is a Foundation Year Doctor in a GP surgery. Sia is 25-year-old woman who has presented with PV discharge and intermittent bleeding. They have been asked to perform a cervical smear and bimanual examination. The patient has already been consented for the procedure.

Case 13

The candidate is a Foundation Year Doctor in the General Obstetrics clinic. They have been asked to examine the pregnant abdomen of a 28-year-old woman, Lucy, who is currently 28 weeks pregnant. She has come in for a routine check.

The candidate should then present their findings to you and please ask the following questions:

The fundal height is 32cm. Is this normal or abnormal?
Please give examples of what may cause this measurement.

Case 14

The candidate is a Foundation Year Doctor based at a GP practice. Gina is a 35-year-old woman who has been sent a letter asking to attend a routine appointment at her GP surgery due to abnormal smear results. The results state:

Mild dyskaryosis, HPV positive.

They have been asked to counsel the patient in view of these findings and answer any questions she may have. They do not need to examine the patient.

Case 15

The candidate is a Foundation Year Doctor based at a GP practice. Celia is an 18-year-old woman who has asked to talk about starting the oral contraceptive pill. The candidate has been asked to counsel the patient regarding the oral contraceptive pill and answer any questions she may have. They have been asked to take a focused history to elicit suitability for the chosen method of contraception. They do not need to examine the patient.

Case 16

The candidate is a Foundation Year Doctor in the GUM clinic. Marc is a 19-year-old man who has come in for a routine STI screen after having had unprotected sexual intercourse with a casual partner. They have been asked to take a focused history and counsel this patient for a HIV test, but they do not need to examine the patient.

Case 17

The candidate is a Foundation Year Doctor in the GUM clinic. David is a 27-year-old man who was diagnosed with HIV in a routine STI check and informed last week at the clinic. He has come back today for follow up. The candidate has been asked to answer any questions he may have, but they do not need to examine the patient.

Case 18

The candidate is a Foundation Year Doctor in a GP practice. Avanti is a 24-year-old woman who has requested an urgent appointment as she has recently discovered she is pregnant. The candidate has been asked to discuss the patient's concerns and how she wishes to proceed with the pregnancy.

They do not need to examine the patient.

Case 19

The candidate is a Foundation Year Doctor in a GP surgery. They have been asked to see Gloria, a 25-year-old Nigerian woman who is intending on starting a family. She is a known carrier of sickle cell disease about would like to discuss how this will impact her pregnancy and risks. They have been asked to counsel her and discuss her concerns.

They do not need to examine the patient.

Case 20

The candidate is a Foundation Year Doctor in a GP surgery. They have been asked to see Heidi, a 30-year-old woman who is 19 weeks pregnant and would like to discuss the whooping cough vaccination. They have been asked to counsel her about the vaccination and the indications and discuss her concerns.

They do not need to examine the patient.

Medicine

Case 1

The candidate is a foundation doctor who has been urgently called to the acute medical unit to assess an unwell patient. The patient has a penicillin allergy and has just been commenced on an intravenous flucloxacillin infusion to treat a case of severe cellulitis. The nurse was extremely busy and did not run through their standard allergy checks before administering the antibiotic.

Shortly after starting the infusion the patient started to complain of feeling unwell. They have developed swelling of the lips and tongue, an urticarial rash, respiratory distress and wheeze.

The candidate should recognise that this is anaphylaxis, and start emergency management as appropriate.

If the candidate asks for observations please supply them with the following information:

	Pre-treatment	Delayed Treatment	Post- Treatment (adrenaline, oxygen, fluids)
Saturations	90% on air	88% on air	98% on 15L NRB
Respiratory Rate	24	28	22
Heart Rate	120	140	130
Blood Pressure	85/40	75/32	100/80
Capillary Refill Time	4 seconds	4 seconds	3 seconds
Temperature	37.4	37.4	37.4
Blood Sugar	5.6	5.6	5.6

You may act as a second pair of hands to assist the candidate if they call for help.

At 6 minutes stop the candidate and ask how they would like to further manage the patient.

Case 2

The candidate is a foundation year doctor who has been asked to assess an unwell patient in the emergency department. The patient has been admitted with a short history of confusion, fever and is generally unwell. The nurse in triage has asked the candidate to assess the patient, as she is concerned.

The candidate should recognise that this patient could have sepsis, and start emergency management as appropriate.

If the candidate asks for observations please supply them with the following information:

	Pre-treatment	Delayed Treatment	Post- Treatment (oxygen, fluids, antibiotics)
Saturations	95% on air	94% on air	98% on 15L via NRB
Respiratory Rate	26	30	24
Heart Rate	115	125	101
Blood Pressure	90/65	72/55	103/70
Capillary Refill Time	4 seconds	5 seconds	3 seconds
Temperature	38.5	38.6	37.9
Blood Sugar	8.4	8.4	8.4

You may act as a second pair of hands to assist the candidate if they call for help.

When the candidate cannulates and takes bloods, please prompt to ask which bloods they would take if needed.

If the candidate requests a catheter set, or attempts to perform the procedure, please move them on.

At 6 minutes stop the candidate and ask how they would like to further manage the patient in particular the "Sepsis 6"

Case 3

The candidate is a foundation doctor who has been asked to assess a patient with haematemesis and melena on the liver ward. The patient is known to have cirrhosis with portal hypertension and varices. The patient has signs of chronic liver disease and evidence of haematemesis and melena on examination.

The candidate should recognise that this patient is having an upper GI bleed (most likely variceal in origin) and start appropriate emergency management.

If the candidate asks for observations please supply them with the following information:

	Pre-treatment	Delayed Treatment	Post-Treatment (antibiotics, fluid, blood)
Saturations	94% on air	94% on air	98% on 15L NRB
Respiratory Rate	25	25	24
Heart Rate	120	125	110
Blood Pressure	81/69	73/62	90/70
Capillary Refill Time	4 seconds	5 seconds	3 seconds
Temperature	36.5	36.5	36.5
Blood Sugar	6.2	6.2	6.2

You may act as a second pair of hands to assist the candidate if they call for help.

When the candidate cannulates and takes bloods, please prompt to ask which bloods they would take if needed.

If the candidate requests the results of a venous blood gas please tell them that the haemoglobin is 65g/L

If the candidate requests a catheter set, or attempts to perform the procedure, please move them on.

At 6 minutes stop the candidate and ask how they would like to further manage the patient.

Case 4

The candidate has been asked to examine the patient and report back their findings. The patient has a history of occupational asbestos exposure and a history suggestive of pulmonary fibrosis. When the candidate examines the patient they find clubbing, reduced chest expansion and bilateral basal fine crackles, which do not change in character on coughing.

At 6 minutes please stop the candidate and ask them to present their findings.

Case 5

The candidate has been asked to examine the patient and report back their findings. The patient has a history of a renal transplantation for end stage renal failure caused by diabetes. She has previously had haemodialysis via a left sided radio-cephalic fistula that is no longer in use.

When the candidate examines the patient they find finger pricks in keeping with blood glucose testing, a left radio-cephalic fistula with no evidence of recent use, a hockey-shaped scar in the right iliac fossa and a with an underlying palpable mass that is non-tender.

At 6 minutes please stop the candidate and ask them to present their findings.

Case 6

The candidate has been asked to examine the patient and report back their findings. The patient has a history of rheumatic fever as a child and has attended for a check up. When the candidate examines the patient they find an irregularly irregular pulse at a rate of 85, a displaced apex beat, a pan-systolic murmur heard loudest in the mitral area that radiates into the axilla. There are no features of heart failure.

If the candidate requests the blood pressure please tell them that it is 135/70mmHg

At 6 minutes please stop the candidate and ask them to present their findings.

Case 7

A 45-year-old lady comes into the emergency department with a 3 day history of poor balance and falls. She was diagnosed with multiple sclerosis 10 years ago. The foundation doctor has been asked to perform a thorough cerebellar examination and present their findings to you.

The patient has an ataxic gait, particularly on heel toe walking. Romberg's test however is negative. There is no truncal ataxia. She also has nystagmus on bilateral lateral gaze and an intention tremor on both sides. Her speech also sounds dysarthric.

At 6 minutes ask the candidate to present their findings.

Case 8

A 45-year-old lady has been admitted to the Acute Medical Unit for treatment for a chest infection. Today she has mentioned to the team that she has been having pain in her hands for the past few months. Currently, the patient is not in pain. The candidate has been asked to complete a hand examination and present their findings back to you.

The patient does not have any nail, skin changes or scars. There is visible swelling over the MCP joints, PIP joints and wrists bilaterally. Temperature is increased over the swollen joints, and they are tender to palpation. The pulses are intact. The patient is able to make the prayer signs, but is unable to fully complete the range of movement. Power and sensation are intact. The patient can perform functional tasks, but they can be painful. She has some nodules on her elbows.

During the examination, as the candidate palpates the joints, the patient grimaces in pain. If candidate notices and offers analgesia, you should acknowledge this and state, "the patient has now been given pain relief, you can continue" and allow the candidate to continue examining.

At 6 minutes please stop the candidate and ask them to present their findings. Show the candidate a picture demonstrating the hand signs of rheumatoid arthritis and ask the candidate to list the deformities present.

Case 9

A 78-year-old gentleman has presented to his GP with a tremor in his hands and the candidate has been asked to examine the patient.
If the candidate goes to examine the lower limbs please move them on and inform them that they only need to examine upper limbs.
If candidate asks the patient to write a sentence please ask them to move on, and give them the relevant mark.
Positive finds are:
Resting Pill-rolling tremor worse on distraction
Increased tone (lead pipe rigidity)
Cogwheel rigidity
Bradykinesia
Shuffling gait
Reduced arm swing
Stooped posture
Difficulty initiating movement
Hypophonia (quiet voice)

At 6 minutes please stop the candidate and ask them to present their findings.

Case 10

A 65-year-old man has attended the emergency department with a 2 hour history of central crushing chest pain. An ECG has been done as well as routine bloods.
The candidate has been asked to interpret the ECG and explain their findings to the patient. The candidate has been asked to voice their interpretation of the ECG out loud. If they do not do this please prompt them to do so.
At 6 minutes please stop the candidate and ask them how they would like to assess and manage this patient.
The candidate should identify that this is an Acute ST Elevation MI. They would assess them using an ABCDE approach. They require oxygen, morphine, nitrates, aspirin and percutaneous coronary intervention (PCI). If the candidate is doing well you may ask them which is the most likely coronary artery to have been affected.

Case 11

The candidate is a foundation year doctor in the emergency department seeing a 42-year old gentleman who has presented with a one-week history of productive cough and shortness of breath.
Provide the candidate with a copy of the chest x-ray showing a moderate unilateral pleural effusion. Please ask the candidate to present the chest x-ray to you, and then proceed to explain the findings to the patient.
Please stop the candidate at 6 minutes to discuss further management of pleural effusions.

Case 12

Joe is a 60-year-old man with known COPD has become drowsy on the respiratory ward.

The foundation doctor on call has been bleeped to review the patient. As part of an ABCDE assessment an arterial blood gas has been done. The actor/helper (nurse) has run the gas and presents the printout of results to the candidate. The ABG shows a decompensated chronic type 2 respiratory failure.

Encourage the candidate to take a few minutes to look at the ABG result and interpret it. When the candidate is ready, ask them to present their findings. Prompt the candidate to state if the picture is compensated or decompensated. Ask the candidate to summarise the next steps in the management of this patient. Ask for common causes for type 2 respiratory failure – commonest cause: COPD, others: reduced respiratory effort (e.g. drug effect), chest wall deformity.

If time allows and if candidate is doing well, ask the candidate to explain the difference between type 1 and type 2 respiratory failure.

Case 13
The candidate is the medical foundation doctor on call. James is a 32-year-old patient, with generalised abdominal pain and vomiting. He has been asking for the results of his blood tests that were taken earlier today. The candidate has been asked to explain the findings of these results to the patient, exploring with him the causes for these abnormalities and deciding on a management plan with the patient.

The candidate must take a brief history, explain that the blood results show changes consistent with excess alcohol intake and formulate a management plan with the patient.

Case 14
The candidate has been asked to set up a syringe driver for a palliative care patient on the ward who is no longer able to take medications by mouth. The main symptom control issue for this patient is pain. The patient already has a subcutaneous butterfly needle in situ.

A colleague has prescribed the following, on the advice of the palliative care team;
5mg diamorphine over 24 hours
10mls water for injection

Note: 5mg of diamorphine is 1 ampule

There will be approximately 21mls in the syringe to be given over 24 hours, therefore the correct rate is 0.88 mls an hour
Paper and a calculator are provided for the candidate if needed for workings out. A nurse is available to double check drugs, fluids and calculations.

Case 15
The candidate is a foundation year doctor working in geriatrics outpatients. Winston is an 85 year old gentleman who is complaining of progressively worsening calf pain on the left hand side, which is now starting to affect his mobility.

The candidate has been asked to perform an ABPI on the left hand side and document their findings on the paper provided. If the candidate tries to take bilateral measurements please move them on.

At 6 minutes please ask the candidate about their findings and their interpretation of these findings.

Case 16
The candidate is a foundation year doctor on the gastroenterology ward. They have been asked to check and administer a blood transfusion to a patient who has just come back to the ward from endoscopy.

The candidate must safely check and prepare the unit of blood for administration, assisted by the ward nurse.

Towards the end of the station the candidate may require direct questioning regarding frequency of observations during transfusion and time limits for product administration after removal from temperature controlled storage.

Case 17

The candidate is a foundation year doctor on a medical ward. They have been asked to take blood cultures from a patient who has just spiked a temperature of 38.1°C.

The candidate will perform this skill on the dummy arm using the equipment provided. The actor will provide the voice of the patient.

Case 18

The candidate has been asked to take a focused history from a patient.

The patient is a 75-year-old retired school teacher. Over the last few weeks he has become increasingly short of breath on exertion. He is only able to move between rooms at home before becoming breathless. 6 months ago he was able to walk to the local shops. He does not feel breathless at rest. Sleeping has become increasingly difficult as he becomes breathless when lying down flat. He wakes up a few times a night gasping for breath. He has now resorted to sleeping in an armchair. His ankles have become swollen over the past few weeks. He has no wheeze, chest pain, cough, fever, palpitations or weight loss. He has no recent ravel history.

His mother had a heart attack in her 60s and his father died of lung cancer aged 82.
He had a large heart attack 6 months ago and required 2 stents. He also has hypertension, and high cholesterol.
His medications include aspirin, clopidogrel, atorvastatin, ramipril, bisoprolol, lansoprazole and GTN. He has a penicillin allergy (rash).
He is an ex-smoker. He smoked 15 a day for 20 years but gave up aged 40. He drinks two glasses of wine a week.
He lives in a house with stairs and is the main carer for his wife who has Alzhiemer's. He does not want to be admitted to hospital as he's concerned about how his wife will manage.
At 6 minutes please stop the candidate ask them to present their findings and suggest a management plan.

Case 19

The candidate has been asked to take a focused history from a patient.

The patient is a 23-year-old man has come to his GP with a history of diarrhoea. He is normally well with no other medical conditions. His symptoms started 4 weeks ago. Initially the patient thought he had food poisoning following a recent holiday to Spain. The patient is opening his bowels 5-6 times per day, and it is often bloody. He often experiences abdominal pain that is worse before he opens his bowels. He has symptoms of urgency, and has had some faecal incontinence. He has lots 3-4kg in weight and is fatigued. He has no history of mouth ulcers, eye or joint pain or rashes.
He has no other medical conditions and does not take any regular medications. He drinks alcohol occasionally, but started smoking a couple of years ago.
He has a family history of type 2-diabetes and his Grandma recently had a stroke. There is no family history of cancer.
He is embarrassed about coming to see the GP and his symptoms are starting to impact on his social life. He works as a bus driver and has had to take time off because of his symptoms.
At 6 minutes please stop the candidate ask them to present their findings and suggest a management plan.

Case 20

The candidate has been asked to take focussed history from a patient. The patient is a 71-year-old lady called Brenda who has presented to the emergency department with collapse.
Prior to the event the patient was sat watching TV. On standing she felt nauseous and light headed. Her husband noted that she was pale. The patient did not experience any chest pain, breathlessness or palpitations.

The next thing the patient remembers is being on the floor. Her husband says she was only unconscious for a few seconds. There was no incontinence, tongue biting or seizure activity noted. She did not sustain any injuries.
She was disorientated and confused for a few seconds only. She made a quick recovery. Her husband was concerned so he bought her to the emergency department.

She has no history of syncope, but over the past few weeks has been feeling dizzy especially when changing position. Last week the patient felt dizzy whilst gardening, but her symptoms resolved after lying down. She has been well otherwise, but admits to not drinking enough fluids.

She has a history of high blood pressure, but this is now well controlled with medications. She used to be on a blood pressure medication that made her ankles swell, but this has recently been changed to bendroflumethiazide.

The correct diagnosis is syncope due to postural hypotension (secondary to dehydration and antihypertensives/diuretics).

At 6 minutes please stop the candidate ask them to present their findings and suggest a management plan.

Case 21
The candidate has been asked to take focussed history from a patient.

The patient is a 65-year-old lady who has presented to the GP with weight loss. She has been losing weight for the past 6 months, but has not been trying to lose weight. She has noticed that her clothes are loose. She has had some diarrhoea; prior to this she had a normal bowel habit. She has noticed that her appetite has reduced, and she often skips meals. She is also a bit irritable, and has been feeling tremulous and experiencing palpitations intermittently.

She has no past medical history and does not take any regular medications. Her brother and sister are diabetic.
She is concerned as her mother died of breast cancer in her 60s, and lost weight in her terminal phase. She is concerned that she may have cancer.
At 6 minutes please stop the candidate ask them to present their findings and suggest a management plan.

Case 22
This is a communication station. The candidate has been asked to explain a diagnosis of Type-2 Diabetes to a patient. Please assess their communication skills.
The patient is a 43-year-old lorry driver, who has been called back to the surgery following some recent blood tests. He is unaware that these blood tests show that he has Type 2 Diabetes. He is overweight and has hypertension and high cholesterol. He is a smoker of 20 cigarettes per day.

His father had diabetes and died of a heart attack aged 75. His father had suffered quite badly with foot problems. The patient is concerned about the possibility of having to inject himself with insulin.

Case 23
This is a communication station. The candidate has been asked to explain a gastroscopy procedure to a patient. They are not expected to consent the patient. Please assess their communication skills.

Patricia is a 52-year old lady attending outpatient's gastroenterology clinic for troublesome and persistent reflux. She is scheduled for a gastroscopy in two weeks' time. The patient is concerned that she may have cancer. She has not had a gastroscopy before, and is concerned about having the procedure and is adamant that she wants sedation. She is planning to drive to her son's graduation on the day of the procedure.

Case 24
This is a communication station. The candidate has been asked to speak to a relative who is upset that their father has fallen whilst an inpatient. Please assess their communication skills.

The patient has had an unwitnessed fall. He was found by a healthcare assistant sat on the floor, and does not appear to have sustained any injuries. His family only found out he had fallen when they phoned the ward to check on his progress this morning. The family are upset and would like an explanation as to why this has happened and what will be done next.

Case 25
This is a communication station. The candidate has been asked to speak to the family of a patient who has been a victim of a serious medication error. Please assess their communication skills.

The patient is Cara, a 72-year-old woman known to have a penicillin allergy. She was prescribed and administered an intravenous dose of Co-amoxiclav earlier today, to which she developed an anaphylactic reaction. She has been managed appropriately and is now stable on HDU.

Paediatrics

Case 1
A 10 year old boy called Paul has come into ED via ambulance with his father after witnessing him having a fit. Paul is currently sitting on a trolley with a GCS of 15.

The FY1 doctor in the paediatric team has been asked to take the initial history.
After 6 minutes stop the candidate whatever stage they are at and ask them to summarise their findings and management plan.

Case 2
An 8 month old boy has been brought in by his parents with a 3 day history of cough reduced feeding and some difficulty in breathing.
The FY1 doctor in the paediatric team has been asked to take the initial history and then summarise their findings back to the team.
After 6 minutes stop the candidate whatever stage they are at and ask them summarise their findings and management plan.

Case 3
A 3 year old girl is brought in by her mother after an episode of shaking all over. The toddler is alert and active but miserable with a fever in triage.

The FY1 doctor in the paediatric team has been asked to take the initial history and then summarise their findings back to the team.
After 6 minutes stop the candidate whatever stage they are at and ask them summarise their findings and management plan.

Case 4
A mother has brought her 14 month old baby girl to the Paediatric Outpatient Department. She was referred by her GP, who was concerned that her growth has been poor.

The FY1 doctor in the paediatric team has been asked to take the history and to summarise their findings back to the team. Please show the candidate the growth chart if they ask for it. If not, please use it to facilitate discussion after the history has been taken.
After 6 minutes ask the candidate to conclude the discussion and ask them to summarise the history, and to discuss their management plan.

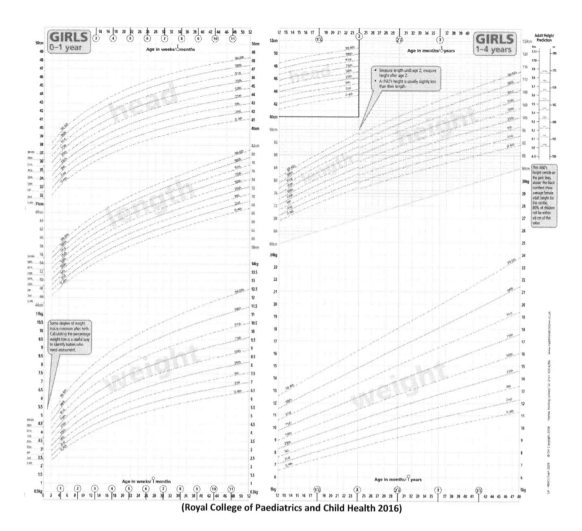

(Royal College of Paediatrics and Child Health 2016)

Case 5

A mother has brought her four month old baby to the local Emergency Department with a burnt arm.

The FY1 in the Emergency Department has been asked to see the child immediately as the nurse has concerns about the burn. They have been asked to take the history, and to summarise back to the team.

After 6 minutes ask the candidate to conclude the discussion and ask them to summarise the history, and to discuss their management plan.   They will need to discuss their next steps, which should include how to escalate in this situation. Please prompt the candidate to suggest what they would do if the mother tries to leave.

Case 6

A 5 day old baby is referred into the Emergency Department by the community midwife, who is worried because the baby has lost 12% of his birth weight.

The FY1 doctor in the Paediatric team has been asked to take the history and to summarise their findings back to the team.

After 6 minutes ask the candidate to conclude the discussion and ask them to summarise the history, and to discuss their management plan.

Case 7

The candidate is an FY1 doctor in Paediatric ED. They have been asked to assess the suicide risk of Alice, a 12 year old girl who has been brought to the ED by her mother after school noticed numerous cut marks on her forearms.

Alice has been seen with her mother already; her injuries are superficial, not of medical significance, and have been dressed. Both Alice and her mother have agreed that Alice should speak to a doctor on her own.

Alice is quiet and shy, but will open up and answer all questions asked if the candidate communicates empathetically.
After 6 minutes ask the candidate to conclude the discussion and ask them to summarise the history, and to discuss their plan for investigations and management.

Ask them:
What do you think Alice's risk of suicide is, and why?
What would be your next steps in management?

Case 8
The candidate is an FY1 doctor in Paediatric ED. They have been asked to take a history from the mother of Oscar, a three week old boy. His parents have brought him to the ED after he had a floppy episode whilst feeding. Oscar's observations are normal, and there are no acute clinical concerns.

The parent will express distress that Oscar could have died, and will want to know what can be done to make sure this doesn't happen again.

After 6 minutes ask the candidate to conclude the discussion and ask them to summarise the history, and to discuss their plan for investigations and management.
Ask them:
Please tell me what differential diagnoses you are considering, and why.
What would be your next steps in management?

Case 9
The candidate is a junior doctor on a post natal ward, and has been asked to perform a routine baby check on a well baby.
After 6 minutes ask the candidate to conclude the examination and ask them to summarise their findings, differential diagnosis, and to discuss their plan for investigations and management.

Ask them: 'Is there is any specific advice you would like to give the mother before she goes home?'

Case 10
A 9 year old child has been referred by their GP to the Paediatric Outpatient Clinic with a 1 year history of recurrent central abdominal pain.

Abdominal examination is completely normal.

After 6 minutes ask the candidate to conclude the examination and ask them to summarise their findings, differential diagnosis, and to discuss their plan for investigations and management.

Case 11
A 12 year old girl has been referred by the GP with raised BP in the surgery today.

After 6 minutes ask the candidate to conclude the examination and ask them to summarise their findings, differential diagnosis, and to discuss their plan for investigations and management.

Case 12
A 15 year old boy with Cystic Fibrosis has been electively admitted to the ward for a course of intravenous antibiotics. He is currently well.

After 6 minutes ask the candidate to conclude the examination and ask them to summarise their findings, differential diagnosis, and to discuss their plan for investigations and management.

Ask 'In addition to the paediatrician, who else may be involved in this child's care?'.

Case 13

A 9 year old girl has increased tone, weakness and hyperreflexia of the upper limbs bilaterally, and in all areas.

After 6 minutes ask the candidate to conclude the examination and ask them to summarise their findings, differential diagnosis, and to discuss their plan for investigations and management.

Ask them: "How they would you differentiate between an upper or lower motor neurone lesion."

Case 14

An 8 year old boy who was born at 28 weeks gestation, with a history of grade 3 IVH has been brought to clinic for his routine follow up.

The candidate is an FY1 doctor in the clinic who has been asked to perform a lower limb neurological examination including assessment of gait then summarise their findings back to their senior. The candidate should perform the whole examination, please ask them to move on if they offer to test lower limb pain sensation.

After 6 minutes ask the candidate to conclude the examination and ask them to summarise their findings, differential diagnosis, and to discuss their plan for investigations and management.

It is most likely this scenario is pointing to a left hemiparesis following IVH. However, you can ask the candidate about other causes of hemiplegia. These will include stroke, head injury, brain tumour, infections, vasculitis, leukodystrophies.

Case 15

Sarah is a 14-year-old girl and has recently been diagnosed with asthma, following an admission to the children's ward with a wheezy episode. She is now well and ready for discharge home.

The FY1 has been asked to explain to Sarah what asthma is, including the lifelong nature of the condition. The candidate should use age appropriate language to explain asthma to Sarah. They should enquire about triggers and ensure Sarah knows when to take medication and seek advice from an adult if she is unwell.

At 6 minutes, stop the candidate and ask them if there is anything further they wish to add.

Case 16

Ben is 18 months old. He was admitted to the children's ward following a febrile convulsion. He had a runny nose and temperature for 3 days before the convulsion. His fever was 39.2C at the time. It lasted 3 minutes and his mother described shaking of both his arms and his legs and Ben was not responding to her. It stopped by itself before the ambulance arrived and Ben has been very well since admission to the ward.

The FY1 doctor has been asked to explain to Ben's mother exactly what a febrile convulsion is. The candidate should give an explanation to the parent, elicit any concerns they have and deal with any queries appropriately.

At 6 minutes, stop the candidate and ask them if there is any further advice they wish to give Ben's parents.

Case 17

Jack is 18 months old and has been diagnosed with a viral upper respiratory tract infection. He attended the ED with a 24-hour history of a runny nose, dry cough and a fever. He is generally well in himself, eating and drinking as usual and playing in the waiting room. His mother wants him to have antibiotics for his infection but these have not been prescribed. The FY1 doctor has been asked to talk to her by the ED nursing staff.

Case 18

A woman at 25 weeks gestation has been brought to Labour Ward with contractions and cervical dilatation. She is expected to deliver in the next few hours.

The junior doctor in the paediatric team has been asked to speak to the mother about the impending preterm delivery.

At 6 minutes, stop the candidate and ask them if there is any further advice they wish to give.

Case 19

A newborn baby has been delivered in poor condition following shoulder dystocia and there is evidence of hypoxic ischaemic encephalopathy. Two hours after birth the baby had seizures which indicated the need to start therapeutic hypothermia and transfer the baby to a tertiary centre for ongoing management.

The junior doctor in the paediatric team has been asked to speak to the parents to explain the need for transfer to a tertiary centre.

At 6 minutes, ask the candidate to conclude the discussion and ask them how they would differentiate between mild, moderate and severe hypoxic ischaemic encephalopathy in the newborn from initial clinical examination.

Case 20

A 7 month old boy has attended ED with bronchiolitis. He is generally well but his condition is complicated by an oxygen requirement and poor oral intake that necessitates admission to the short stay ward.

The FY1 doctor in the paediatric team has been asked to explain to the family the diagnosis of bronchiolitis and the need to admit to the ward for further management.

After 6 minutes ask the candidate to conclude the discussion and ask them to name 2 investigations they would consider performing in this case.

Case 21

The candidate will be expected to demonstrate to a parent how to use an inhaler with a mask and spacer and how to clean the spacer and mask. They should introduce themselves and confirm who they are speaking to. They should elicit parent's prior knowledge. They should acknowledge the parents anxiety.

They should use one of Iris's teddy bears / dolls to demonstrate to how to use an MDI with an age appropriate spacer and mask. They should explain how to clean the spacer and mask. They should summarise their discussion. They should offer the parent written information. They should ask if parent has any questions and also offer parent opportunity to have a further discussion before discharge.

Case 22

A mother on the postnatal ward was told yesterday that her newborn son shows signs of Down's Syndrome. She is awaiting the results of a genetic test to confirm the diagnosis. She is very worried and has lots of questions she would like answered. The FY1 should tell the mother the immediate concerns (to rule out congenital cardiac anomaly, check for hypothyroidism, to establish feeding). The FY1 should outline long term problems. The FY1 should explain about referral to community paediatrics and the MDT. The FY1 should offer to chase results, get seniors to come back to talk to mother and offer written information. The FY1 should also direct the mother to Down Syndrome support groups.

Case 23

Benjy, an ex 32 week premature baby on the Special Care Baby Unit is now 8 weeks old and due his first set of routine immunisations.

The FY1 doctor on the team has been asked to obtain verbal consent from his mother and then perform the task using the equipment provided.

During the practical component, ask regarding landmarks in infants for intramuscular injections.

If the following has not been mentioned prior, at 6 minutes, ask the candidate to complete the procedure and ask:
Can you think of any complications of intramuscular injections you would mention to the parents?
What side effects of vaccinations would you warn the parents to expect?

Case 24

A 4 year old boy being treated for pneumonia on the children's ward has become unresponsive. He was admitted that day and is being treated with intravenous antibiotics. He has been gradually deteriorating and from his observation chart it would appear that the patient is septic.

The FY1 doctor has been fast-bleeped to urgently assess him as the rest of the team is attending a neonatal emergency. They should initially open the child's airway, assess for signs of life and responsiveness, before following the cardiac arrest algorithm. The candidate should ask for a cardiac arrest call (2222, Paediatric Cardiac Arrest) to be made.

The initial rhythm (once the pads are placed) is PEA and so adrenaline should be given followed by chest compressions being quickly re-commenced. At next assessment the rhythm remains unchanged and so reversible causes must be considered. After a further 2 minute cycle the rhythm is VF, at this stage the candidate must prepare for and then give an asynchronous DC shock. This successfully converts the patient back into sinus rhythm and the candidate should then discontinue CPR and state they would give post cardiac arrest treatment, including referral and transfer to PICU.

The mother is understandably distraught and initially angry that the doctors have not seen her son sooner. Ask the candidate how best they would deal with that situation?

After 6 minutes please stop the candidate and ask them to summarise their initial treatment and further management.

Case 25

The candidate will describe the fracture seen in the radiograph to the medical student and then discuss differential causes as well as their management plan.

The candidate should go through systematically how they would interpret and present a radiograph of a fracture. They must start with ensuring they have the correct patient film (patient name, hospital number and DOB) followed by stating the date, film type and adequacy. It is essential they advise that it is a 'left distal shaft radial fracture', with a transverse pattern and a degree of angulation.

After describing the fracture, the candidate should give their differential causes including: fall/trauma or non-accidental injury. They will then give a management plan including:

Analgesia
Senior Review
Safeguarding check
Surgical- likely need manipulation under anaesthetic
Non-surgical- back slab + below elbow cast

Please stop them after 6 minutes and ask them to discuss their differential causes and management plan.

General Practice

Case 1

A 60 year old gentleman, Peter, has been asked to see a doctor as the practice nurse noticed his blood pressure was elevated.

The candidate, is acting as the foundation year doctor Doctor, and has been asked to take a brief history from the patient.

After 6 minutes, please stop the candidate and ask:

"Please summarise your findings and discuss how you would like to investigate and manage this patient."

If they ask, give them the examination findings below:

Examination findings: Mr Pritchard is well, but overweight. His weight today is 93kg. His BMI is 30. You specifically measure his blood pressure, the best of three readings was 152/92.

Questions to ask if there is time:

What is the first-line treatment you would initiate if hypertension was confirmed?

What would you consider if this didn't work?

Case 2

Amanda a 50 year old lady presents to the General Practice complaining of palpitations.

The candidate, is acting as the foundation year doctor, and has been asked to take a history from the patient.

After 6 minutes please stop the candidate at whatever stage they are and ask them to present the case with their primary differential diagnoses. Following this ask them what their next steps regarding investigations and management will be.

If they ask, give them the examination findings below:

Examination findings: Mrs Adams is comfortable at rest and does not look like she is in any discomfort. Her observations are within normal ranges. However on palpation of her pulse, it feels irregularly irregular. All other systemic examinations are normal.

Questions to ask if there is time:

What are the common causes of Atrial Fibrillation?

What is the CHA_2DS_2VAS Score?

Case 3

A 70 year old woman Diana, has presented to the GP surgery complaining of increased breathlessness and cough.

The candidate, is acting as the foundation year doctor Doctor, and has been asked to take a history from the patient.

After 6 minutes please stop the candidate at whatever stage they are and ask them to present the case with their primary differential diagnoses. Following this ask them what their next steps regarding investigations and management will be.

If the candidate asks the patient to demonstrate inhaler technique inform them that the patient's technique is adequate.

If they ask, give them the examination findings below:

Examination findings: Observations stable, afebrile, saturations 92% on air. The patient is mildly dyspnoeic but there is no visible cyanosis. There is air entry on both sides of the chest with widespread wheeze on auscultation. All other systemic examinations are normal.

Questions to ask if there is time:

What would the spirometry results of a patient with COPD show?

What other primary care interventions could improve the control of the COPD?

Case 4

Jack a 60 year old man has presented to the GP surgery with a 2 month history of persistent cough.

The candidate, is acting as the foundation year doctor, and has been asked to take a history from the patient.

After 6 minutes please stop the candidate at whatever stage they are and ask them to present the case with their primary differential diagnoses. Following this ask them what their next steps regarding investigations and management will be.

If they ask, give them the examination findings below:
Examination findings: Mr Jackson looks comfortable at rest, but cachectic, on inspection there is obvious finger clubbing, his chest is clear on auscultation and percussion, normal expansion bilaterally, no lymphadenopathy. All other systemic examinations are normal.

Questions to ask if there is time:
What are the different types of lung cancer? How do they present differently and what is their prognoses?
What are the complications of lung cancer?

Case 5

A 33 year old woman, Bekah attends the GP practice with a headache. The candidate, is acting as the foundation year doctor, and has been asked to take a history from the patient.
After 6 minutes please stop the candidate at whatever stage they are and ask them to present the case with their primary differential diagnoses. Following this ask them what their next steps regarding investigations and management will be.

If they ask, give them the examination findings below:
Examination findings:
Louisa is comfortable at rest. Her observations are all in normal range, including her blood pressure.
She has no significant neurological signs on a full upper and lower limb and cranial nerve examination. All other systemic examinations are normal.
Questions to ask if there is time:
What are the diagnostic criteria for a migraine?

Case 6

Colleen has presented to the GP surgery as she is worried about her husband's progressing confusion.
The candidate, is acting as the foundation year doctor, and has been asked to take a history from the patient's wife.
After 6 minutes please stop the candidate at whatever stage they are and ask them to present the case with their primary differential diagnoses. Following this ask them what their next steps regarding investigations and management will be.
Questions to ask if there is time:
What will a referral to memory clinic provide for this patient?

Case 7

A 38 year old lady Philippa, has presented to the GP surgery complaining of feeling unwell. It is noted from recent letters that she has recently been diagnosed with multiple sclerosis following two admissions to hospital under the Neurology team but has not seen her GP since her diagnosis.
The candidate is an foundation year doctor in a GP practice and have been asked to carry out a consultation with Philippa, discuss her symptoms and address any concerns she may have.
After 6 minutes please stop the candidate and ask them to summarise the consultation and assessing patients understanding.

If they ask, give them the examination findings below:
Examination findings:
Philippa is comfortable at rest, observations are normal. Chest is clear with good air entry bilaterally. Throat is red with swollen tonsils, no pus. All other systemic examinations are normal.
Questions to ask if there is time:
What is the classification of Multiple Sclerosis?
What medications can be used acutely and to prevent relapses?

Case 8

A 45 year old gentleman Harry has presented to the GP surgery as he would like to cut down on his alcohol intake.
The candidate, is acting as the foundation year doctor and has been asked to take a history from the patient.
After 6 minutes please stop the candidate and ask them to present the case with their primary differential diagnoses. Following this ask them what their next steps regarding investigations and management will be.

If they ask, give them the examination findings below:

Examination findings:

Harry is comfortable at rest and is not confused, with normal observations. There are no peripheral signs of chronic liver disease including dupytrens contractures or spider naevi. His abdomen is soft and there is no tenderness and no evidence of hepatomegaly or jaundice. No evidence of peripheral neuropathy.

All other systemic examinations are normal.

Questions to ask if there is time:

What is Wernicke's encephalopathy and Korsakoffs?

What are the signs of alcohol withdrawal?

Case 9

A 37 year old gentleman Sam has presented to the GP surgery complaining of rectal bleeding.

The candidate, is acting as the foundation year doctor, and has been asked to take a history from the patient.

After 6 minutes please stop the candidate at whatever stage they are and ask them to present the case with their primary differential diagnoses. Following this ask them what their next steps regarding investigations and management will be.

If they ask, give them the examination findings below:

Examination findings:

Sam is comfortable at rest. Digital rectal examination is uncomfortable for the patient and there is no evidence of haemorrhoids. All other systemic examinations are normal.

Questions to ask if there is time:

What is the classification for the degree of haemorrhoids?

What is the surgical treatment of haemorrhoids?

Case 10

A 50 year old woman Sarah has presented to the GP surgery after having found a lump in her breast.

The candidate, is acting as the foundation year doctor, and has been asked to take a history from the patient. After 6 minutes please stop the candidate at whatever stage they are and ask them to present the case with their primary differential diagnoses. Following this ask them what their next steps regarding investigations and management will be.

If they ask, give them the examination findings below:

Examination findings:

Sarah is comfortable at rest with normal observations. On examination of the breasts, there is some mild dimpling of the skin on the left with nipple inversion. There is a small hard fixed lump in the upper quadrant that seems slightly uncomfortable. All other systemic examinations are normal.

Questions to ask if there is time:

Where are the main sights of spread from breast cancer?

What types of breast cancer are there, and which have a worse prognosis?

Case 11

A 64 year old gentleman Winston has presented to the GP surgery complaining of blood in his urine.

The candidate, is acting as the foundation year doctor, and has been asked to take a history from the patient.

After 6 minutes please stop the candidate and ask them to present the case with their primary differential diagnoses. Following this ask them what their next steps regarding investigations and management will be.

If they ask, give them the examination findings below:

Examination findings:

Winston is comfortable at rest, does look very slim. His abdomen is soft and non tender, with no palpable bladder. Urine dip shows 4+ blood and is a rose colour.

All other systemic examinations are normal.

Questions to ask if there is time:

What is the TNM staging for bladder cancer and how does that affect the treatment given?

Case 12

A 55 year old woman Geeta has presented to the GP surgery complaining of feeling unwell.
The candidate, is acting as the foundation year doctor, and has been asked to take a brief history from the patient.

After 6 minutes please stop the candidate and ask them to present the case and propose their next steps regarding investigations and management.

If they ask, give them the examination findings below:
Examination findings:
Geeta is comfortable at rest, with normal observations. Her abdomen is soft and she has mild suprapubic tenderness. Her urine dip result with her that she just performed with the nurse. It is positive for moderate nitrites and leucocytes. There is no blood present.

All other systemic examinations are normal.

Case 13

A 42 year old gentleman Praveen has attended the GP surgery for a routine diabetic follow up but he is complaining of feeling funny in the last few weeks.
The candidate, is acting as the foundation year doctor, and has been asked to take a history from the patient.

After 6 minutes please stop the candidate at whatever stage they are and ask them to present the case with their primary differential diagnoses. Following this ask them what their next steps regarding investigations and management will be.
If they ask, give them the examination findings below:
Examination findings:
Praveen is comfortable, current BM 7.8. Observations are normal.
All other systemic examinations are normal.

Results:
HbA1c has been stable – last performed 4 months ago 42mmolmol (7.0%)

Questions to ask if there is time:
How is a formal diagnosis of Type 2 Diabetes made?
What are the complications of diabetes?

Case 14

A 38 year old gentleman Spencer has presented to the GP surgery with a rash that is seen on both elbows on the flexors surfaces and is raised with dry scaly plaques, in keeping with active psoriasis.
The candidate, is acting as the foundation year doctor and has been asked to take a history and examine the patient.

After 6 minutes please stop the candidate and ask them to present the case with their primary differential diagnoses. Following this ask them what their next steps regarding investigations and management will be.

Case 15

A 59 year old gentleman, Mr Hugo, has presented to the GP surgery with a small mole. It has a dark central raised region with a lighter irregular border that appears itchy with some evidence of bleeding.
The candidate, is acting as the foundation year doctor, and has been asked to take a history from the patient.

After 6 minutes please stop the candidate at whatever stage they are and ask them to present the case with their primary differential diagnoses. Following this ask them what their next steps regarding investigations and management will be.
Questions to ask if there is time:
What are the different types of skin cancers, how do they present differently?
What are the different type of treatment for skin cancer?

Actors instructions

ENT 108

Anaesthetics & Critical Care 114

Orthopaedics & Rheumatology 124

Psychiatry 131

Surgery 145

Emergency medicine 151

Obstetrics & Gynaecology 160

Medicine 168

Paediatrics 174

General Practice 181

ENT

Case 1

You are a 6 year old boy with a 2 day history of left sided muffled hearing. Onset of symptoms was right after playing in the playground with other kids. The child is normally very inquisitive and tends to put things either into his various orifices (this particular info should only be provided if asked directly).

The child can still hear sounds and whispers, but very distorted in the left ear. Also complains of associated intermittent left otalgia, minimal discharge from the ear (slightly blood stained and non-offensive), and a 'weird' fullness in the ear.

If asked directly, the child can reveal that whilst playing with his friend, they wondered if a piece of plasticine will fit in their respective ears

Case 2

You are a 35 year old man with a 5 day history of discharge from the left ear with associated tenderness when the pinna is pulled, tenderness over the bony prominence below/behind the ear, and muffled hearing on the left side
You have never had this problem before, and besides having your adenoids and tonsils removed as a child, are otherwise fit and well.

If asked directly, volunteer that; the discharge is offensive, yellow, sometimes blood stained, is persistent, often leaves yellow crusts on your pillow and associated with headaches.

You smoke 40 cigarettes a day and have done so for 20 years. If the candidate asks you if there is a family history of ear problems or family history of medical problems in general, ask them if they want to know about any specific conditions. Essentially, unless asked directly, do not volunteer the information that your dad and his dad died of a large cancer inside the nose
If the candidate does not mention cancer, you should act very worried about the possibility of this being cancer. Ask the candidate of it is possible for cancers in the nose to cause ear problems

Case 3

Two actors may be required for this station; one is the patient, the other is the mother

You are a 6 year old boy with bleeding from the left ear. You were playing in the playground when your best friend inserted a pencil into your left ear. The bleeding started as soon as you removed the pencil.
The ear was incredibly painful initially, but since the school nurse gave you some Calpol, you feel much better. The blood was bright red, there was a lot of it, bled for about 15 minutes, but thankfully, the bleeding has stopped.
Since the bleeding stopped, you have noticed that your hearing from the left side is muffled, and you have a funny sensation in your left ear, best described as 'something poking your ear hole'.
You have no temperatures, no pus from the ear, no neck swelling, no redness of the external ear or canal, etc, no signs of an infection
Your mum can confirm that you are have suffered in the past with multiple ear infections on the right side, have had a grommet inserted into the right side, and are now partially deaf on the right side. The fact that you may potentially lose hearing on the left side is extremely distressing for your mum, and when your mum asks if there is a chance your left ear/sided hearing may be permanently impaired, you also get very distressed.
Mum can also confirm that you are otherwise fit and well, up to date with vaccinations, and besides the steroid ear drops you take for the right ear, you do not take any other regular medications, and have no allergies
**Mother:
Ask specifically for the possibility of your child being permanently deaf on the left side. If the candidate attempts to deflect the question, you can get increasingly aggressive with the questioning until you get a clear answer. If the candidate claims that there is no chance of this, you can get very distressed and request to speak to a more senior doctor than a FY2. If the candidate suggests that permanent impairment is a possibility, then point out that this may mean that your child is permanently deaf (bilaterally); expect a clear demonstration of empathy at this point.

Case 4

You are a 30 year old male attending a GP practice. For the past year you have noticed a lump behind your left ear, it's normally not painful but occasionally can be and sometimes it leaks fluid which is yellow and occasionally blood stained. As it has persisted you have come to the GP to find out what it is.

You are otherwise well and have never had any hearing problems before.

Examination findings:
The lump is behind the left ear, it is fixed to the skin but not to any underlying structures
There is no pain
There is no mastoid tenderness
There is no erythema
Examination of the canal is NORMAL

Case 5

You are a 56 year-year-old male builder and the reason why you came to see the doctor is because your wife has been nagging you for ages that you can't smell properly! You've never had a good sense of smell and always put it down to smoking so you don't really see the point of coming in at all.

You concede that it's probably getting worse but you're not bothered about it too much. The only thing that concerns you is that you're finding it increasingly hard to take part in the local pub's annual cider tasting competition because your sense of taste has deteriorated as well. You frequently have colds and a blocked nose even in summer but always put is down to the fact that you work outdoors.

You suffer from asthma and take the blue inhalers on occasions. You have high blood pressure for which you take amlodipine and diabetes for which you take metformin. Your mates complain that you snore very loudly when you travel with them to the construction sites!

Case 6

You are a 54 year old woman with a 2 week history of erythema around her nose.

You noticed a mild redness around your nose when you came back from holiday in Spain. You initially thought it was sunburn, but it has got worse and spread from your nose to your cheeks.

Your face feels quite puffy and sore. You have been feeling quite run down and tired recently. The rash itself is not tender. If directly asked, state that your joints have been hurting recently, especially in your hands. You have no past medical history. No regular medications. No known allergies. You take HRT for Menopause. You live with your husband and 2 children. Smoke 10/day for the last 20 years and minimal alcohol. You are a housewife

No accurate family history, but you do remember a great aunt who always had a red face and was wheelchair bound before she died.

Your primary concern is that it may be cancer.

Case 7

You are a 46 year old man attending a GP practice. For years your partner has complained about your noisy breathing, especially at night. In addition to this you feel as if your right nostril is always blocked. As it has persisted you have come to the GP to find out what it is.
You are otherwise well.

Case 8

You are a 65 year old woman attending a GP practice. You have noticed this lump on the inside of your left nostril which has been growing over the last 3 months. It has bled intermittently. You are a lifelong smoker of 20/day but otherwise well. You are concerned it is cancer.

Case 9

You are a 12-year old boy who has been fit and healthy previously. You have a healthy family, and have no allergies. You do not drink alcohol and do not smoke or take recreational drugs.

A week ago you were playing hide and seek with your parents and accidentally were head-butted during the game on your nose. You had instantly a nose bleed that stopped with pressure within a few minutes. You carried on playing and had no further problems that day, except for a mild swelling of your nose. The swelling progressed gradually then it had regressed over the last few days. However, the regression of the swelling has allowed you to notice that the bony part of your nose is squint towards the left hand side. Also, you have been troubled for few days with a worsening blockage of your nose.

Since yesterday, you have developed headaches all over your head and intermittent fevers but no vomiting, nausea or vision problems. Apart from the bleeding you had after the incident, you have had no further bleeding or any nasal discharge. You and your family are extremely concerned about your nose deformity and want it to be sorted so it does not affect your cosmetic appearance on a long term basis.

The candidate should be considerate, polite and professional.

He/she should introduce him/herself appropriately, explain what he/she intends to do, and wash his/her hands before and after the examination.

He/she should check what areas in your body are painful to be considerate towards these during the examination.

The candidate should ask you if you have any questions, and then should explain his/her findings and management plan to you and your family in lay terms.

Case 10

You are a 19-year-old young male who was on a night out and was assaulted (ie: punched in the face) by two other guys. You just had a pint of beer and were not drunk. There was no other trauma and you feel fine and calm.
You don't think you lost much blood but it is still oozing slightly. You used a paper tissue to sustain the bleeding with good effect.
You did not lost consciousness and fully remember what happened. You do not have any other symptoms such as headaches or dizziness

Case 11

You are a 58 year old bricklayer attending GP with progressive difficulty in swallowing for the past 6 weeks. You previously ate a full normal diet but now find that solid food, such as meat, sticks in the throat and you have only been able to eat soup for the past 1 week. You can drink fluids although sometimes this causes you to cough and choke a little bit. Your appetite is reduced. Swallowing is not generally painful

You do not know exactly how much you weigh but your trousers are a little looser than last month. In the last week you have also noticed a small, firm, non-tender lump on the left side of your neck and pain in the left ear. No other ear symptoms. You have no difficulty in breathing and walked half a mile to the surgery today.

You take Amlodipine for high blood pressure and have no drug allergies. You have smoked 10-20 roll-up cigarettes every day since you were 17 years old and drink 2 pints of strong lager most evenings after work. You live with your wife of 35 years who thinks your voice is more hoarse than usual.

If asked, you are worried this might be a tumour as your father had throat cancer and died aged 55.

Case 12

You are a 20 year old student attending the GP practice with progressive difficulty in swallowing and worsening pain for the past 5 days, particularly on the right side.

You can feel large swellings under the jaw on both sides of your neck which are tender to palpate and have pain throbbing to the right ear. You have no ear discharge or loss of hearing. You have no difficulty in breathing but cannot open your mouth as wide as normal and your voice is altered ("Hot Potato voice"). In the last 24 hours you have been able to drink 1 litre of water but have not eaten since yesterday.

You have well controlled asthma and play Rugby 7s for your university. You have been taking regular Co-codamol from the pharmacy. You use a salbutamol inhaler regularly and avoid NSAIDS as they make you wheezy. Penicillin gives you a rash and swollen lips. You are a non-smoker and drink alcohol 1-2 times per week.

You are concerned that you are meant to be playing rugby at the weekend in an important Cup competition

Case 13

You are a 29 year old drama teacher attending the GP as you have problem with your voice. You first noted this 3 months ago when you were producing and acting in a musical for 5 consecutive nights whilst feeling run down and suffering with a cold. It happened suddenly and you could not even perform on the last night when you lost your voice almost completely. You now find your voice quality gets more husky as the day goes on and when you teach evening classes you find it hard to project your voice adequately and the throat feels sore and strained.

Your voice is at its best first thing in the morning, although not perfect, and you noticed it was significantly better when you took 2 weeks off work for a relaxing holiday recently.

You smoke 5 cigarettes at the weekends, drink alcohol 2 nights per week. You drink approx. 1.5 litres of water a day and several cups of caffeinated tea. Your breathing is fine and you perform yoga twice a week.

You take the oral contraceptive pill and an over the counter vitamin supplement. You use a steroid inhaler for asthma. You have an allergy to latex, causing a rash. Alcohol and spicy foods give you gastric reflux. You have never had any surgery or a thyroid disorder.

You are concerned you may need surgery to your voice box and are nervous that your voice will never be the same again. You rely on your voice for work and you like to perform at open-mic nights but find your singing voice is very unreliable now.

Case 14

You are a 71 year retired secretary attending the emergency department with difficulty in breathing. This happened suddenly today at 1.30pm when you were eating in a restaurant with your family.

You finished your starter but whilst eating a rack of lamb your denture broke and you think you have swallowed either the denture or a piece of lamb bone. Since then you are making harsh rasping sound whenever you breath in and out.

You have pain at the level of your 'Adam's apple' which is worse when you try to talk or swallow. You are spitting out your saliva into a bowl.

You have previously had an anaphylactic allergy to shellfish and your daughter ate crab at the meal.

You are a non-smoker and drink in moderation. You had coronary artery bypass surgery 8 months ago and take Aspirin, Simvastatin, Clopidogrel and Ramipril.

Case 15

Patient information –
36M, in ED resus. Trauma call patient; Motorbike versus lorry with significant facial injuries.
No known past medical, drug or allergy history.
He had morphine from the ambulance crew, and was been given a dose of intravenous Co-Amoxiclav on arrival in Resus.
Developed symptoms 15 minutes after the Co-Amoxiclav.
Initial assessment:
GCS E4 V2 M6
Tachypnoea (Resp rate 34)
Dyspnoea with increased drooling

Moderate bilateral air entry on auscultation
Patient appears well perfused, has a flushed sweaty face, and with distended neck veins + a swollen bloody protruding tongue
Further assessment:

GCS E2 V1 2   Resp rate 8
Reduced stridor   Minimal air entry bilaterally

Cyanosis involving the lips, reduced use of the accessory muscles, reduced chest movement
Nil change in neck swelling
Use of accessory respiratory muscles noted, with a marked effort of breathing

Case 16

You are a 79 year old retired Post Office worker attending the GP with a feeling of a lump in throat and progressive difficulty in swallowing over the past 5 months. Food seems to get stuck in the throat and occasionally you have to regurgitate it. You have noticed that occasionally you can feel a smooth soft swelling in the neck slightly to the left side. You were able to feel it this morning after a breakfast of tea and toast but it doesn't seem to be there now. Your husband complains that at times your breath smells and you get embarrassed by a gurgling sound that sometimes happens at meal times.

You have no pain on swallowing but have osteoarthritis affecting your neck and shoulders making it difficult to flex and extend your head. You have no difficulty breathing or talking although you have had 3 episodes of a chest infection in the last 6 months and had to be admitted to hospital for a pneumonia once.

You have well controlled hypertension and you take iron supplements. No allergies. You quit smoking 50 years ago and drink alcohol once per week at the most.

You are concerned that you have lost 5kg in the last 5 months and are worried you may have a cancer of the oesophagus.

Case 17

You are a 22 year old woman who attends the emergency department (ED) with sudden palpitations and a progressively growing neck swelling.
You have noticed in the middle of your neck a swelling that has been gradually growing over the past four weeks. The swelling is not tender and does not affect your voice, swallowing or breathing. Over the past month you have been troubled with many symptoms that are increasing in number and in severity. You have been troubled with marked irritability, sweating of palms and feet, and trembling of your hands. Despite having an excellent appetite, you have lost over half a stone in weight over the past month. Your periods have not changed, however your relationship with your boyfriend is strained due to your bad temper.

You have booked an appointment next week with your GP due to the neck swelling, and an appointment with the opticians as you have been getting blurring and double vision over the past two weeks. Tonight, you woke up with a sudden feeling of palpitations that you thought were due to you being anxious. However, your palpitations persisted for longer than an hour, so you attend ED. You have tremor in your hands and are feeling very anxious, short of breath and light-headed.

You have not had trauma, foreign travel, or illnesses recently. Your medical history includes resolved childhood asthma and an appendicectomy at the age of 13. The only medicine you take is the oral contraceptive pill; you are allergic to latex.

You work as a freelance artist, smoke only marijuana occasionally, and drink 30 units weekly of alcohol. Your mother has systemic lupus erythematosus and you lost your father to a heart attack.

The candidate will take a history from you about your symptoms in 7 minutes. Remember that you are very anxious, shaky-handed and short-tempered.

Case 18

You are a 45 years old man who is being seen at the ENT clinic for a lump that has been gradually growing over the past two months in the right side of your neck. Apart from the lump you feel otherwise well in yourself and have had no issues with your breathing, voice, swallowing or weight. You have a firm non-tender swelling on the right hand side of your neck that doesn't move with your swallowing. Your examination will otherwise reveal no abnormalities.

You are very worried that the lump is cancerous as you lost your father to an oesophageal cancer 2 years ago.

The candidate should be considerate, polite and professional. They should introduce themselves appropriately, explain what they intends to do, and wash his/her hands before and after the examination. They should check what areas in your body are painful to be considerate towards these during the examination. The candidate should ask you if you have any questions or concerns, and then should explain their findings and management plan to you in lay terms and in a considerate manner towards your anxiety.

Case 19
You are an 84 year old lady with a 2 hour history of complete loss of vision in the left eye.

This morning whilst having coffee with your daughter, you noticed a sudden loss of vision in the left eye. 'Like the light switch was turned off in the room, but just with one eye'. You can only see the difference between light and dark. It has stayed like this since it began about 2 hours ago so you have been brought into the emergency department straight away by your daughter.

There were no preceding flashes of light or floaters in the eye and your other eye is completely fine. There is no pain in the left eye and no double vision, but you have had a headache for the past few days. It starts from the left temple, and radiates to the jaw and scalp. It is a dull ache that isn't really helped by either paracetamol or ibuprofen, it's there all the time and it is made worse when you have something to eat. Yesterday you had a couple of similar episodes, however they only lasted 30 seconds or so, so you ignored it.

No past problems with your eyes with the exception of having both cataracts removed 10 years ago. "In my younger days I was a bit short sighted but since I've had my cataracts done, I only need to wear my glasses for reading". You've been feeling generally run down for the past 6 weeks with aches and pains over the shoulders and back of the neck. Combing your hair has been more of an effort and when you get the brush on your scalp it has been a bit sore. "If you'd asked me a couple of months ago how my general health was I'd have said I was fit as a fiddle, but over the past few months I've been really feeling my age, with aches and pains and feeling generally run down." You haven't seen your GP about this.

No regular medications. You are allergic to penicillin – years ago it caused a rash.
You live alone, don't drive and are independent with activities of daily living.

Your mother was blind in one eye in later life but you don't know the cause. All children and grandchildren have normal, healthy eyes.

Your primary concern is that your symptoms are due to a stroke. Your sister recently died following a stroke. "Will I get my sight back?"

Case 20
You are a 24-year old lady who over the last couple of days has noticed gradual blurring of the right vision. You can still read large signs but struggle with reading smaller print.

The eye has also become slightly painful on eye movements there is no discharge or trauma.

You have never had anything like this in the past. You are otherwise fit, take no regular medications, have no allergies, no family history and do not smoke or drink.

Anaesthetics & Critical Care

Case 1

You are a 52-year-old man and are expecting to have keyhole surgery today to repair an inguinal hernia in your right groin.

You are worried about your operation, and are keen to speak to an anaesthetist. 5 years ago you had key-hole surgery in this same hospital to have your gallbladder removed, and when you woke up afterwards you had a very sore throat and were told it had been difficult to insert a breathing tube. You were kept in hospital overnight for observation, but allowed home the next day. If asked, you were not admitted to ICU.

You are hoping to be reassured that this won't happen again today, and even wonder if you can avoid a general anaesthetic all together. You will be satisfied if the doctor explains that they will get a more senior colleague to speak with you about different methods of securing a breathing tube, or performing a spinal anaesthetic instead.

The doctor taking your history may ask you to open your mouth or make other simple facial expressions. If you are asked if you have any dental work, you will report that you have two crowns on your upper incisors.

You know you have put on weight since your last anaesthetic, and volunteer that you are a bit embarrassed that the admission nurse has documented your BMI as 34. If asked, you report that you take Ramipril 5mg a day for high blood pressure, smoke 10 cigarettes a day and drink 3-4 pints in the pub on a Friday. You are not allergic to anything.

Case 2

You are a 78-year-old man presenting for surgery to repair an inguinal hernia that has been causing pain.

You have previously had heart trouble and had a heart attack two years ago after which you had two stents inserted into the arteries supplying your heart. Following this you recovered well and currently live alone in a house with stairs and take your dog walking for a couple of miles each morning. You sleep with one pillow, don't have swollen ankles and have no other medical problems. You were last seen in the cardiology clinic around 6 months ago and were discharged back to primary care. Your last echo around this time was 'fine'.

You have no known respiratory disease, diabetes or stroke.

You had a general anaesthetic in 2000 for a knee replacement and had no problems.

You currently take a beta blocker, aspirin, a statin and ramipril. You have no allergies. You don't smoke and drink very occasionally at bridge club.

You are a little worried as you have heard having a general anaesthetic is very dangerous for someone who has had heart trouble. You feel quite fit but you would like to make sure everything has been done and no further tests are required. Speaking to a consultant anaesthetist would help allay your fears.

Case 3

You are a 44-year-old woman who has had a breast lump that you noticed 6 months ago. The hospital has performed a needle biopsy under local anaesthetic and you have been assured the lump is benign. The surgeons have recommended removal for more formal testing and peace of mind, and you are attending today for the operation under general anaesthetic.

You have had a general anaesthetic in the past for an appendix operation and had no problems.

You have been treated for asthma since you were a child, and are known to the respiratory team in the hospital, seeing them every 6 months or so. At your last appointment the consultant added in a tablet medication to help control symptoms. You use a purple inhaler (Seretide) twice daily, and a blue inhaler (Ventolin) when required. You also take a tablet (montelukast) once daily. This allows you to continue exercise regularly. You have never smoked.

You have been to the Emergency Department multiple times because of asthma attacks, and on one occasion had an admission to the Intensive Care Unit (ICU) after a reaction to a pain medication. After using diclofenac for an ankle injury your wheeze came on severely and you required 2 days on a ventilator. It was a very scary experience for you, and you are very worried about these types of drugs (NSAIDs) and need reassurance they won't be used. You want to make sure the allergy is recorded on your notes. As long as you can be reassured you will be happy to continue to general anesthetic.

Case 4

The candidate is to take the role of a Foundation Year1 in Anaesthetics, while you are a student ODP. You have asked the candidate to explain to you why Waveform Capnography is used, and to help you understand six different capnography waveforms.

After their initial explanation of capnography, show them each trace in turn. If prompting is required to move through the station, for each waveform ask;
What does this waveform show – is it abnormal?
What clinical problem(s) could produce this waveform?
What can we do to identify or correct the problem(s)?

If they are unable to complete a waveform, allow them to move onto the next.

Capnography Waveforms

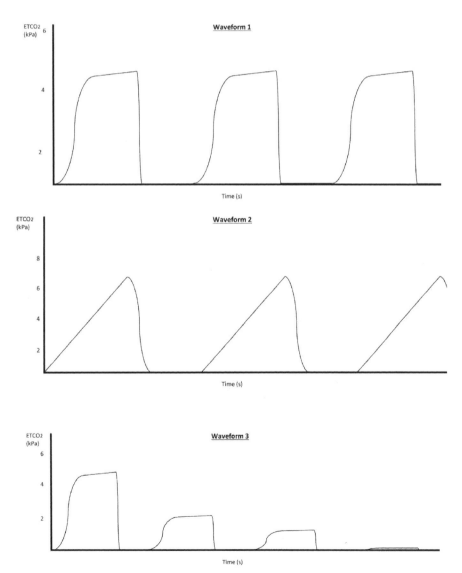

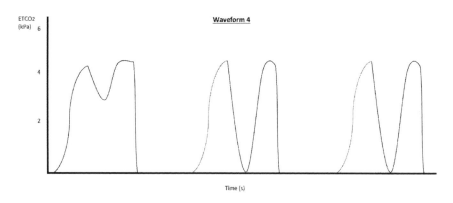

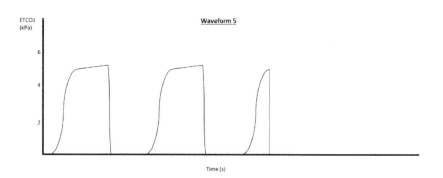

Case 5

You are a Registrar covering the Emergency Department. You have performed an arterial blood gas on Richard, a 28 year old male who has presented to hospital acutely short of breath. He is currently having 60% oxygen via venturi mask.

The Foundation year 1 Doctor has been asked to to interpret the blood gas and present their findings to you.

When they have finished, you should ask them the following questions:

What they would like to do next?

What tests they would like (if any)?

What their treatment would be if the CXR showed consolidation of the Right Middle Lobe?

What changes may they see on the arterial blood gas if the patient was tiring?

How they would treat the lactic acidosis?

What arterial PO2 they would expect with an inspired oxygen concentration of 60% in a healthy subject?

Case 6

As per examiner brief

Case 7

You are an experienced staff nurse who has asked the candidate to see Samuel, a 53-year-old man whose GP has referred him for investigation of ascites.

You are concerned that your admission observations reveal of heart rate of 120 and blood pressure of 75/40.

Direct the candidate to make an assessment of the mannequin. Initial findings will be as follows;

A: Talking in full sentences, but complaining of feeling light headed and nauseated.

B: RR 26, SpO2 96% on air, otherwise normal.

C: Cold, clammy peripheries up to shoulders. Central capillary refill less than 4 seconds. Regular radial pulse rate of 120/min, blood pressure 75/40.

D: Responds to voice/GCS 14 (eye opens to voice.) Pupils 3mm, equal and reactive, BM 5.

E: Temperature 36. Spider Naevi over chest wall. Distended abdomen (ascites). Malaena on bed sheets.

As the station progresses, the patient will continue to bleed and their condition will deteriorate with falling conscious level and worsening haemodynamic instability.

If the candidate asks for further history, the patient takes no regular medications, but has drank excessive alcohol for over 10 years. He currently drinking 1L of vodka and 10 cans of super-strength lager per day. His GP referred him to the medical team this morning for investigation of ascites. If questioned about bowel habit, the patient will report 2 days of large amounts of offensive, black, runny stool.

You are an experienced nurse who is able to assist the candidate in initiating any treatment which they feel is appropriate.

Case 8

You are a staff nurse working on the medical ward. You have called the Foundation Year 1 doctor to see a patient who you found unconscious in bed.

He is a 72-year-old man being treated for pneumonia. He also has a history of hypertension and Type 2 Diabetes. He has eaten little today due to nausea but has received his regular medications (Amlodipine and Insulin). He has no allergies and no relatives available for a collateral history.

You will assist the doctor with any requests and provide appropriate results.

Results

Observations

> Respiratory rate - 24
> Heart rate – 116bpm
> Blood pressure – 96/64mmHg
> Temperature – 37.9°C
> Oxygen saturation – 91% on room air

Examination findings

> A   - Airway patent with no abnormal sounds
> B   - Equal chest expansion bilaterally
>   - Trachea central
>   - Dull percussion note in right base
>   - Bronchial breathing in right lower zone
> C   - Cool, clammy patient with generalised pallor
> - Palpable central and peripheral pulses – regular rhythm with tachycardia
>   - Normal heart sounds
> D   - AVPU on alertness scale; GCS – 6/15 (E1V1M4)
>   - Capillary blood glucose – 2.3mmol/L
>   - Dilated pupils, equal and reactive
> E   - No signs of trauma or injury
>   - Normal abdominal examination
>   - No focal neurological deficit

Case 9

You are the paramedic who brought Lena, a 19-year-old woman to the Emergency Department resus. Her mother called for an ambulance having discovered her daughter unconscious at home.

Direct the candidate to perform an examination of the mannequin and treat any problems they identify.

If they seek evidence of poisoning or overdose, hand them empty packets of amitriptyline, which Lena's mother takes for back pain. State that the mother is concerned her daughter may have self-harmed, as Lena has been low in mood since failing her university exams.

An ABCDE examination will reveal:

A: Snoring, which improves with simple airway manoeuvres and an airway adjunct
B: RR 10, SpO2 96% on air, otherwise normal
C: Warm peripheries, radial pulse normal volume, regular at 120 beats per minute, BP 90/50, CRT 2 seconds.
D: Responds to pain, GCS 7 E1V2M4. Pupils 6mm, equal and reactive. BM 5.
E: Temperature 37. Nil of note.

Following the initial assessment, the candidate may ask you to perform certain tasks or administer medications.

We would expect them to request;

Senior Help – in particular they may state they need an anesthetist to manage the airway. Tell them you have bleeped for assistance, but there may be a delay in help arriving.
Oxygen – 15L via a Non Re-Breathe Mask.
Airway Adjuncts – they may request either oropharyngeal or nasaopharyngeal airways; offer a selection of sizes so they can demonstrate correct sizing. Offer to take over the maintenance of airway manoeuvers, e.g. jaw thrust.

IV Access – they may also request blood tests, including Paracetamol/Salicylate levels.

Arterial Blood Gas - after a delay for processing show them results with pH 7.22, PaCO2 6.8 kPA, PaO2 25 kPA, HCO3 20, BE -3.5, Lac 3.0

ECG – produce a 12 lead ECG showing a prolonged QRS interval; ask the candidate to explain the findings to you.

Drugs and IV Fluids – in particular they may request Sodium Bicarbonate.

National Poisoning Information Service – they may ask you to consult "Toxbase" for information on amitriptyline overdose, tell them the nurse-in-charge is looking for this.

Case 10
You are a senior staff nurse in charge of the bay on a medical ward. You have been looking after Jonny during your last two shifts. He is receiving 500mg levofloxacin IV twice daily to treat his pneumonia (he is penicillin allergic) and has been doing well. As far as you know he had been seizure-free for over a year, and was administered his normal doses of sodium valproate on the ward last night and this morning. His seizure started abruptly 7 minutes ago, with generalised tonic-clonic pattern when he was lying in bed. He hasn't bitten his tongue, but does have a clenched jaw and an erratic breathing pattern.

You have alerted the patient's own medical team, but haven't initiated a priority call. After 5 minutes of seizures you administered a single dose of buccal midazolam (10mg) and applied oxygen through a reservoir mask, but have given no intravenous medications, as they are not prescribed. The patient is still on his back, and you haven't managed to move the patient into a lateral position yet.

His cannula is patent and working well. You would like to know what to do next, in particular which medications should be prescribed and given. You think this is status epilepticus and are worried about what to do if the seizures do not terminate with initial treatment.

Case 11
You are an experienced charge nurse in the Resus area of the Emergency Department. You brought the patient Tim through from the Majors area after he dropped his blood pressure and became drowsy. He has no airway compromise, and is breathing at a rate of 26 breaths / min. He has a Glasgow Coma Score of 13 (E3, V4, M6), but is unable to give a clear history at the moment. You haven't yet managed to put an oxygen mask on him to administer oxygen.

The patient has no significant past medical history apart from an enlarged prostate. He takes no medicines and has no allergies. He has been suffering from nausea and vomiting for 18 hours, with some left loin pain. It was mildly tender on that side when the ED doctor examined him briefly. The patient has no abdominal distension or rebound tenderness, and has normal bowel sounds. He had his bowels open normally this morning.

On arrival in the ED the patient's temperature was 38.9°C with rigors. It is still elevated at 38.4C (he has been given paracetamol). He became muddled and drowsy in the main majors area, and has been moved into resus. He has a bolus of 250ml crystalloid infusing at the moment, with nothing else prescribed. He has had no antibiotics. Blood results are pending (FBC. UE, CRP), but he did not have any blood cultures or serum lactate sent when he was cannulated.

You are fully trained to perform IV cannulation, urinary catheterisation and blood tests, and administer treatment as requested. If the candidate does not initially offer a diagnosis of sepsis, enquire about their differential diagnosis. Offer to apply an oxygen mask and prepare antibiotics if a request for these is not forthcoming.

Case 12

You are a staff nurse who has asked the candidate to see Dan, a 28 year old awaiting wash -out of an infected elbow effusion. He complained of feeling unwell as you were completing your drug rounds - he feels light headed, anxious and "just not right."

Direct the candidate to make an assessment of the Mannequin. Initial findings will be as follows;

A: Talking in full sentences, but complaining his lips feel "puffy".
B: RR 24, SpO2 96% on air, central trachea, equal chest expansion, resonant percussion note throughout, mild bilateral wheeze.
C: Warm peripheries, central and capillary refill less than 2 seconds, regular radial pulse rate of 110/min, blood pressure 90/50.
D: Alert/GCS 15. Pupils 3mm, equal and reactive, BM 5
E: Temperature 36.7. An infusion of 2g of Flucloxacillin is in progress. No rash, but face and chest look flushed.

If the candidate asks for further history, the patient is normally fit and well, has no known allergies, and was admitted this morning with an infected elbow infusion. You have just commenced his first dose of IV flucloxacillin.

His last set of observations before complaining of feeling unwell showed a RR of 16, SpO2 of 99% on air, heart rate of 90 and blood pressure of 115/80.

Following the initial assessment the candidate may ask you to perform certain tasks or administer medications. Please state that you are happy to do so, but ask specifically for drug doses and route of administration.

We would expect them to request;

Adrenaline: This should be given as 0.5mL of 1:1000 adrenaline **IM**, and can be repeated if needed every 5 minutes.
If they don't volunteer a specific dose and route for adrenaline, please show them both the 1:1000 and 1:10 000 Minijets and ask them to tell you which one to give and via which route.
Oxygen: 15L via a Non-Rebreathe Mask.
IV fluids: 500 or 1000ml of crystalloid, either Normal Saline or Hartmanns Solution.
Chlorphenamine: 10mg IV.
Hydrocortisone: 200mg IV.

The patient should complain of feeling more unwell and on re-assessment the candidate will find:

A: Stridor, struggling to speak
B: Widespread wheeze, reduced air entry
C: HR 140, BP 60/30
D: Eye opening to voice
E: Lip and tongue swelling, urticarial rash over chest wall

If they have not already done so, we would expect them to summon urgent help and administer or repeat IM adrenaline, as well as request any of the measures above which are outstanding.

After a second appropriate dose of IM adrenaline, tell the candidate that the patient is showing signs of improvement.

NB: If high dose adrenaline (0.5-1mg) is wrongly administered intravenously, the patient should should develop short lived but profound tachycardia (>180) and hypertension (200/110).

Case 13
Patient:
You are a 76-year-old female who has been brought into the ED having been found at home. You are confused and don't remember the last few hours. You don't understand what is happening.

Daughter:
You have come into hospital with your mother who you found very unwell and drowsy in her home earlier today when you popped round for a visit. Your mother had a part of her left lung removed a year ago. She completed her 3rd cycle of chemotherapy over a month ago and had been doing quite well, though she has been very fatigued during her treatment. Before all this her mother had always been in good health with no other previous medical problems. She only takes paracetamol occasionally for aches and pains and a water tablet called frusemide which her GP gave her for swollen legs. She is not allergic to anything, is an ex smoker and drinks no alcohol. You are very concerned about how confused your mum seems and are convinced that the cancer must have come back and spread to her brain.

Case 14
You are a nurse in the Emergency Department. You have sought help from one of the Foundation doctors to manage a patient who appears to be choking in the waiting room.

Use the following information to guide the candidate through the station, which should be conducted on a resuscitation mannequin:

The patient is conscious initially and is coughing in order to relieve a partial airway obstruction. The candidate should initially encourage coughing and observe for signs of deterioration.

After a short time, tell the candidate that further coughing efforts are silent and that the patient is showing signs of respiratory distress.

The candidate should deliver back blows and abdominal thrusts in order to relieve the airway obstruction.

Allow the candidate to perform 2 rounds of 5 back blows and 5 abdominal thrusts before informing them that the patient appears to have lost consciousness.

The candidate should then check for signs of life and, having confirmed cardiac arrest, they should summon the arrest team and start basic life support with your assistance.

Case 15
You are the nurse on the cardiology ward. Your patient, Adam is a 65 year old man admitted with SOB and pleuritic chest pain, has just collapsed
The candidate will check for signs of life – inform them there is no pulse or breathing
The candidate will perform CPR on the mannequin
Connect the defibrillator when asked
Assist with ventilation if asked by the candidate
At the first rhythm check the defibrillator should show VF
After one shock and 2 minutes CPR, the defibrillator should show a rate of 120bpm with no pulse (PEA)
After 1mg adrenaline and a further 2 minutes CPR, the rhythm is a sinus tachycardia and there is a palpable carotid pulse indicating ROSC.

Case 16
You are a 25-year-old man who was knocked off your bike and landed on your back. You can remember the incident clearly but now can't move your legs. You are very worried. You also feel a little short of breath and light headed. You have some pain between your shoulder blades but nowhere else.

You are in perfect health and not taking in medications regularly. You do not smoke or take an recreational drugs and drink socially only. You are personal trainer and exercise daily whilst currently training for an ultra marathon. You are terrified you may never be able to work or compete again.

Case 17
You are Lisa, a 25 year old woman who is 36 weeks pregnant with your first child. As you near your due date, you are becoming increasingly anxious about childbirth, particularly about how you will manage with the pain.
You have several girlfriends who have had epidurals during labour and a few of them went on to have caesarian sections. This has worried you as you've also heard that epidurals can prolong labour. Last week you read a terrible story online about a woman who sustained nerve damage following an epidural and she couldn't walk for 6 months. All these things have really put you off the idea of having one, but you are also terrified of being in pain.
Your partner's mother used to be a midwife and she has told you that in her day women just got on with it and didn't make such a fuss. You're finding that your partner isn't being particularly supportive either, which is making you feel worse.
At your routine midwifery appointment, you decide to ask to speak to a doctor about the options available to you for pain relief during your labour. In addition to exploring the options, you would like to know whether epidurals make you more likely to need a caesarian or prolong your labour.

Case 18
You are a 4th year medical student in the first week of your Anaesthetics rotation. Today you are placed on a list with a Foundation Year doctor who you hope will be able to talk you through the drugs that are commonly used in anaesthetics - there seem to be hundreds and you're finding it all a bit confusing!
Ask the candidate if they could tell you what each of the drugs is used for. When they have gone through the drugs ask what is meant by the term 'balanced anaesthesia'. You have a misconception that the drugs used to put the patient to sleep at the start need to last for the whole operation. Ask the candidate 'how do you make sure you give them enough to keep them asleep all the way through? What if the operation takes longer than expected?

Case 19
You are to undergo an OGD after a referral from your GP who is concerned about your history of worsening abdominal pain. The procedure has been explained briefly by your doctor, and you are aware of the indication for it.

You have also discussed it with your friend, who recently had a bad experience during an OGD, as he was awake during the procedure and did not tolerate it well. You are now worried that you will have a similar experience.

A nurse has kindly asked one of the doctors to speak to you about the procedure. You are a non-smoker with no allergies, and drink alcohol socially. You have also been taking antacids over the counter as they relieve your pain. You recently started working as a taxi driver and concerned about being off work. This information is to be provided only when asked directly.

Case 20
You are a first year midwifery student attending the labour ward as part of your clinical experience. This is your second week, and you have been present at a number of normal deliveries but are now going to observe an elective Caesarean section in theatres for the first time. The patient hasn't arrived in the theatre yet, and you want to take the opportunity to ask the anaesthetist about the planned anaesthetic.

You initially have some confusion as you thought all operations are carried out under general anaesthetic and can't believe that the proposed anaesthetic is an awake regional technique. After realising that this is a standard technique you are very inquisitive about the process. You would like to know about the reasons women might select this type of anaesthetic rather than a general anaesthetic, as you would much rather be asleep for any operation. You would also like to know what checks should be carried out prior to performing a spinal.

You know that epidurals are sited in the back and require a lot of clarification as to why a spinal is different to an epidural. Aim to have elements of the process repeatedly explained by the doctor, and ask if you can help by preparing the (incorrect) epidural equipment, such as adhesive tape and epidural drug-delivery pump.

If the doctor becomes impatient, or fails to explain things adequately to your level of understanding this only adds to your level of confusion, and you may become flustered and upset.

Case 21

You are a third-year medical student on an anaesthetics attachment. It is your first day in the anaesthetic room and would like some teaching on the basics of oxygen delivery. You have been on medical and surgical placements in hospital, so have seen different types of masks used to give patients oxygen, but don't feel confident as to which device should be used when. You would like to ask the Foundation Year1 doctor the names of each of the devices, and some clarification as to their usage.

In particular, enquire about the what the tubing should be attached to (you have seen different gas supplies on the wall, and cylinders used as well). For each device you'd like to know some of their advantages and disadvantages. Review the examiner's instructions at this point, as some content will be covered during direct questioning from the examiner.

Case 22

You are Betty, an 80 year old lady who has undergone a left total hip replacement under general anaesthetic. You came around from the anaesthetic 2 hours ago and felt ok initially, but have developed increasingly severe pain over the last half an hour.

You are currently experiencing 5/10 pain in your hip at rest and 6/10 pain when you try move your leg.

PMH:
Osteoarthritis, Hypertension, Hypercholestrolaemia, Peptic ulcer

DH:
Allergic to penicillin- rash
Co-codamol 30/500 1-2 tablets QDS
Amlodipine 5mg
Simvastatin 40mg OD
Omeprazole 20mg OD

Case 23

You are a 60-year-old woman who was admitted for mastectomy for breast cancer. Your post operative pain has been managed quite well using IV morphine PCA and you are keen to transition to oral medication so you can be freed up from the some of the wires! You feel some discomfort around the wound and nowhere else. If you had to score your pain out of ten you would say '2' at rest and '5' when you cough or try to get up.

You have a little nausea and feel a bit 'bunged up'; you haven't opened your bowels in 3 days. You have taken ibuprofen before with no problems and have been eating and drinking well so far.

You have no allergies and have not taken oral morphine before.

You have no other co-morbidities.

Case 24

You are an experienced recovery nurse who is competent in checking and administering blood products. You should check the patient's identity, prescription, and the blood unit label with the candidate.

You are particularly aware that patients should undergo 3-point confirmation of identity prior to proceeding (Name, DOB, and Unit Number)

You remember on previous occasions using a special blood giving-set. The unit has been appropriately prescribed to run over a duration of 3 hours.

You have just performed observations on the patient. The patient's pulse rate is 78 beats per minute, blood pressure 133/81 mmHg, respiratory rate 19, and temperature 36.3 degrees centigrade. The patient's cannula is patent and working well.

The porters brought the blood unit to recovery (out of the blood bank fridge) 20 minutes ago. You would like to know what to do if the transfusion takes longer than the prescribed three hours as you are aware of guidance to complete transfusion within four hours of the blood product leaving controlled temperature storage.

Resources
Patient Band with 3-point ID: Name, DOB, Unit Number
Mock up of blood component label: with 3-point ID, blood type, date, +/- Unit Number.
Relevant section of blood product prescription chart (patient info and section with prescription)

Case 25
You are the nurse on the GI ward, and are concerned that this patient who has just returned from a colonoscopy is drowsy and making snoring sounds.
You have noticed from the colonoscopy notes that she has received 100mcg of fentanyl and 4 mg of midazolam.

If asked, you report that her respiratory rate is 6 breaths/minute, and her SpO2 on room air is 90%.

The candidate should try to get a response from the patient, the patient will grimace and make some flexion movements with her upper limbs, but won't open her eyes and will continue to snore. (GCS 6 E1V1M4)

If the candidate performs the initial airway manoeuvers correctly and applies 15L of oxygen via a non-rebreathe mask, you may inform them that the SpO2 is now 98%.

To move the candidate through the station, tell them that the patient is still snoring when the nasopharyngeal airway is inserted. They should move on to insert an oropharyngeal airway. If this is inserted correctly, tell them that the snoring has stopped. If they ask, tell them that the chest and abdomen are moving in synchrony, that the mask is misting/they can feel breath on their cheek. However, re-enforce that the respiratory rate is only 6 breaths/minute. If they do not move on to assist the patient's breathing with the self-inflating bag, prompt them by stating the respiratory rate is now 4 breaths/minute and that the SpO2 is 92%.

The final task the candidate should perform is the insertion of an iGel, if they do not move on to perform this themselves you may prompt them – "do you want to insert a Supraglottic Airway Device? That would free our hands from holding the mask."
You may assist the candidate by passing them any pieces of equipment which they ask you for. They may also ask you to squeeze the self-inflating bag, or assist with mouth opening or jaw thrust during insertion of the Supraglottic Airway Device/iGel.

If you are asked to summon help, or obtain specific drugs such as naloxone or flumazenil, assure them that you have made the request and that these things are on their way.

Equipment Requirements:

Mannequin with working airway anatomy and lungs which will expand.
Non-rebreathe O2 mask
Face Mask and Self-Inflating Bag
Nasopharyngeal Airways in Sizes 6, 7 and 8.
Lubricant gel
Oropharyngeal Airways in Sizes 2, 3 and 4
iGel Supraglottic Airway Devices in Sizes 3, 4 and 5

Orthopaedics & Rheumatology

Case 1

You are a 40-year-old rugby player attending the orthopaedic clinic with a troublesome shoulder. You have had multiple episodes of dislocation always during rugby matches. Most of these episodes have been treated with reduction on the field however the most recent episode last week required sedation in the emergency department.

Your main concern now is the ongoing feeling that the shoulder is unstable. The shoulder is dislocating with minimal force and recently you have been apprehensive to do weights or put your arms above your head for fear of dislocation. This is now affecting your work as a labourer. You have not experienced any numbness or weakness in the arm following these injuries.

You are otherwise fit and well, no previous illnesses or operations.

You are worried about the need for surgery.

Case 2

A 70-year-old male, retired builder has presented to orthopaedic clinics with bilateral hip and groin pain for months – now worsening in the past few weeks.

You have noticed the pain for a few months but in the past few weeks this has significantly worsened. When asked directly this pain has been noticed when trying to play with your young grandson. You get constant dull aching pain in both hips and groin region with no radiation down the leg. The pain can be at day or night but is worse after prolonged activity such as walking, climbing stairs and getting in and out of a car. You have no back pain, no weakness in either leg and no giving way.

You are a retired builder with a history of hypertension, T2DM and you are an ex-smoker. You have a family history of arthritis.

You are worried about the need for surgery.

Case 3

You are a 47-year old female has been referred by her GP to the orthopaedic hand clinic with a 3-month history of right hand and wrist pain which has failed to settle with activity modification and splinting.
You have noticed that the pain in the hand and wrist is particularly severe overnight and can wake you at night. Other exacerbating factors include using the telephone and typing on the computer. Over the last few weeks you have noticed pins and needles and altered sensation in your thumb tip and index finger. This can occur at night and required you to 'shake' your hand before it feels normal again. These symptoms prompted use of a split from the GP but no improvement.

You have had similar symptoms 3 years ago around the time of birth of you daughter which resolved spontaneously. You have no other past medical history but a strong family history of hypothyroidism. You have no allergies. You are a current smoker but consume no alcohol. You are married and have 2 children and have completed your family.

You have had trouble in functioning at work due to pain when typing and writing and your grip feels weaker. Fortunately, your employers have been very accommodating and understanding.

You are worried about the need for surgery.

Case 4

You are a 25-year-old male who works as an accountant. You have been experiencing increasing lower back pain and bilateral buttock pain over the past 9-months. Your symptoms are progressive and haven't resolved despite using regular anti-inflammatories (Ibuprofen) or compound analgesia (Co-Codamol) which was prescribed by your GP. You haven't noticed any episodes of swelling affecting your peripheral joints. You have suffered with Achilles tendonitis which you had attributed to regular running. Unfortunately, due to your symptoms you have been unable to partake in physical activity over the past 6-weeks.

You have had trouble with rising from bed in the mornings due to your pain and stiffness. Additionally, you find it difficult to wash and dress in the mornings and you have been late to work on a number of occasions over the last few weeks. You have also felt increasingly fatigued but associate this with increased stress at work. Your employers are concerned by your declining performance. Your job is desk-based and you find it difficult to maintain a comfortable position after working at your desk for over an hour.

You have seen your GP on 4 occasions over the last 12 weeks. You are troubled by your symptoms and are concerned by their failure to resolve. Your late father had "a bad back" at a young age but you are unaware of the underlying cause.

You are known to have a past history of uveitis which was treated successfully by ophthalmologists 3 years previously with no recurrence. Your sister has Crohn's disease and your brother cutaneous psoriasis. You have no allergies. You are a non-smoker and are tee-total. You are single with no partner.

Your main concern relates to your difficulty in participating in regular sport and exercise.

Case 5
You are a 75-year-old female who is retired. You have been experiencing increasing thoracic and lumbar back pain over the past 2 months. You thought this was related to simple 'wear and tear' arthritis and ignored the symptoms initially. You don't like troubling your GP and have tried to self-medicate and manage your symptoms with over-the-counter Ibuprofen, 200mg TDS but this has failed to settle your symptoms fully.

Your pain has suddenly worsened over the past 48 hours and this prompted you to attend the emergency department. You have experienced 10kg unintentional weight loss over the past 4 weeks, a loss of appetite and feel increasingly fatigued. Neither rest nor activity worsens your pain but you experience pain at night which disrupts your sleep.

You are embarrassed to disclose to an episode of faecal incontinence that you experienced prior to your attendance appointment and that it has been difficult for you to pass urine over the past 24 hours. You will only reveal this to the candidate if asked directly. You have also noted a change in sensation around the perianal region. Your mobility is affected and you feel your legs are weaker and 'heavier' than previously.

You have no significant past medical history of note. You are an ex-smoker (you gave up 10 years ago but smoked over 20 cigarettes per day for over 30 years). You have had a chronic cough for 4 months but haven't sought medical attention for this. You consume no alcohol. You live at home with your husband. You are otherwise fit and well with no prescription medications and you have no allergies.

Your main concern relates to your neurological symptoms and your recent decline in health, you have a feeling that there is a sinister cause of your symptoms.

Case 6
You have presented to your GP with a 3-month history of generalised muscle and joint pain. As this is an examination station, you are not allowed to provide a detailed clinical history for the candidate. You are allowed to interact with the candidate if they ask if you your name and age or if you experience any pain during the examination. You must however answer 3 specific questions (see below) that are part of the GALS examination.
Do you have any pain or stiffness in your muscles, joints or back?
Can you dress yourself completely without any difficulty?
Can you walk up and down the stairs without any difficulty?

The candidate should seek permission to examine you. If you are in extreme pain, you must inform the candidate and examiner.

Case 7
You have come to see an Orthopaedic surgeon for an appointment about your weak and restricted shoulder movements. You had a previous episode of right shoulder dislocation while playing rugby in your 20's. Your right shoulder is weak particularly when trying the lift forward and to the side above shoulder height. Whilst there is discomfort at extreme ranges

of movement pain is not a major symptom. You are able to get your hand behind your back easily and most shoulder movement are preserved.

The candidate will introduce themselves and explain the process of the examination. They will instruct you with actions they wish to perform which may include standing and sitting or lying on the bed. Please follow the candidate's instructions You are allowed to answer their questions before the examination starts.

During the examination your shoulder to not be acutely tender to palpation. You are able to do a full range of movement in the shoulder with the exception that when lifting out to the side you experience weakness through the mid-range of motion. You fail to fully abduct your arm against resistance and have some weakness to external rotation.

Case 8
You have come to see your GP for an appointment about your painful left hip. The hip pain has gradually worsened over the course of 2 years which no preceding injury. The pain is a dull ache and you feel it both in the side of the hip but also into the groin crease. You are currently unable to garden or walk more than a mile without stopping due to this pain.

The candidate will introduce themselves and explain the process of the examination. They will instruct you with actions they wish to perform which may include standing, walking and lying on the bed. Please follow the candidate's instructions You can answer their questions before the examination starts.

During the examination you are able to walk with moderate pain in the left hip but getting on and off the examination couch difficult. The left hip is not tender to touch. Your hip feels stiff and you are unable to bring your knees to your chest due to stiffness. The worst pain is when the candidate rotates the hip, particularly internal rotation.

Case 9
You have come to see your GP for an appointment about your painful left knee. You injured your knee playing football 4 weeks ago. At the time you remember a twisting injury, and sudden pain and swelling but you were able to continue walking. Since then the knee is painful over the lateral (outer half) of the knee and occasionally locks in one position.

The candidate will introduce themselves and explain the process of the examination. They will instruct you with actions they wish to perform which may include standing, walking and lying on the bed. Please follow the candidate's instructions You are allowed to answer their questions before the examination starts.

During the examination you are able to walk but get pain in the outer half of the knee when turning. The left knee is tender to touch in the lateral (outer half) of the knee but not elsewhere. Your knee is not stiff and has a normal range of movement but when twisting tests are done you feel acute pain.

Case 10
You are a 40-year-old female patient presenting to the emergency department with severe lower back pain of acute onset when diving into a swimming pool. You have had back pain for 6 months and previously been seen by physiotherapists with some benefit. This acute pain presents with a central lower back pain and pain radiates down your right leg. If asked the nature of the pain you should describe it as a sharp, shooting pain running down the back of the leg. You feel that there are pins and needles sensation in the right foot but you can walk and have not noticed any weakness.

The candidate will introduce themselves and explain the process of the examination. They will instruct you with actions they wish to perform which may include standing, walking and lying on the bed. Please follow the candidate's instructions You are allowed to answer their questions before the examination starts.

During the examination, you are able to walk with moderate pain. The key examination finding should be acute sharp shooting pain when your right leg is lifted straight off the bed. When sensation of the foot is being tested you can feel light touch but not as strongly as the other side. You have normal power in the foot and ankle.

Case 11
A 70-year-old female patient presents to see you in a GP clinic appointment complaining of bilateral pain around the big toe and difficulty with some footwear. This pain has been a problem for a long time but worsened over 6 months.

The candidate will introduce themselves and explain the process of the examination. They will instruct you with actions they wish to perform. Please follow the candidate's instructions. You can answer their questions before the examination starts.

During the examination you are likely to have to present your feet. The candidate will make comments about the observed signs of the feet. Further examination will require the examiner to palpate foot and ankle at which point you will describe pain on palpation around the big toes affecting the joints. You have no specific pain or tenderness during examination of your other digits.

Case 12

You are a 40-year-old female patient presents to the emergency department with severe neck pain of acute onset after a low energy collision as the driver of a car. Your neck pain is constant, severe and radiates down your right arm. On and off you report tingling sensation in the arm.

The candidate will introduce themselves and explain the process of the examination. They will instruct you with actions they wish to perform which may include standing, walking and sitting on the bed. Please follow the candidate's instructions You are allowed to answer their questions before the examination starts.

During the examination you are able to move both arms through a normal range of movement with the exception of restriction of right shoulder movements due to pain. You have good power in the upper limbs and are able to resist the examiner when asked. You have reduced but intact sensation over the outer aspect of the shoulder but otherwise good sensation in the rest of the arms.

Case 13
Image for interpretation

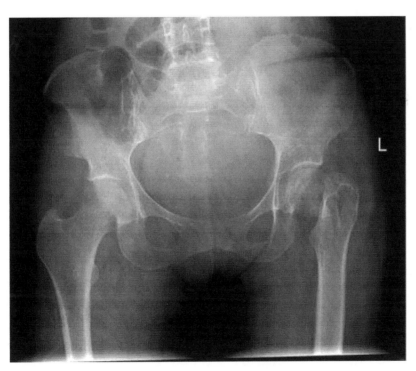

Case 14

You are a new CNS working with the metabolic bone team. You saw a complex patient yesterday in clinic and discussed him with the consultant at the time. The consultant suggested that send off a few investigations. You now have the results but are not entirely sure how best to interpret them. The consultant is on leave but another member of the medical team is around to provide advice.

The patient has known end stage renal failure and is on peritoneal dialysis. They have had some mild non-specific generalised aches and pains recently but no evidence of arthritis.

You have several questions for the doctor

What is the likely diagnosis?

Would calcium supplements be helpful

Should you give them vitamin D supplements and if so which kind

Are there any other types of drugs that could be helpful?

If drugs don't work what would be the next step

The appropriate answers should be:

Secondary hyperparathyroidism in a patient with known end stage renal failure

Start a phosphate binder – usually calcium supplements such as calcichew

Treat with a vitamin D analogue (alfacalcidol or calcitriol) – the candidate must ensure that they specify the right kind of vitamin D preparation

Consider a calcimimetic drug (cinacalcet)

If the above isn't working, consider referral to endocrine surgeon for parathyroidectomy

Case 15

No actor is required for this station

Case 16

You are a 25-year-old fit and well man involved in a road traffic accident whilst riding your motorcycle. You were thrown from the bike and managed to get up yourself at the scene. You have walked since the accident and have taken off your own helmet. You have walked into the Emergency Department as you have a painful neck. You do not have any symptoms of numbness or weakness in any of your limbs and no other parts of your body are painful. You have been brought through to the resuscitation area of the ED and are standing next to the bed holding your neck.

You know where you are, the time and are not confused. You recall all the events surrounding the accident. You are not combative and comply with the candidate's instructions.

Assistant's Instructions:

You are not to provide any advice to the candidate. If the candidate requests that you manually immobilise the patient's neck then you are to place one hand on either side of the patient's head with your fingers touching the shoulders holding the head in a stable position. You are to maintain this position until asked to stop by the candidate.

Case 17

You are in extreme pain following an operation on your tibial fracture earlier today. The pain is the worst you've ever felt and you are getting pins and needles in the leg. You have had lots of extra morphine pain relief without success.

The candidate will ask some basic questions then proceed to examine your leg. Due to the nature of the condition the examiners will feedback the positive findings to the candidate.

Case 18

You have been involved in an RTA. The candidate will describe to the examiner with demonstration steps to assess your injuries. You do not need to do anything to assist this scenario.

The candidate will ask some basic questions then proceed to examine your leg. Due to the nature of the condition the examiners will feedback the positive findings to the candidate.

Case 19

You are a 19 year old man who has been stabbed in the arm 2 hours ago. You can report to the candidate that you have felt that the affected hand is cold and numb to the touch.

The candidate will ask some basic questions then proceed to examine your leg. Due to the nature of the condition the examiners will feedback the positive findings to the candidate.

Case 20

You are a 95-year-old lady who has been brought up to the orthopaedic ward from accident and emergency. You are normally a nursing home resident and following a fall you were found by her carers on the floor. You are in pain but disorientated in time and place and unable to fully answer any questions from the candidate.

The candidate will ask some basic questions then proceed to examine your leg. Due to the nature of the condition the examiners will feedback the positive findings to the candidate.

Case 21

You are a 56-year-old man who fell from a ladder at a height of 3m whilst painting the outside of your house. You landed on both your feet onto tarmac. You were unable to get up at afterwards and your partner called for an ambulance. The ambulance crew arrived rapidly and put a cervical collar with blocks on and placed you on a stretcher and brought you to the resuscitation part of the ED.

You are aware of where you are and what happened. You can talk normally and your breathing feels normal. You have pain in both your feet and your back only. You don't have any pain in your neck, chest, abdomen or pelvis. Apart from the pain in your feet your legs feel otherwise normal. When asked if you have any pain you are very focused on the pain in your heels.

Case 22

You have fallen whilst drunk last night and been admitted the hospital with a broken right ankle. After a brief visit from the on-call consultant this morning you were informed that you are awaiting an operation to fix your broken ankle on today's trauma operating list. The consultant had to move on to the next patient and told you another doctor would return and explain it to you.

You didn't get much sleep last night as you were brought up very late from the emergency department. Your pain is under control and although you feel a bit worse for wear you are no longer drunk. You would like to know how long the operation will take and what is involved. You are alarmed by the fact that some serious risks are listed by the doctor but accept that they are part and parcel of the treatment you require once explained to you

You are currently at university and do tend to drink a bit too much and you smoke socially. You take the oral contraceptive pill but no other medications and are in general good health. You have never had an operation or anaesthetic before. This is making you very nervous about today. It doesn't help that you are tired and hungry as you were not allowed anything to eat and drink in preparation for the operation.

You have already been up on a set of crutches this morning with the physiotherapist and you found it very hard work but managed it safely.

When asked if they can put a mark on the correct leg prior to the operation you ask why that is necessary considering you have a plaster on your leg and only one of your ankle is bruised and swollen!

Case 23

You have fallen whilst drunk and been admitted the hospital with a broken ankle. You underwent surgery yesterday to fix the broken bone with a combination of metal plates and screws. It was explained to you that you need to be in a plaster and cannot put any weight through that leg for the next 6 weeks. You will be walking with crutches.

You hadn't thought about Deep Vein Thrombosis (blood clot in the leg veins) until the nurse giving you your enoxaparin injection in your tummy last night explained what it was for (to reduce the risk of DVT). You have since been looking on the internet and are concerned that you are at risk. This has worried you as your parents neighbour had died two years ago after developing a blood clot (you don't know the specific circumstances of this). You also think that your aunt may have developed a blood clot after a period in hospital but seemed to recover ok. You are currently at university and do tend to drink a bit too much and you smoke socially. You take the oral contraceptive pill but no other medications and are in general good health and good physical shape (i.e. not clinically obese).

The doctor will attempt to assess your risk of developing a DVT by asking you some questions and will explain methods by which the risk can be reduced. You can help steer the consultation appropriately by asking pertinent questions such as:
Do you think I am at risk of getting a DVT?
What can I do to prevent it?
You are not particularly needle phobic but don't like the idea of being 'stabbed' every day and you are not keen on wearing the stocking in bed at night as they make you hot.

Finally, (if there is time) you were hoping to fly out to Spain for a holiday with friends next month and you would like to know if this is a good idea.

Case 24
You are a 78-year-old woman who recently had an innocuous fall at home onto your left hand. Unfortunately, you fractured your wrist and it has been put in a cast. The orthopaedic team were happy with the alignment of the fracture but were concerned that it didn't take much force to break the bone. They suggested that you see your GP to start a type of medication called a bisphosphonate.

In fracture clinic they didn't explain anything about these medications but you have done your own research online and are quite concerned about the potential side effects. You have read that they can "rot your jaw" and even can cause unusual hip fractures in some cases. You are baffled why anyone would think these medications are a good idea as it sounds like they do more harm than good. You just need to be more careful at home and avoid falling.

Initially you will be quite adamant that you don't want to start the medication but with proper explanation of the risks and a sympathetic ear you will be willing to try it. A friend of yours has osteoporosis and is given a medication that they take by injection once every 6 months called denosumab. Can't you have that instead?

Case 25
You are a 30-year-old woman and have been experiencing joint pain and swelling that has developed gradually over the past 8 weeks. It has been affecting your hands, wrists and knees bilaterally. You saw a different doctor in clinic two weeks ago who arranged some investigations including blood tests and an ultrasound scan. One of the things that the previous doctor mentioned they were considering was rheumatoid arthritis.

You don't know a great deal about rheumatoid arthritis but would like to know more. You would like to know about the condition and if anything you have done might have caused it to develop (if asked, you are a non-smoker).

You think that your grandmother had rheumatoid arthritis and she was very disabled by the condition. In particular, her hands were quite deformed. You are worried that this might happen to you.

You would like to know what treatments are available for the condition and if there will be any side effects from the treatment. You hope to start a family one day and are concerned that you will pass the disease onto your children. You currently work in an office and are concerned about the impact of the disease on your job. You also are a keen cyclist and wonder if you should give up cycling.

Psychiatry

Case 1
Background
You are a 45-year-old supermarket cashier called Annabel. You have been forced to come to see your GP by your sister who is concerned about excessive tooth brushing. You brush your teeth approximately 20 times per day, and have been doing so increasingly for the past 6 months, but more so in the past 2 weeks.

Your behaviour
You are anxious, rubbing your hands, embarrassed to be there. You are keen for reassurance. You are generally cooperative, but you do not feel you need to seek any help yourself, and are looking at the door as you are eager to leave the consultation.

Your history of symptoms
You admit this is bizarre behaviour, but cannot help worrying. You have tried to take your mind off brushing your teeth, but nothing works. You feel the behaviour is justified by the "trillions of germs" in the environment that enter your body through your teeth. These are your own thoughts, and all started six months ago, when one of your friends fell ill after contracting a heart condition (infective endocarditis) secondary to a dental infection.

You have a ritual involving a specific order of turning the taps on, washing your toothbrush in a particular way 10 times, brushing your teeth for 5 minutes, followed by mouthwash. This ritual improves your anxiety levels momentarily. You try to resist repeating the rituals, but this is difficult.

On direct questioning about symptoms of anxiety, you acknowledge these symptoms in yourself. Much of this anxiety is centred around your job. Concerns have been raised by how long it takes you to check items customers have bought. You are worried you may lose your job, and feel guilty and hopeless. When it all becomes too much, you feel your heart racing, you feel clammy and get butterflies in your stomach.

You do not have any previous medical or psychiatric history. As a child, you wouldn't step on cracks or walk under ladders. You do not take any medication. When asked about allergies, you say you are allergic to the "pesky germs" in the environment. You live alone, but your sister lives nearby. There is no family history of mental illness. You do not drink alcohol or smoke, and have never taken illicit drugs.

Your mental state
Your symptoms "get you down" but you are not low all the time. You generally sleep OK" but often wake up with worry. Your appetite and energy levels are also "OK." Your ability to enjoy things is "normal."

Questions and actions
Throughout the consultation: Do you think something is wrong with me doctor?

Case 2
Background
You are 37-year-old man called Rafael. Your elderly father has a long standing history of bipolar disorder and has recently been detained under Section 3 of the Mental Health Act (1983). You have come to the hospital today and speak with the consultant as you are not happy with some of things you have witnessed on the ward.

Incident
Yesterday when you were on the ward you could see a group of nurses sat in the office chatting. And when your father knocked on the door he was ignored for several minutes. When somebody did answer the door, your father told the nurse that he wanted to go for a cigarette, but was told he would have to come back later because it was 'handover', this left your father quite agitated and distressed, which made you very angry.

You think it's very rude that the nurses all sit in the office having a chat and ignoring the patients. In your mind, the nurses should be trying to calm the patients down rather than distressing them even further. Additionally, you noticed that the linen cupboard was very dirty and that your father's bedding hasn't been changed for several days. You have taken pictures to prove this.

You are thinking about suing the trust for negligence or at least going to the press with the photos and telling them about this incident.

Behaviour

When you learn that you have to speak to the trainee doctor you start to get increasingly irritated and pace up and down. You are initially reluctant to sit down and speak to the trainee doctor. You feel very annoyed that you have to talk to a trainee that is younger than you are, who may not be able to make any useful decisions. You doubt they know much about your father. You think it is unacceptable that the consultant is not on the ward to hear your concerns and that your father's care has been left in the hands of a trainee doctor. You are feeling very upset and quite angry, a confrontational or defensive approach from the doctor is likely to heighten your anxiety and increase the volume of your voice.

If you feel that the candidate has taken you seriously and listened to your concerns, you start to feel calmer and less worried about your father.

Case 3

Background

You are a 25-year-old lady called Phoebe who has self-presented to the emergency department after deliberately cutting parts of your body (upper arms, upper legs and stomach). You have been seen by the emergency department registrar who felt that no stitches or other medical interventions were required.

Your behaviour

You have attended the emergency department voluntarily to have your cuts assessed as you thought they might need stitches. However, once you were informed this wasn't necessary, you wanted to go home immediately and are annoyed that you now have to wait to see a psychiatry doctor. You are prone to becoming irritable and angry when you feel people aren't listening to you properly, or don't truly care about your needs. If the candidate doesn't act sensitively towards you, you threaten to walk out of the consultation. At first you are guarded with your information, giving only one word answers, but if the candidate gains your trust you reveal the more intimate parts of your life story.

Your history of symptoms

You have been self-harming since the age of 12. This started as superficial cuts to your wrists using razors. You then started to cut other parts of your body such as the tops of your legs, arms, and neck, but you like to keep this hidden so you wear long sleeved clothes and a scarf. Cutting gives you a feeling of release of tension. You have carried out other forms of self-harm such as swallowing bleach and batteries. You have taken several overdoses in the past, of about 10 paracetamol tablets on each occasion with a bottle of vodka. One of the overdoses followed a break-up with your ex-boyfriend and you were admitted to a psychiatric unit.

You grew up with your mother and father. However, your father raped you repeatedly between the ages of 5 and 10. The abuse stopped because your father committed suicide. You tried to tell your mum what was happening on more than one occasion but she didn't believe you. You have a volatile relationship with your mum and you are convinced that she doesn't truly love you.

You didn't enjoy school. and left when you were 16. You were suspended several times due to acts of unprovoked aggression and violence towards school teachers, and were nearly expelled twice for throwing chairs at other students. Your friendships never lasted long and there was a period when you were verbally bullied. Your school reports also said that you were prone to lying, for example telling everyone that you were rich and that your dad was a famous actor who had been killed in a car crash. You now work at call centre but your boss is threatening to sack you as you have had frequent days off work for stress.

You find it difficult to trust people, particularly men. You are in a relationship with a female at the moment (although you don't label yourself as gay). It's a "rocky" relationship and you have frequent arguments and break-ups. You are convinced that she will leave you and think she is probably having an affair.

There are times in your life when you feel sad and empty. These tend to be triggered by something that reminds you of the rapes, such as a particular song that you may hear on the radio. During these times you carry out self-harm.

You have not experienced any unusual symptoms such as hearing voices or seeing things that other people can't see. You don't have any preoccupation with religion or ideas that your thoughts are being tampered with. You are not currently feeling suicidal and did not intend to end of your life with this current episode of self-harm.

You have no medical conditions and are not on any regular medications. You don't have any allergies. You drink a couple of bottles of wine and some "shots" at the weekend when out with your friends. You occasionally use ecstasy.

Case 4
Background
You are a 23-year-old lady called Ling. Your friend has brought you into the hospital today; you do not understand why he is concerned. You gave birth 6 weeks ago to your first child and are worried that your baby will be taken away from you.

Your Mental State
Your appearance is unkempt and you have a closed defensive posture. Your behaviour is irritable. Your speech is slow and disjointed; you sometimes find it difficult to recall thoughts. You feel low in mood and hopeless as a mother. You hear voices that only you can hear telling you that you are a terrible mother. You randomly shout in response saying "I'm not a bad mother, I'm trying my best!". The voices sometimes command you to end it all and you find it difficult to resist this temptation. You are not experiencing any visual or tactile hallucinations. You do not believe there is anything wrong with you. You refuse any medication or treatment and accuse the doctor of working with social services to take your son away.

Your history of symptoms
Your friend is concerned about your recent behaviour as he found you locked in your bathroom with your child. The voices have told you that you are unfit to be a mother and that social services are monitoring you through radio waves. You have not been able to sleep or eat for weeks but are full of energy.

You had a planned pregnancy, however during the pregnancy you split from your partner and have not heard from him since. Towards the end of the pregnancy you were admitted to hospital with bleeding and had an emergency caesarean section at 30 weeks, which was a very traumatic experience. You have not bonded with your baby as he was kept in hospital due to medical complications and came home 2 weeks ago. Since he has come home you have struggled to take care of him alone and have barely slept. The nurses say that he is underweight. You have tried to breastfeed but he fusses so much that you have given up trying to feed him more than once a day.

You have no personal history of mental illness. You were adopted so do not know if you have a family history of psychiatric illness. You have no other significant medical history, regular medications or drug allergies.

You have not harmed yourself yet, but you have been tempted to end it all like the voices tell you to. You have not made any clear plans yet. You feel like there is nothing that will prevent you from trying to commit suicide and say "everyone will be better off without me." The voices have not told you to harm your baby and you do not have the temptation to do so.

You used to drink ½ a bottle of wine a day but stopped when you found out you were pregnant. You used to work in a shop. You have no support at home apart from a friend who lives with you.

Case 5
Background:
You are Mark, a 27-year-old man who has been taken into the emergency department by the police on Section 136 because you were found to be agitated in the city centre.

Overall impression:
You are overtly anxious, suspicious and paranoid about everyone around you. You are angry at the staff, but also scared of them, because they are all 'part of it'. You have been under a lot of stress lately; you weren't causing trouble in the city you were just trying to help. You can be irritable, especially if you don't think the candidate is empathetic. You are dressed in dirty walking gear and trainers and have a large bag with you full of things you might need 'just in case'. You talk quickly,

your eye contact is poor and your legs are constantly fidgeting because you are nervous. You have difficulty concentrating on the conversation.

Thoughts and beliefs:
On further questioning you tell the doctor that your stress is because of the difficulties you are having with your neighbours. It all started with a petty argument about the bins and escalated from there. Since then they seem to have something against you and have been making your life hell.

You believe that they are putting cameras everywhere in your house and around the city disguised in ordinary objects to keep an eye on you. You have had to throw away your TV, radio and lots of other items because of this. Today, you were trying to destroy some of these cameras hidden around the city. They are very well hidden and even though you think you can see a camera you can never actually find one. You have also covered your ceiling with tin foil to protect you against the radiation that they are sending down onto your flat. You have had thoughts about attacking your neighbours in order to protect society but you don't think the police would believe you.

You sometimes feel like your thoughts become muddled, and that is probably due to the radiation. However, you do not think that anyone is putting thoughts into your head, blocking or taking your thoughts.

Perceptions:
You can hear your neighbours talking about you, these voices are not in your head, they are clear and they are coming though the walls or down the pipes. There are 2 voices, one male and one female, but they aren't the real voices of your neighbours, that's because they use a disguise. They often say bad things about you, and talk about their next plan. The voices don't talk directly to you, they don't command you to do things and they don't comment on what you are doing.

Mood and affect:
You have been understandably extremely anxious, and you constantly have to be prepared which is very stressful. Your sleep is erratic and your appetite is poor, due to all the stress the neighbours are causing you. You haven't left the house lately because you think they are waiting for you to do so, in order for them to install more cameras. You couldn't possibly be that predictable, which means you've had to make excuses not to go to work at the local supermarket. Despite all this you don't feel down, depressed or suicidal in any way.

Cognition:
You have not had any problems with your memory, you are not confused and you are orientated to time, place and person. You are annoyed that the doctor would ask you about these things 'I'm not stupid'.

Insight:
You have no insight into your mental state. You have absolutely no doubt that this is all true, but you don't know why everyone is so against you. You think that some of the staff at the hospital could be 'in on it' too so you are keen to get out as soon as possible. You try and convince the doctor to let you go so you can get to safety. You are not willing to stay and not willing to receive treatment because there isn't anything wrong with you.

Case 6
Background
You are a 32-year-old housewife called Annie with 2 young children of 3 and 5 years old. You have come to see the GP because your eldest daughter has recently started school and you haven't been able to take her there yourself because it makes you feel too anxious.

You think it all started 3 weeks ago you when you were dropping your daughter off at school and you suddenly became really unwell. During this episode you felt dizzy, sweaty, couldn't breathe properly and had pain in your chest. You thought you were having a heart attack and it felt like you were dying. Luckily, a passer-by called an ambulance and the paramedics arrived quickly. You were only in hospital for a few hours before the doctors discharged you with the diagnosis of a panic attack, but you don't think this can be true because your symptoms were real. This all happened near the school entrance with lots of parents around and you felt humiliated by the experience. You're embarrassed to talk about it, and are terrified that if you leave the house it will happen again, and potentially cause serious harm to your health. A few months ago you had 2 similar episodes in the supermarket, but these weren't as severe and resolved after 4 to 5 minutes.

Since the event you have been unable to take your daughter to school due to feeling anxious when you get near the front door. This makes you think you're are a bad mother and you feel extremely guilty. You haven't left the house since the episode and, upon reflection, you realise you have hardly left the house in the last 6 months. You often make excuses to avoid social occasions, do your shopping online and rarely take your children out. However, you think this is because you have 2 young children who take up all your time and they prefer playing in the garden rather than the park.

You have always been quite a shy person and never liked going to events with crowds or big social occasions. Nevertheless, you did used to enjoy meeting up with your close friends and family and taking your children to the local swimming pool but you haven't done this for a few months now. You spend your days playing games with the children in the house. You often can't get to sleep because you are worried about these attacks. You do sometimes feel hopeless and find yourself crying for no reason, but you have never self harmed or thought about suicide. You don't drink alcohol or take drugs, and have no past medical history or drug allergies. You smoke 10 to 20 cigarettes a day, and have noticed that you are smoking more than usual at the moment. You haven't had any problems with concentration and your energy levels and appetite have been normal. As a child you had a normal upbringing and never had any problems at school.

Your husband is very supportive and encouraged you to see the doctor because he thinks you are on edge all the time and have trouble relaxing. He took the day off work to come with you today because you were scared to leave the house alone.

Behaviour
You have very poor eye contact, spending most of the consultation looking down into your lap and are very shy. You are very fidgety, sat on the edge of the chair constantly rubbing your hands together or fiddling with the edge of your clothing.

Questions and actions
You do not volunteer information unless directly asked, answer minimally. You are extremely anxious and need lots of reassurance, but you become more open if you feel the doctor has put you at ease.

Case 7
Background
You are a 43-year-old male called Liam who was diagnosed with paranoid schizophrenia 5 years ago. You have tried 2 different anti-psychotic medications (olanzapine, aripiprazole) and neither seemed to 'make any difference' even at maximal doses. Your symptoms have worsened recently and you came to see the consultant in clinic today because you have been hearing voices more frequently. The consultant recommended that you should try a new 'atypical' anti-psychotic. You have been informed that one of the foundation doctors will need to discuss the medication with you, but you don't know why.

You have been hearing voices in your head for many years. You can hear multiple voices talking to each other, saying horrible things about you and laughing at you. Most of the time you find ways to ignore them but sometimes they don't stop and recently you have damaged a car due to frustration and this got you into trouble with the police. They make you feel worthless and guilty making it difficult for you to be happy in life. You have never injured yourself or thought about committing suicide.

You have no past medical history, have never been admitted to hospital, and have no known drug allergies. There is no family history of medical problems.

Your behaviour
You are quiet and reserved. Poor eye contact throughout and mildly distracted. You are not very interested in what the doctor has to say and you're not sure why you need to try another tablet. You have limited insight into your condition and don't think that another tablet will help you.

Questions and actions
If asked 'do you understand?' just nod in agreement. Although, on further questioning it is quite apparent you don't understand and are in need of further clarification. You are quite reluctant to try a new medication, especially one with lots of side effects, but at the end of the consultation you agree to try the medication.

Case 8

Background

You are a 20-year-old university student called Summer who was brought to the emergency department by your parents following a period of unusual behaviour. You were subsequently admitted to the acute psychiatric ward under Section 2 of the MHA (1983).

Your behaviour

You cannot keep still, and often lean close to the doctor in rather a provocative manner. At times you offer to place your healing hands on their body. At other times you get up and pace around the room in an excited manner. Your eye contact is very intense and your facial expression appears euphoric.

Your rate of speech is very fast and loud. At times it is difficult for the doctor to get a word in edge-ways and you often go off on a tangent about other topics which don't relate to the question you were originally asked. At times you may respond to messages from God that you are being sent. You get irritated when the doctor tries to bring you back to the subject. You are easily distracted.

Your history of symptoms

Over the past few weeks you have become more and more irritated by your family members who are always trying to "cramp your style". Lately you have been feeling happier than you have ever felt in your life with a great deal of energy, but for some reason your family seem worried and forced you to come to the emergency department. You think they are jealous of your "healing powers."

You are relishing student life and share a house with several other psychology students. Lately you have been feeling so excited that you haven't slept for several days. You are up all night writing long essays about your powers. Your mind races with fantastic ideas. You have an insatiable appetite. You are feeling more confident in your looks than ever before, and love wearing skimpy outfits as you love the attention you get. You have spent all of your student loan and savings on new clothes, jewellery and make up. You have slept with several different men over the last few days, some of whom you met when "out and about". You feel "in love" with the world and give out money to anyone you think may need it. You're not interested in drugs or alcohol as these would just "slow you down".

You can see the TV in 3D and have x-ray vision which allows you to see inside people's bodies. This allows you to be a healer and you believe that this is a power that has been bestowed on you by 'God'. You are feeling incredibly optimistic and know that you have been 'blessed' with the ability to heal all suffering in the world. God is sending you messages, telling you to use your healing powers on everyone you meet.

On one occasion you were picked up by the police because you were using your healing powers on people at the local shopping centre. The Police didn't understand that you have special powers. You were released after questioning and do not have a criminal record.

Yesterday you splashed out on a brand new car using your credit card as you have spent all your savings. You drove several hours from university and dropped in on some family friends in the middle of the night to tell them about your special powers and to heal them of their health problems. It must have been them that called your parents.

You have no medical problems that you know of and don't take any regular medications. If asked, you admit that in the past you have had periods of feeling very low in mood to the point where you haven't wanted to leave the house for several weeks. Last year you were briefly admitted to hospital due to feeling suicidal and taking a paracetamol overdose. You think this was mainly due to a break-up with your boyfriend. You are therefore particularly enjoying the way you feel at the moment and have no insight that your current mood could in fact be pathological. You can't understand why your parents are so worried about you and you describe your mood as "fantastic". You have no thoughts of suicide of self-harm at present. You are adamant that you don't need any medication as "feeling this good can't be a bad thing".

If asked about your personality before the depression, you say that your mum has always called you "over emotional" since you were a child. However, you have had a happy childhood and have not experienced abuse of any sort. Your mum tells you that you had an aunt who "wasn't right in the head" and committed suicide when she was in her 40's.

Case 9
Background
You are a 30-year old lady called Charmaine who has recently been admitted to the inpatient psychiatry ward following your first episode of mania. During this episode you went on a huge gambling spree and spent your entire life savings, you became socially and sexually disinhibited and aggressive towards family members and friends.

Your consultant has recommended initiating lithium therapy. The foundation doctor on the ward would like to talk to you about starting this new medication. Your current mental state is calm and lucid and you are able to take in and weigh up the information given.

You don't know anything about the drug and have never heard of it before, however are keen to find out as much as possible to help you make your decision and help you get back to your job as a teacher.

You are in a long-term relationship and are planning on having children in the near-future, although you're not currently "trying". This is something that is very important to you. If the candidate mentions any potential risks to a developing baby, you are shocked.

You have no physical health concerns other than mild asthma, and you have no known allergies. You are not on any regular medications, except for a salbutamol inhaler which you rarely use. You have a family history of hypothyroidism on your mother's side and your father had an MI aged 50. You have never smoked, drink 2 to 3 glasses of wine a week and have never taken any illicit drugs.

Case 10
Background and behaviour:
You are a 29-year-old senior nurse called Paul working on the Endocrine ward. You have recently had an incident where a colleague posted an insulting image on your Facebook account saying that you were a 'home-wrecker'. This is the first time anyone has asked you about your feelings and you are willing to share it. You make little eye contact and speak in a detached manner.

History of symptoms:

You have had 3 very rocky relationships with members of staff over the past 2 years which has led to you being alienated from the other nurses and gossiped about. One of these relationships provoked a divorce between two senior doctors who have been working at the hospital for many years.

You feel isolated and that no one likes you. You have not been sleeping well and have been taking lorazepam and anti-histamines which you have stolen from the drugs cupboard. You have been drinking a bottle of wine a night to help 'ease the pain'. You do not take recreational drugs.

You were diagnosed with anxiety and depressive disorder as a teenager. You have been in admitted to the psychiatric unit for taking a diazepam overdose when you were 21 following breaking up with a boyfriend. You were glad at that time to have survived. You have no history of self-harm. You have difficulty making friends at work and live far away from your family and old university friends. You have no past medical history or regular medication.

Your self-esteem is rock bottom, and the only thing you enjoy is looking after your patients. You have found it very difficult to remember jobs however, and over the past week there have been errors in patient care. For example, you gave one patient another patient's medication as they shared the same surname. You became tearful because you have forgotten that patient A was going home and that you have not prepared transport. You have no history of hallucinations or delusions.

When asked about suicide you explain that all this pain you feel is not worth being 'in this reality' and that you would rather be 'on the other side.' You have gathered a supply of lorazepam at home which would be enough to end your life. You have not written a suicide note or made a will because 'who will care to read it?' You think you'll take the pills when you have driven to a secluded area in the nearby national park so that no one will find you. You have thought about doing this in the next few days.

Case 11

Background

You are a 17-year-old boy called Taylor of stocky build wearing jogging bottoms and a T-shirt. You have been forced to come to the GP by your mum who keeps nagging you for spending too time in your room and not joining the family at meal times.

Your behaviour

You are annoyed that you have wasted valuable time coming to the GP surgery in order to convince your mum that you are not abnormal. You are keen to get this consultation over with so that you can prove to her she is wrong. Throughout the consultation you are embarrassed and can easily become defensive saying "why does it matter?'

Your history of symptoms

You care about your body and appearance; you want to maintain good health and that is your priority at the moment. Sometimes you slip up and eat a little too much (you become a bit embarrassed when talking about this). You admit to eating up to 5 chocolate bars, 6 muffins and 5 donuts on the last occasion. During these periods you feel totally out of control. In order to compensate you have been doing exercises in your room.

Your daily exercise regime lasts 3 hours and 25 minutes: it involves running on the spot, skipping, star jumps, weights and other fat burning exercises. When asked what you eat normally you explain that you try to have a banana for mid-morning snack and porridge for lunch. Sometimes you do get hungry and then you have one of your *slip ups* but you always take laxatives following these episodes to help get rid of all the toxins which make you feel disgusting and fat. You'll then add an extra hour onto your training session the next day. You have been doing this up to 2-3 times a week for the last 6 months. Your mum doesn't believe any of this and is worried that you are always alone. She doesn't trust anything you're saying and it's not fair!

Otherwise you try to work hard at school but get easily distracted with gossip from other students. There's a girl you really like at school but you haven't had the confidence to ask her out as you want to get thinner first. You were bullied at primary school for a number of years about your weight. You do like learning, however, and hope to become a doctor someday but are not sure if you are clever enough and feel that you might not get into medicine if you're too fat. You insist that you do not take illicit drugs, smoke or drink alcohol. You are a little stressed at the moment with all that's going on. You don't sleep very well and have been waking up early in the morning but you have not had any thoughts of suicide and have never self-harmed. You do not have any previous medical history and have no family history of mental illness. You are not on any regular prescribed or OTC medications and have no known drug allergies.

Case 12

You are a 48-year-old lady called Violet who is currently an inpatient in the mental health unit. You have schizoaffective disorder and have had multiple admissions to the mental health unit and tried many different antipsychotics. 1 week ago you were started on a new injection which was helping. Over the last 48 hours you have become very unwell. The candidate is a foundation doctor in the emergency department who has been asked to examine you.

You are sweaty, clammy and look unwell. You feel so ill that you can barely talk or move. You only make occasional groans and incomprehensible words in response to questions and you have your eyes closed unless spoken to. You are very confused about where you are.

Your arms and legs are so stiff they feel like lead pipes and you are hardly able to bend them. It takes quite a lot of force from the doctor to bend or move your arms and legs. Also you have a severe tremor in both of your hands. You are able to follow instructions but it takes a lot of effort for you to move.

You are heart is beating very quickly and your blood pressure has dropped. Your breathing is heavy and laboured. You have had some urinary incontinence but you are too confused to be embarrassed about it. Currently you are in a hospital bed in Resus and everyone is busy rushing around you and, understandably, you feel very distressed and are trying to take the oxygen mask off repeatedly.

Case 13
Your background:
You are a 52-year-old female called Roya who has come into see the GP because you have been feeling low every day for the past 2 months.

Your behaviour:
You are hunched over and making little eye contact. Speak quietly initially until the candidate has made a good rapport with you. You may begin to cry when you are speaking about the difficult events you have experienced.

Your history of symptoms:
Three months ago you lost your job at a clothing factory. You have found it hard to find another job. You feel like the situation is hopeless and this has extended to other parts of your life. You are beginning to feel as if things are never going to get better. Your mood is worse in the mornings. You no longer enjoy things as you used to. You used to like going to the cinema, reading books and being with your family but recently you haven't enjoyed these activities. Your energy levels are "ok... I guess". Your concentration is really poor at the moment and you are finding it hard to focus in job interviews, follow TV programmes and keep a track of storylines in books. You do not feel guilty and you haven't noticed any changes or slowing down in your body movements.

Although you feel worried and anxious occasionally, this has not changed. You do not have worrying thoughts running through your mind. You do not experience any symptoms of panic or worry that something bad is going to happen. You do not have suicidal thoughts and you would never to do anything to hurt yourself or others. You have clear thoughts for the future including wanting to get help for your low mood and trying to find a job. You do not have psychotic symptoms such as delusions or hallucinations. You have no medical problems and you do not take any medications or have any allergies. You don't drink alcohol for religious reasons and have never tried drugs. You do not smoke.

You are divorced and have two children who are 15 and 18 years old. You are currently unemployed. You have never experienced any previous mental health problems such as depression or elated mood. Your mother suffered with depression before she passed away and had antidepressants that helped her.

Your mental state:
Your appetite is ok and you haven't lost any weight. Your sleep is often disrupted and you are waking up at 4-5am every morning unable to get back to sleep. Your libido hasn't changed and you aren't currently in a relationship.

If asked admit that you feel that you are suffering with depression, you are interested in help with this including antidepressants or therapy.

Case 14
Your background:
You are a 21-year-old male called Ahmed. People are watching you and monitoring your every movement through a microchip that has been implanted in your brain. They know where you are going and what you are thinking.

Your mental state:
You are dishevelled, with messy hair and your jumper tied around your head. You are sitting in the corner of the room on the floor muttering and appear to be talking to people who aren't in the room. You don't notice the doctor as they walk in. When they attempt to engage you, you can come and sit on the chair but continue to keep responding to voices. Appear to be actively responding to voices whilst looking at corners of the room (e.g. "yes," "you're right," "ok") and say that they are confirming that we are all being controlled by a central group of elite professionals. You do not know who the voices are but there are two males, and you know they are "safe" and "can be trusted".

Your history of symptoms:
You were in the middle of the busy street trying to tell the public about the people who are watching you, when you were arrested by the police. These voices have been going on for months. They do not talk to you, but talk about you, they describe what you are doing in a running commentary fashion, like a movie. They do not tell you to do things, such as harming others, and you think you would be able to resist it if they did instruct you.

Although you do not think anything is wrong with you mentally, you admit to having had two previous psychiatric admissions. Both were initially under Section 136, followed by Section 3. You were only discharge from your last admission 2 weeks ago and have stopped taking your medication (olanzapine, mirtazapine) and have started smoking cannabis again. You feel that cannabis helps to make things clear such as the messages from the voices. You started smoking cannabis when you were 15 and smoke 4-5 joints every day apart from when you were in hospital.

You do not have any thoughts of hurting yourself or others. You have no medical problems. You do not drink alcohol or take any drugs apart from cannabis. Your brother has paranoid schizophrenia and is currently in hospital. You believe this to be part of the conspiracy. You live at home with your parents. You have never had a proper job and are receiving benefits.

You do not believe that you have a mental health illness and firmly believe that there is a conspiracy involving you and your brother. You do not want help from psychiatric services and do not need medication.

Case 15

Background:
You are a 78-year-old man called Albert and you have booked an appointment at the GP surgery because you have become more forgetful. You live with your wife and 45-year-old daughter who have both insisted you visit your GP.

History of symptoms:
Your memory problems initially started about 1 year ago when you noticed that it was difficult to find words. This has persisted, and over the past six months, your memory problems have got markedly worse. Your daughter had to remind you to visit the GP surgery today, as you completely forgot about it. You missed an appointment with the opticians and forgot to go to a friend's birthday party, which you feel embarrassed about. You've also noticed that you keep losing your keys and can never remember where you've put them. On one occasion you even left the taps running and the sink overflowed. Your daughter was very unhappy. On another occasion, an incident happened when your wife gave you your usual morning insulin injection, left for the shops, and your daughter nearly gave you the same dose again shortly after as you completely forgot you had already taken it. Luckily your wife returned before it was given and you didn't receive any extra insulin. Since then, your wife and daughter always check with eachother before giving your dose. This incident made you feel stupid, embarrassed and upset. But you know your family were just trying to look after you.

You used to be able to visit some friends nearby, but since you had a near-miss when driving, your wife doesn't want you to drive. You don't drive much, but sometimes you still use the car to go to the shops when your daughter or wife aren't around. You're starting to feel fed up and low, and think you're becoming a burden on the family. You used to enjoy playing bridge but now struggle to keep focused on the game. You've generally lost interest in your old hobbies and are struggling with disturbed sleep (waking in the night, restlessness). You now sleep in a separate room to your wife as she finds it so unsettling.

You have type 2 diabetes, high blood pressure and had a "mini-stroke" four years ago. You take some tablets for your blood pressure and diabetes, and insulin injections with your meals. You're drink an occasional shandy approximately every other evening and have never used recreational drugs. You used to smoke, but stopped 30 years ago. You smoked about 10 per day for 20 years. You have no history of mental health problems. You were reluctant to attend today but know that it is best to have things checked out.

Your mental state:
You are still eating well and you have not had any thoughts of suicide and wouldn't end your life, because of your family. You're very close to your wife and daughter and despite the issues with your memory there have not been any big arguments recently. You've never been aggressive or violent towards them. You have not had any paranoid thoughts of experienced any hallucinations. At the back of your mind you're worried because your dad had Alzheimer's disease.

Case 16

Background:
You are a 70-year-old wife of Reginald "Reggie" (92 years old). Your name is Alexandra. You have come in today at the request of the medical team to give a summary of the events leading up to your husband's admission. You are wearing designer clothing, sunglasses and do not maintain good eye contact. You are impatient, appear bored and have a distaste for hospitals and the NHS in general.

History of symptoms:

The maid found Mr Hammond on the floor of the garage yesterday evening with a golf club in his hand. He was rousable but very confused. She called the ambulance who took him to the emergency department, where he was admitted under the medical team. Reggie has been behaving strangely for the past 2 to 3 days. He has been saying that the journalists have been writing about him, accusing him of unspeakable things. When asked what exactly, he gave a terrified, haunted look and hobbled off. He has been clutching his abdomen at times, and the maid said he was incontinent of urine, which is new. He had a hip operation 6 months ago and was recovering well with the help of Leon his private physiotherapist.

He has an irregular heart beat, benign prostatic enlargement and regularly suffers from constipation. He has no history of confusion and his memory is normally good. He has been taking co-codamol since the hip replacement, as well as rivaroxaban and tamsulosin daily and laxido as required.

He walks with one stick but is able to wander around the garden, with an exercise tolerance of 30 to 40 metres. He often spends his weekends at the local cricket club where he is the Senior President. On weekdays he reads in the library or at the members only whisky bar in town for which he is an honorary member. In other words, he does not show much excitement for time spent with you, and your relationship has become increasingly distant over the last 2 to 3 years.

The night before his admission you heard him rumbling around his bedroom, moaning and making an absolute racket throughout the early hours of the morning. In the afternoon the day after, Leon who had been visiting you socially, advised you to see if he was alright and he was fast asleep. On waking him he seemed to be quite lucid initially but then went back to that incessant rubbish about the newspaper journalists. He also called you Judie, the name of his vile, interfering daughter. The maid also noted that he needed help getting up from the toilet yesterday as his legs felt like jelly, and that she also noted incredibly strong smelling urine. He has eaten little in the way of food over the past few days and didn't drink his usual glass of whisky yesterday afternoon, which is unusual for him.

Does this mean that you should take control his health care as he now no longer has his mental faculties? You are very keen to let nature take its course. You don't think it would be fair to him - to prolong his life.

Case 17

Background

You are a 78-year-old man called Clifford. Your daughter has insisted that you come to see the GP today. You were at home this morning when she visited and she was concerned that you forgot to turn the hob off after you made breakfast. You have forgotten to turn the hob off 4 times in the past two months; you don't cook anymore and can't remember turning the hob on this morning. You think she is overreacting, as you would have realized the hob was on eventually and she should mind her own business.

History of symptoms

You have had some problems with your memory over the last 6-12 months, but you don't think it is anything out of the ordinary for your age. You often lose your keys, but think this is normal for anyone. If asked you have been locked out of your house several times recently, but your daughter keeps a spare set of keys. You sometimes forget your neighbour's names but you remember family members and do not forget faces.

Your daughter comes over to help you with cooking and cleaning as you have been getting slower at housework, she mentioned that sometimes when she comes over you seem confused for a few hours but then go back to normal. During these periods she said that you cannot remember her name or where you are. Your daughter keeps sending you to the GP, who often thinks you have a UTI, but the tests are always negative. You get defensive when asked if you can wash and dress yourself, and reject the idea that you need any help.

You have type 2 diabetes and high blood pressure for which you take Amlodipine OD and Metformin BD. Five months ago you got a dosset box to help you take your medication. You have been taken to the emergency department on 3 occasions after a fall at home, but you have never been admitted into hospital with any injuries. Over the last 2 months you have noticed you spill your tea more because you have shakes, your grandkids have said you are moving around slower as well. You do not drink or smoke, you've stopped driving 2 years ago after getting lost on your way home to the supermarket.

Your Mental State

Your appearance is unkempt and you have poor eye contact with the doctor. You are reluctant to talk to the doctor as you are upset to be there for no reason. You are rude to the doctor and threaten to leave the appointment. Your mood has been low for a long time, no suicidal thoughts. Your speech is slow and disjointed as you have difficulty remembering certain words. You see rabbits in your bedroom, your daughter claims to not see them, but you know they are there as they make noises eating their carrots under your bed. This keeps you up all night. You do not have insight to your condition – you think your daughter is overreacting and you want to go home.

AMTS

Name – Correct	Age – Incorrect
Date of birth – Incorrect	Time – Correct
Current monarch – Correct	Dates of WW1 – Incorrect
2 objects – Correct	2 people – Incorrect
Count backwards – Incorrect	Address – Incorrect

Total = 4/10

Case 18

Background

You are a 15-year-old girl called Grace who is currently studying for your GCSEs. Your Mum has taken you to the emergency department after she found you crying in your room next to an empty packet of paracetamol.

Over the last few weeks there have been a few things that have made you upset and angry. You and your boyfriend have been arguing and on two separate occasions he's called you a "fat bitch" and "not worth it". Because of this you are constantly worrying that he's going to break up with you. On top of this you are getting behind with your homework and recently underachieved in your mock GCSEs. Your Mum is putting a huge amount of pressure on you to do well in your exams and it's making you feel like a failure.

Two hours ago, in the spur of the moment, you took 18 paracetamol tablets from the bathroom cupboard and drank half a bottle of wine you found in the fridge to "make it all go away". You didn't think this would end your life and you did not write a suicide note. You immediately regretted it and text your boyfriend what had happened, hoping it would make him feel guilty. Your mum was in the next room but didn't hear you at the time. You left the wine bottle and the packet of tablets next to you rather than trying to hide them. You have never done anything like this before but feel you have been pushed into feeling this way, and that "everything is getting too much". In the past few weeks you have thought about harming yourself in some way to make your problems go away but have not acted on these thoughts. You wouldn't want to end your life because you have great family and friends and you're looking forward to going to college next year.

You enjoy shopping with your friends, spending time with your boyfriend and going to school, most of the time. You have no problems sleeping, no weight loss and your appetite is normal. You sometimes smoke cannabis with your friends and rarely drink alcohol. You have two older brothers (John 18, Paul 22) who are both at university. A few weekends ago, you went to stay with John to experience university life; you got very drunk and took a drug that all of his friends were doing called 'Black Mamba'. It made you feel psychedelic and like you saw neon coloured flowers and animals all night.

You have never been in trouble with the police. You have no known medical problems, and don't take any regular medications or have any drug allergies. You are not known to the mental health services, and there is no family history of mental illness. You don't think that you're depressed and don't want any further treatment. You are really embarrassed about what happened. You deny self-harm or suicidal ideation, and are sure this won't happen again. You don't know why your mum is making such a 'big deal out of it'.

Behaviour and appearance

You are wearing your school uniform and you usually wear lots of make up. You are usually quite chatty and confident but today you are withdrawn and embarrassed by your actions so spend most of the consultation looking down at your hands fiddling with your jewellery/clothes. You aren't sure about the answer to lots of the questions so you just shrug and say 'I don't know'.

Case 19

Background:

You are a 15-year-old young girl called Natalia who has come to the emergency department with a deep cut on your forearm, which was self-inflicted. The foundation year doctor has been asked to come and speak to you in more detail about it. You cut yourself today after a row with your mother. You were very angry and did it impulsively. You didn't intend to cut yourself deeply and had no wish to end your life or attend hospital. You suffer from depression and mood swings, and you are known to a Children and Adolescent Mental Health Service (CAMHS). You have regular meetings with your care coordinator, who you are due to see next week.

History of symptoms:

You always cut yourself superficially on your arms and legs, and you have never self-harmed by any other means. This is the first time you have ever cut yourself deeply enough to require any intervention or attendance to ED.

You have been cutting yourself on and off since the age of 12. You can't remember why or how you started, but you find it helps when you are feeling distressed or out of control. It provides momentary relief. You usually cut yourself at least once a week and this has not changed recently. You also used to bang your head repeatedly on the wall until you got a bruise but you haven't done this for a few years. You have never blacked out.

You have no medical conditions and do not take any regular medication. You live with your parents, who are both teachers, and you have a boyfriend who is supportive. You attend a mainstream school which is going well. You see the school counselor occasionally when you feel stressed. Your parents know about your mental health problems and one of them accompanies you to your appointments with the CAMHS team and your social worker. They know about your cutting and your Mother came with you to A&E today. No-one else in your family has any history of mental health problems or self-harm. You do not use any drugs but you do binge-drink at the weekends when you are with friends. You do not drink alone. You were born at full term and there have been no developmental concerns (walking and talking at all the normal times).

Your behaviour:

You are rational and not distressed; you have calmed down after the altercation with your mother. You feel embarrassed. You have no plans to cut or hurt yourself now or in the immediate future, although you acknowledge that you will continue to cut yourself superficially as a form of relief. You do not feel severely depressed. You have never experienced any delusional or paranoid beliefs, and you have never heard voices or seen things that aren't there. You would like to go home. You do not want to come into hospital.

Case 20

Background:

You are a 16-year-old schoolgirl called Sam who has been referred to see a child and adolescent psychiatrist by your GP.

Behaviour:

You are looking down toward your feet at the start of the interview. You are shy and have crossed your arms on your lap. You didn't want to come and see a psychiatrist and you feel worried about making things worse. Initially speak quietly and timidly, looking at the ground. As the foundation doctor makes you feel at ease start speaking more loudly and coherently. You should look sad and may be tearful at times when speaking about the difficulties you have encountered.

History of symptoms:

For the past four months you have been bullied at school by a group of 4 girls who you used to be friends with. You are larger than the other girls and it started with name-calling such as "fatty, piggy, supersize". This has escalated and now they are writing horrible messages on your social media page. Recently someone hacked into your social media account and wrote a message on your timeline saying "I am such an unhappy slut. I might as well kill myself". Over 40 people liked this before you managed to take it down. They have created an online page called "We hate Sam" and over a 100 people have joined. At school other students have started ignoring you and laughing behind your back. You have no friends. So far the bullying has been psychological only. But the bullies have threatened to hurt you physically if you tell anyone. You haven't reported any of this to anyone and you wish the situation would just "go away". You have started skipping school to avoid the bullying, which is why your mum made you see the GP, but the online bullying means you can never escape. You are not sure if you are depressed but you would like help to feel "back to normal".

You do not have suicidal thoughts and you would never to do anything to hurt yourself. You have clear thoughts for the future including wanting to become a painter one day. You do not have psychotic symptoms. You do not have any medical problems, regular medications or allergies. You do not smoke, drink alcohol, or take drugs. You were born at full term and there were no developmental concerns (walking and talking at the normal times). You attend mainstream school. Your parents divorced when you were 7 and you now live with your mother, step-father and their new 9-month old baby. Home has been busy with the new baby. You see your biological father every other weekend. You describe a happy childhood, despite your parent's divorce. You are not known to the child and adolescent mental health services, or social services. No family history of mental illness or suicide.

Mental state:
As a result of the bullying you have started feeling low all day every day for the past three months. Your mood is at its lowest when you are about to go to school. Whilst you still enjoy watching TV, reading books, painting and being with your family, you feel tired all the time. You have disturbed sleep and find that you are waking up at 4am every day. You have been overeating, as food has become your only comfort and friend. Your concentration has become poor and your grades at school are getting worse. Your self confidence is rock bottom and you feel the situation is hopeless. You do not feel guilty as you recognize that the bullying isn't your fault.

Surgery

Case 1

You are a 72-year-old man named Charles, who is attending Emergency department due to the sudden onset of a severe pain in your abdomen. You have had some grumbling type pains for several months and thought it was indigestion.

This afternoon when you were reading the paper when a sudden pain started in the centre of your abdomen that made you double over, feel very faint and almost lose consciousness. It is a very sharp pain and at its worst is 9/10 in severity. The pain is also felt in your back. The paracetamol that you had when it came on has not touched it and you are beginning to feel hot and sweaty as well as very nauseous. Nothing appears to be making it better or worse and you are feeling increasingly anxious about what it might be. You have been opening your bowels normally and have not lost any weight recently.

Generally you are quite fit and well and are a retired Civil Servant who still finds time to play regular golf. You live at home with your partner and travel extensively. You remember your GP years ago putting you on a medication for high blood pressure but you stopped taking it because you didn't like the taste and have never been back. You are not currently taking any regular medications and have only had one operation in the past where they removed your gallbladder. You are an only child and remember that your father had a sudden death when you were young but that your mother never explained why.

You are intermittently very distressed because of the pain. Try to get the doctor to tell you what he thinks is going on and question whether you are going to die?

Case 2

You are a 22-year-old history student named Lisa. For the last 12 hours you've been experiencing severe abdominal pain. The pain woke you up from your sleep. The pain started in the right iliac fossa and you can feel it below your belly button too. The pain is quite sharp; it's 7 out of 10 and seems to come in waves but never totally goes away.

The pain started very suddenly. You took some paracetamol earlier and that seems to have helped with the pain a bit. Lying still makes the pain feel a bit better as well. Walking makes it worse. The pain is making you feel sick and you've lost your appetite. You have not vomited. You had one loose bowel motion this morning.

You have some mild increase in urinary frequency but no dysuria. You've passed urine 5 times in the last few hours. Your boyfriend drove you to hospital and the car journey felt uncomfortable. You don't feel feverish; you've got no joint pain or muscle soreness. No one else at home is unwell. You've not travelled abroad recently or eating from takeaways.

You've recently had a sexual transmitted disease check-up, which was negative. You have one male sexual partner. You have no vaginal discharge. You are not currently using contraception. You're mid-cycle and normally have a regular 28-day cycle. You don't think you're pregnant.

You had a laparoscopy under the gynecologists last year for a similar pain and were told you had endometriosis. You haven't had any other operations. You suffer with hay fever and take an antihistamine in the summer but you can't remember the name. You have asthma and use a blue inhaler. You don't have any drug allergies.

You're a non-smoker drink alcohol socially and don't use illicit drugs. You live with your boyfriend You have no relevant family history and no other symptoms.

Case 3

You are a 70-year-old man named Alex, you made an appointment with your GP today because of 2 days of worsening central abdominal pain and 24 hours of persistent vomiting.

The pain is much worse on movement and you are most comfortable laying flat. It is a moderately severe constant pain. You were mostly concerned by the fact that you have been vomiting everything you try to swallow. The rest of the time you are vomiting bile and have not been able to take your regular medications. You feel that this is just a stomach bug and don't understand why the GP sent you to hospital, you only wanted a medicine for the vomiting.

You had also developed an increased frequency in opening your bowels in those 3 months. You last opened your bowels 4 days ago. When probed you realize that you have not passed wind for at least a day, maybe more.

You suffer from high blood pressure, diabetes and atrial fibrillation. You had polyps removed from the bowel 4 years ago. You are on many medications but cannot remember their names. You are not aware of any specific illnesses in the family.

You have smoked 10 cigarettes a day for at least 50 years. You don't drink alcohol and used to work as a HGV driver. You admit to have been very unhealthy in your working years.

If asked you have noticed reduced appetite for a while and have gone down at least 3 notches on your belt in the past 3 months.

If asked about other symptoms: you have noticed only- pallor of the face, shortness of breath on walking and increased lethargy.

Case 4

You are a 62-year-old gentleman named Simon, who has been experiencing pain on passing stool for the last week. This pain is mild and is more of a discomfort on defecation. As soon as you pass stool the pain disappeared. You have noticed that your stool has been getting harder. You have been having increasing difficulty-passing stool for the past 2 months, which has been getting worse. You have to strain more and have a feeling that you have not passed everything that is inside.

You have not noticed any bleeding. 10 years ago you had episodes of rectal bleeding and underwent a colonoscopy. This revealed a polyp that was removed.

You have lost 5 kilograms of weight in the last 3 months but should only mention this if asked directly. You did not plan on losing this weight but view it as a good thing as you are overweight.

You also suffer with high blood pressure and take 10mg of amlodipine once a day for this. You do not have any allergies.

Your father developed bowel cancer and had to have part of his bowel removed before he passed away from pneumonia. You smoke 10 cigarettes a day. You drink alcohol socially. You live with your wife and are fully independent.

You are worried that this could be cancer as your father had it before he died and are scared that you could need an operation.

Case 5

You are a 68-year-old lady named Jenny, who is panicking after having vomited a large amount of blood this morning. You vomited around 1 pint of blood this morning and immediately called an ambulance. You had a second episode of vomiting in the ambulance bringing up a further half a pint of blood. The blood looks dark red with no clots and nothing mixed in. You have never experienced anything like this before.

You are not in any pain, only scared about the experience and think you are dying. You feel dizzy, especially when you stand up and have stayed on the hospital bed not moving because of this. You have not opened your bowels today. You have not noticed any blood in your stool and it does not look black, although it has looked a bit darker in the last two weeks. You have not passed any urine this morning.

You did not have any episodes of vomiting prior to this. You have not had any reflux or any symptoms of heartburn. You have not had any pain in your abdomen recently. You have not been involved in any trauma. You have no signs of infection and have not been losing any weight.

Only give this information if asked directly. You have been drinking increasing amounts of alcohol ever since your husband passed away of pancreatic cancer one and a half years ago. You drink around 1-2 bottles of wine a night.

You do not have any other medical problems and are not on any regular medications. You have no allergies that you know of.

You live alone since your husband passed away. You have a daughter who moved to Australia 3 months ago. You do not smoke. You drink alcohol as mentioned above.

Case 6

You are a 41-year-old mother of three. You've come to hospital today because you can no longer tolerate the pain in your upper abdomen. The pain is severe, constant, and you can feel it like a band travelling under your right ribs to your back. The pain is worse with eating and hasn't settled since your burger and doughnut last night. You feel nauseated and have vomited several times.

Co-codamol has helped bring the pain down from an 8 to a 6. There are no positions that help you get more comfortable.

You have dark urine and pale stools. You feel feverish and unwell. You had an episode of shaking and shivering last night. You've been feeling hot and cold all day today. No one else at home is unwell. Bowel open normally this morning. No urinary symptoms. Mild headache. You feel very thirsty and extremely itchy.

You had a similar episode 2 years ago, which only lasted 12 hours. Two years ago you went to the GP who gave you omeprazole and organized an USS. He said you had gallstones but nothing needed to be done. Since then you've had intermittent pain which feels like trapped wind normally after eating a big meal but goes away on its own and doesn't last long. This time the pain hasn't gone away. You don't think the omeprazole helps. You've gone yellow and this is new, which is extremely worrying. You've had an appendectomy before. You've been told you're overweight and you developed diabetes in your last two pregnancies.

You only take Omeprazole and are allergic to Penicillin. You're a stay at home mother. You smoke 10 cigarettes a day and don't drink alcohol. You have no other symptoms and no relevant family history. Take all other details from your own experience.

Case 7

You are a 68-year-old gentleman named James, who has come to hospital unable to move your left leg. You are able to move your hip but cannot move it at all at the knee or below. This started suddenly, 4 hours ago and you have not been able to move it at all during this time. Your leg is very painful throughout the entirety of the lower leg. The pain does not radiate anywhere and is a very severe, constant pain rating 10/10. Your pain is so severe that unless the candidate offers you pain relief you should be obstructive with giving the history until this is offered.

The appearance of your leg has changed as well. It looks paler in comparison to the other side. However not mottled. When you have touched your leg it has felt very cold. You think your leg has gone numb but it is hard to tell due to the amount of pain.

You cannot walk at all. Before this happened you could walk about 50 metres but would have to stop and take a break due to pain in your calves. Once you rested for a while these pains would disappear.

You have multiple co-morbidities. You have had 2 TIAs (mini-strokes) in the past. You suffer from high cholesterol, type 2 diabetes, ischaemic heart disease and high blood pressure.
You take the following medications:
Amlodipine 10mgOD, Metformin 500mg BD, Bisoprolol 5mg OD, Ramipril 5mg OD, Aspirin 75mg OD, Atorvastatin 10mg ON, GTN spray PRN

You smoke 20 cigarettes a day, drink 1 pint of lager a day on average and live alone.

Case 8

You are a 75-year-old gentleman named Jonathan, who has noticed blood in your urine. There is no pain. You don't have any pain but are worried that you may be bleeding internally and so you have come to your GP. You noticed the blood a couple of weeks ago when your urine started getting darker than usual. The urine cleared up over the next day and so you took no notice of it. A couple of days later however you noticed it again and called the GP practice for an urgent appointment. You have never experienced anything like this before. Now you have noticed red clots and are feeling lightheaded.

You have had problems with your waterworks in the past. Reduced capacity to hold onto your urine and having to wake up middle of the night to urinate several times. You have also noticed that your stream is not as strong as it used to be with terminal dribbling. You do not have any other medical problems and are not on any regular medications. You have no allergies that you know of. You live at home with your wife and dog. In the past you used to work in textile manufacturing company. You do smoke and drink alcohol occasionally.

Case 9

You are a 27-year-old man named Martin who works as an actor in a theatre company. You have come to hospital complaining of a dull ache in the back of your left testis. There is no radiation but you have noticed that your left testis is larger than your right one. You feel a dragging sensation on the left side when you stand up. This ache has been on-going for 3 month and has only moderately improved with simple analgesia.

You can't remember any injury to your testis however do note that you have been feeling feverish recently and having night sweats. You have normal waterworks and bowel habits. Your mother has noticed that you're becoming thin and your clothes do not fit as well.

On further questioning you do remember your mother telling you that you had problems with your testes as a child and had an operation to "bring the testes down". You have had no other operations and are normally fit and well.

You do not take any regular medication and have no allergies. You are a smoker (smoke 10-15/day) and drink regular alcohol. You are sexually active but have no stable partner.

Case 10

You are a 49-year-old lady, very anxious, complaining of having a 3-month history of right breast ache and bloody nipple discharge.
Over the last month, you have noticed a lump in the right breast; increasing in size, irregular shape of your breast with crusty red skin changes. As well as lower dull backache and decrease in appetite.

Only give this information if asked directly. You have been losing weight unintentionally over the last month.

You suffered from early periods and are now menopausal. You do not have any other medical problems and are not on any regular medications. You have no allergies that you know of. You are fit and active but smoke 20 cigarettes a day with occasionally drink alcohol. You are very concerned about what might be going on as it is having significant impact on your life. You have been too scared to seek medical advice. Your sister and mother have suffered from breast cancer.

Case 11

You are Jack an 80-year-old man who had an emergency repair of a hernia 2 days ago. The nursing staff believes you are confused and have asked one of the foundation doctors to assess you.

You believe you are at the local golf club, not in hospital. You believe it is 1958. You assume the gentleman who speaks to you is a young club member and not a doctor as he may suggest. The doctor is likely to ask you about physical symptoms such as pain and shortness of breath however you maintain a disengaged affect with little cooperation with questioning. They may go on to ask specific questions about your age, date of birth, the time and the year. You may find such questions ridiculous and impertinent unless they are proposed in a reassuring and sensitive manner

Initially you are happily confused and this should continue if the doctor attending you maintains a relaxed and reassuring manner. If there are any non-reassuring aspects to their manner or they become frustrated then you may find this confusing and therefore distressing and become increasingly agitated.

The confused affect should continue for the duration of the scenario and is a test of the candidate's stamina in maintaining patience with a floridly confused patient.

Case 12

You are John a 60-year-old photographer from London. You have been having intermittent bleeding from your back passage for 2 months and have attended the surgical assessment unit for a flexible sigmoidoscopy. You are extremely concerned that the bleeding may be due to cancer.

You know little about the procedure apart from that it involves a camera and your back passage. You worry that it will be painful, embarrassing and that a camera passing up your back passage could cause damage. You are also anxious that you could have the test and find out that you might have cancer particularly because a friend has recently been diagnosed with colon cancer.

You would appreciate an explanation of the procedure, what benefits and risks there are and what you need to do to prepare and recover from it. If there are any less invasive alternatives you would like to be told about them so that you can know what other options you may be able to choose.
Because of your concerns about cancer you really want to be investigated as soon as possible. You would also appreciate some reading materials so you can look into this further in your own time.

Case 13
You have received a call an hour ago from your ex-husband explaining that your son is being rushed into emergency theatre for a serious injury. You are very upset about the current situation. Extremely anxious and annoyed that a doctor has not called you at once about your son.

You want to see your son now. You want to know exactly what operation your son is having, complications and is there a risk of him dying? Treatment after splenectomy for patients, will anything change?

First words should be "why was I not called about this before he was taken for his operation?" If the explanation is good and they apologise explaining it was an emergency then you should then calm down.

You're concerned that whenever your son is with your ex-husband he always ends getting injured. *If prompted, mention that you have gone through a difficult divorce recently, brought about because he is always stressed and drinks too much. Ask what the candidate will do with that information and ask them to keep it to themselves.*

Ask when can you take Tom home? Claim your child is always safe with you. Throughout remain very anxious and wait on silence pauses and warm to candidate if they show empathy.

Case 14
You are the ITU registrar. The foundation doctor has been asked to refer an unwell patient to you. You have had a stressful day due to a colleague calling in sick, increasing your workload so are quite blunt with the candidate. You should grudgingly accept the explanation from the candidate, especially if they stress that they are worried about the patient. They will then explain the severity of the patient's pancreatitis.

You should become more approachable if it becomes clear that the candidate has the patient's best interests at heart. You should ask the candidate why they are referring to ITU – what can ITU offer the patient that cannot be done on the ward?

Ask what treatment have they given the patient so far? Ask for recent blood tests and together create a treatment plan of IV fluids, analgelsia and strict fluid chart. Explain that ITU is almost full and there are several patients that have been referred. You should agree to go and review the patient on the ward and see whether you think they are suitable for ITU.

Case 15
You are a 71-year-old male named Ahmed, you are very stoical and are in sound mind after crashing your car. You understand that you are going to need a chest drain for a pneumothorax as you are a retired GP. You take no regular medication and have no allergies.

Ask the candidate what painkillers they are going to give you before they start.

Case 16
No actor required for this station

Case 17
No actor required for this station

Case 18

You are a 25 year old student who was playing a game of "can rip" with your friends and sustained quite a deep cut to the back of your hand. You have completely normal sensation in the hand and can move it freely. If asked about whether you have had a tetanus jab recently, answer that you "don't know what that is". You have no known allergies and no medical problems.

You are very needle phobic. Challenge the doctor at some point to whether he really has to do this to you.

Case 19

You are a 50-year-old man who has had severe upper abdominal pain for the last 4 hours. You are breathing quite fast and are dehydrated and thirsty. You have pain when your abdomen is pushed all over your abdomen. The pain makes you contract your abdominal muscles. The worst pain is in the upper abdomen.

Follow the instructions of the doctor examining you.

Case 20

You are Rafa, a 78-year-old male, having presented with a lump that appeared suddenly this morning following lifting heavy boxes into a van. You have presented because there is a large lump approximately the size of an orange that has appeared in your groin. It is tender to touch. You will be asked your identity and whether you consent to an examination of the lump to be performed. If the candidate fails to ask about a chaperone please prompt that you are not happy to proceed without one.

Case 21

You are Clarissa a 49-year-old who has noticed a non-tender lump in your right breast. Do not offer any information to the candidate but you can respond to questions asking you whether you would like a chaperone and if you are in any pain, and be responsive to their instructions.

Case 22

You are a 35-year-old woman named Susan, who attended her GP surgery complaining of anxiety and fatigue.

You have not noticed any skin or nail changes. You have not had any palpitations and not noticed any pain or swelling in the neck. You have not been feeling overly warm or cool recently and are dressed appropriately for the weather.

You should not feel any pain on examination. You should be asked to swallow sips of water and stick out your tongue by the candidate during the examination.

Case 23

You are Thomas, a 54-year-old gentleman, who has presented complaining of an abnormal lump and dragging sensation in your left testis.

Do not offer any information to the candidate, however you can respond to questions asking whether you would like a chaperone and if you are in any pain.

Case 24

You are a 25-year-old man, named Ben, who has just been knocked off your motorbike by a car turning out from a side road. You have significant pain in your neck and feel quite short of breath.

Follow the instructions of the doctor examining you.

Case 25

You are Bernadette, a 72-year-old woman, who has come to vascular clinic complaining of pain in your calves when walking. Do not offer any information to the candidate however you can respond to questions asking whether you would like a chaperone and if you are in any pain.

Emergency medicine

Case 1
You are a staff nurse in the Emergency Department. You are able to assist the candidate and you know where all the equipment is kept. You are not able to perform tasks unless clearly instructed to by the candidate.

Case 2
A manikin will usually be used for this scenario.

Case 3
You are a newly qualified nurse on the general medical ward. Mr Jones was admitted today with chest pain. He was awaiting a repeat troponin (cardiac blood test) and had been given ACS treatment in the meantime.

He had a heart attack about 3 years ago and you are unaware of any other past medical history.

5 minutes ago he had developed central crushing chest pain then became unresponsive with no pulse or respiratory effort. You started chest compressions and called for a colleague to put out a cardiac arrest call.

When the doctor arrives you are anxious but are able to hand over all of the information above. Your college has brought the defibrillator however they are unable to stay.

From here on you follow the instructions given by the candidate.

Case 4
You are a 19-year-old man who has anaphylactic reactions to peanuts. You have forgotten your epipen on this evening out and didn't think you would need it. You have eaten a kebab, which has been cooked in peanut oil and immediately have started struggling to breathe with lip swelling and a widespread rash. You can't speak apart from pant and wheeze loudly.

By the 2nd round of re-assessment you are starting to feel a bit better and still panting but can say 4 word sentences. However, you feel your heart is racing and can't stop shaking.

By the 3rd stage of re-assessment, you fall asleep and start snoring and wheezing loudly.

Case 5
You are a 35-year-old salesman who is just back at work after a weekend away in the country. You noticed a bit of chest tightness and wheeze since the start of the weekend at the hotel and have had to use your inhalers more frequently. You have been taking the blue inhaler every couple of hours since last night and ran out of it at work. You also forgot to take the purple inhaler that you normally do each morning because you left it at the hotel.

You have had asthma since adolescence but it has been quite well controlled. The wheeze developed in your teens and you were prescribed a blue inhaler to help. You were started on a long acting purple inhaler the following year after your wheeze re-emerged. Your peak flow was last checked over 10 years ago and it was roughly 550 at best.

In the past 10 years you have only had to have nebulisers and steroids once in the hospital and did not stay the night. Your asthma is otherwise well controlled and you are compliant with medications using the purple one daily and blue before exercise.

You are supposed to be moderately breathless during the scenario, but doing this is quite difficult so it is important to try and say no more than 4 or 5 words before you take an extra breath or pause.

Case 6
You are a 22-year-old university student who has been brought into the ED with a 12-hour history of abdominal pain and vomiting. A doctor is going to examine you and try to make an initial diagnosis and initiate a management plan.

You were diagnosed with type 1 diabetes when you were 19. You initially found your insulin difficult to manage but now you find it much easier, although you do occasionally forget to take it. You have not needed any emergency admissions since your diagnosis and see your GP regularly for a medication review. You had your appendix removed age 7. You are otherwise entirely fit and well.

Drug history

Insuman rapid 9 units before breakfast
Insuman rapid 9 units before lunch
Novorapid 10 units before dinner
Levemir 10 units before dinner
No known drug allergies.

You were at a friend's BBQ yesterday and spent all day in the sunshine drinking beer. You're a vegetarian and there wasn't really any vegetarian options so you didn't eat much - for this reason you haven't taken any insulin since 9 am yesterday (it is now 2 pm). Do not volunteer this information unless directly asked.

You started to feel a bit unwell at 7 pm and went home. You felt nauseated and had a mild stomach ache but think this was because you had been out in the sun all day and had drank 5 bottles of beer which is quite a lot for you. You went to bed but awoke at 2 am feeling very sick and with abdominal pain. You have been profusely vomiting since (>30 times). You are vomiting yellow/green fluid with no evidence of blood. Your abdominal pain is generalised with no focus, a constant cramping sensation that does not radiate anywhere and has been mild throughout (3/10). Your bowel habits and stool are normal. You were initially passing urine often but are now passing very little.

You appear to be in mild discomfort and have a rapid breathing pattern. You are feeling drowsy and only provide the information outlined above if directly asked. Your abdomen is mildly tender when pressed. No focal area of pain.

Nurse's instructions

You are a band 5 nurse so have a good level of experience and can independently place monitoring and fulfill the requests the doctor has.

Case 7
You are a staff nurse in the Emergency Department. You are able to assist the candidate and you know where all the equipment is kept. You are not able to perform tasks unless clearly instructed to by the candidate.

Case 8
You are a 62 year old lady with a past medical history includes congestive cardiac failure, chronic kidney disease, hypertension and gout. You have blood tests four times a year and your kidney function has always been relatively stable according to the consultants.

You have not had any change in medications but have been unwell for 5 days with diarrhoea and vomiting and hardly been able to keep anything but small sips of water down. You have continued to take your medication though as you know you should never miss them.

Yesterday you had 'an unusual beating in the chest' and general muscle pains so the GP sent you for a blood test. You had a phone call from GP surgery asking you to go to the hospital urgently as one of the blood markers was raised. You have been taken to the resus room and a juior doctor is about to review you.

Case 9
On your way to work this morning you noticed that you were short of breath, which is unusual for you. You didn't think much of it until you were climbing the stairs on the way into the office and it became worse and was associated with some left sided chest pain. It is this that is worrying you most and prompted you to come into the ED.

You have had a slight cough that is not productive since yesterday. You have not coughed up any blood. You do not feel like you've had any fevers or sweats. The pain was sharp in nature and when questioned tell the candidate that it is worse when you took a deep breath in. It did not radiate anywhere. At it's worst it was 7/10 but at rest and at the moment you don't feel any pain. You are having some difficulty talking in long sentences. You have not taken any painkillers. Both your shortness of breath and chest pain are worse when you exert yourself.

Reveal these details only if asked directly:
You came back from holiday in New Zealand 2 weeks ago. You noticed some swelling of your legs on the flight but since being back you left leg has returned to normal but your right is still swollen and is starting to become painful.

Your other medical complaints consist of only anxiety for which you take an antidepressant. You have never had any operations. You are also taking the oral contraceptive pill. You have no allergies.

If directly asked about your family history explain that your dad had a heart attack three months ago and you are very worried that this might be a heart attack. He is 48 years old. There is no family history of DVT or PE.
You work in a property development firm which is mostly behind a desk. You exercise regularly, gave up smoking 3 years ago and drink socially 1-2 times per week. You have never taken any recreational drugs.

Case 10
You are a 24-year-old professional dancer who has attended the emergency department with a headache.

You have had it for 24 hours and have had to miss work this morning. It came on yesterday morning while you were warming up for a rehearsal and gradually became more painful and hasn't eased up since. You have had a few bad headaches in the past two months (similar in nature and lasting 5-6 hours) but this one has lasted longer and just before it came on you noticed your vision wasn't quite right and your hands felt tingly. Although this resolved within 10 minutes it really worried you.

Site	Right side of your head. No focal area of pain.
Onset	During a morning rehearsal 24 hours ago. Came on gradually, progressed over an hour and then peaked in severity and has stayed at the same intensity since.
Character	Pressure/throbbing sensation
Radiation	None
Associated symptoms	Just before the headache came on you noticed spots in your vision and your hands went tingly - this resolved within a few minutes. You have felt sick since the morning it started but have not vomited. No experience of visual loss, blurred or double vision, zig-zag lines, vertigo, weakness, speech disturbance, loss of consciousness or fits. No unusual smells. No fevers, neck pain or rash.
Timing	Not worse at any particular time of day.
Exacerbating/ Relieving factors	Any activity makes it worse, you feel better if you lay down. Paracetamol seemed to help a little. You haven't tried anything else. No light sensitivity, mild noise sensitivity.
Severity	6/10. You slept OK last night but could not attend work this morning.

You are normally fit and well, you have had an ankle injury for the past 2 months for which you have been taking codeine daily, as you have needed to perform despite the injury. This has been much better over the past week so you have not taken any codeine for several days. You also started taking the contraceptive pill (Microgynon®) four months ago to help ease your periods. Your last menstrual period was 3 weeks ago. Your only family history is your mum's stroke. You live with friends, smoke 7-10 cigarettes/day, drink alcohol 2-3 times per month and take no recreational drugs. No recent foreign travel. You are quite stressed at work but no more than usual, you are expected to perform three times a day and often miss meals and don't hydrate as well as you know you should.

You are concerned that you may be experiencing the early symptoms of a stroke. You know that your mother had a headache and problems with her vision a few days prior to having a stroke, which left her unable to move her right side. She was only 62 when this happened. You expect to have a head scan or that you might need to take aspirin to prevent a stroke - as you know that your mother now takes this to prevent a stroke. If the doctor explains why you do not need a scan and fully addresses your concerns then you are content to proceed with the plan they present.

Case 11
You are a 45-year-old man who has attended the Emergency Department following a head injury. You were building a new shed in the garden when you hit the back of your head on a wooden beam.

You have no other injuries and there is no boggy swelling. You did not lose consciousness at the time, however have been feeling unwell, nauseous and dizzy since the injury. If the candidate asks you about vomiting, state that you have not vomited after the accident. You can remember all events leading up to and after the injury and you did not have a seizure. If asked you also mention that your walking and speech has been unchanged since the injury. There hasn't been any clear fluid or blood from either your nose or ears.

You took some painkillers at home as you had a headache but when your wife returned home a few hours later, she was concerned as you looked pale, had a lump at the back of your head and a persistent headache. She told you to attend the ED to get a scan to check for bleeding.

You are previously fit and well and don't take any medication. You have no allergies. You work as a manager on a building site and if prompted by the candidate disclose that you are worried about bleeding in the brain as you have done some reading on the Internet. You would like a quick scan before going home.

If the doctor tells you there is no indication for a CT scan of your head, you become annoyed. However if the candidate explores your concerns and explains the guidelines and indications for a scan then you are reassured. You return to being pleasant if the doctor also provides written head injury advice in the form of an information leaflet and adequate safety netting.

Case 12
You do not want to talk to the doctor. You have been low in mood for about 6 months now. You attempted suicide with the intention of ending your life. You still feel low in mood and you are still having suicidal thoughts. You should initially give one-word answers and make it very clear that you do not want to talk. The candidate should be able to identify this and make an effort to put you at ease. They should ask open questions and give you time to talk. If they are clearly making an attempt to create a rapport you should start to open up and talk to them more.

You have been planning this suicide attempt for a month now. You have researched how much paracetamol to take in order to end your life and have been collecting tablets for a week. You chose last night as the appropriate time as it was your ex-girlfriend's birthday. You broke up 6 months ago and this is when your low mood started. You drank 1 litre of vodka before taking the tablets. You took about half of the tablets you had bought and then vomited and passed out because you were so drunk. Judging from the packets your friends found around you, you estimate that you took around 40 tablets at 8pm, each one containing 500mg of paracetamol. You did not take any other tablets.

You do not use recreational drugs. You had no intention of being discovered and told your friends you were staying at your parents' house. They have been worried about you lately so rang your parents to check, and when they realised you were not there, they rushed to your house and found you. You had left a note to your family and another to your girlfriend explaining why you felt you had to do this. It was very much your intention to end you life. You still feel as though you don't want to live. You feel stupid that you didn't even manage to kill yourself and given the chance you know you'd try again and do it right next time.

You have been feeling hopeless and worthless since you broke up with your girlfriend. You do not see the point in living if you can't be with her. You cannot think of anything to look forward to in the future. You have never been depressed in the past and have never attempted suicide before. You have not been taking care of yourself lately, have been drinking daily, have called in sick to work a number of times and have not really been eating. You have insight into your condition and you know that you are depressed but you have such a low opinion of yourself that you don't feel like it's been important enough to seek help.

You do have a good network of friends and a supportive family but you have not wanted to burden them with your problems so have isolated yourself from them recently. You know they are worried but you feel it will be better for you and them if you were not alive and not around to bring them down. You don't have children.

The candidate may explain to you that you will need to stay in hospital for medical treatment and you will need to talk to the psychiatric team. At this stage you are too apathetic and low in energy to object. You don't want to have to go over the events again but at the moment your response is: 'whatever, I don't care any more.'

Case 13

You are a 54-year-old man who has presented to the emergency department with fresh red blood coming from the back passage/bottom. You find it hard to quantify the amount of blood. It is mixed in with stool and seen on the toilet paper. Your bowel habit has been slightly constipated recently. You have been going less often and have noticed in the last month that your stool is darker, almost black in colour! This is the first time you have noticed any blood. You have not noticed any mucous in the stool. You deny having any abdominal pain.

You have not vomited but feel nauseated and have been eating and drinking less generally for the last 2 months as you have been less hungry than usual. You have lost a stone over this time but it was unintentional.

You have not had fever or rigors but currently feel clammy.

You deny any urinary symptoms, change in urine colour or yellowing of skin or eyes. You are passing flatus as usual and do not have abdominal distension. You haven't been feeling dizzy, tired or short of breath recently.

You have no other issues such as joint pain, rashes, or obvious lumps in neck/axilla/groin.

You have a previous medical history of a mild heart attack two years ago, which is medically treated with daily aspirin, bisoprolol and simvastatin. You have no known drug allergies. You have no other medical history but did have an operation on your haemorrhoids four years ago.

Your mum died from ovarian cancer, aged 80 and your Dad is still alive and well. Your paternal grandmother died of a heart attack. There are no other medical issues you are aware of in your family.
You currently live with your wife and are fully independent. You do not smoke but enjoy a drink regularly - you drink 2 pints of Guinness a night and also drink around about a bottle of whiskey each weekend. You work as a pub landlord.

You have no idea what has caused this episode but are very concerned it could be cancer and keep asking if the doctor thinks that is what it is.

Case 14

You are a 25-year-old man who has presented to your local hospital having had a collapse.

You had just been at the gym and were sat at the bus stop on your way home, you stood up as the bus was approaching and started to feel light headed. Then you noticed your vision going darker and felt that you felt you were spinning. The next thing you knew the man sat next to you at the bus stop was asking if you were ok, and you were on the ground. He called the ambulance.

The man told you that you passed out and did not hit your head. You did not lose control of your bladder or Bowels. You did not bite your tongue. The man looking after you told the paramedics that it didn't look like you had a seizure. You were out for no more than 30 seconds. You have had this once or twice in the past and just put it down to fainting.

You have been feeling well recently but had forgotten to take your water bottle to the gym this morning and pushed yourself a little harder than normal. You are now feeling well and have not had chest pain.

You are otherwise fit and well. You take no regular medications. You have no allergies. You have no significant illness running in your family, no one has any heart problems or epilepsy. You have not been abroad recently. You have occasional alcohol binges "big nights out". You occasionally take MDMA but haven't in the last 3 months.

Case 15

You are a 66-year-old female who has come to the emergency department as you have been feeling unwell for the past week and have not been able to see your GP.

You returned from visiting your children in Australia just over a week ago and felt unwell the day after your return. You have been coughing for days, more recently bringing up thick green sputum. You have been off your food and have had a few bouts of loose stool. In the past 24 hours you have felt short of breath and this morning you awoke feeling very cold and unable to get warm - you were shivering continuously and so decided to seek emergency care.

The candidate will perform an examination of your chest. You feel breathless and have an increased breathing rate. You don't have any pain.

Case 16

You are a 69-year-old woman who has been brought to the Emergency Department by ambulance after collapsing outside your local shopping centre. Please allow the candidate to examine your cardiovascular system.

If the candidate asks, you are not in any discomfort however please make it clear if they cause you any pain.

Case 17

You are a 65-year-old man brought into ED resus via ambulance. You called 999 as you experienced sudden onset left sided chest pain and shortness of breath.

A - You are able to talk and respond to the candidate, albeit breathlessly.
B - You are breathing fast and shallowly. You feel much worse when you are   laying flat.
C - You feel sweaty, clammy and nauseous.
D - You are fully conscious and aware of who and where you are.
E - When the candidate reaches this stage you should stop responding as you have now lost consciousness

Case 18

You are a 30-year-old man who has come to the ED with a 12 hour long episode of worsening right sided back and abdominal pain, you point and hold your right side just below your ribs. During the consultation you are obviously in pain, cannot sit still and cannot get comfortable.
The pain is severe and gripping in nature, coming in waves. It started slowly but progressed rapidly. It moves all the way down to your groin. You feel sick and have vomited once.
If asked specifically, you have noticed:

- An increased frequency, no blood and no pain on passing urine
- no change in bowel habit
- no fever
- no other symptoms

During the consultation you frequently make comments about how much pain you are in and that you would like it to stop.

You are otherwise fit and well, on no regular medications. You do not smoke or drink. You are an avid gym goer and drink regular protein shakes. You remember your dad being hospitalised when you were younger for kidney problems.

Case 19

You are a 39-year-old gentleman who presents to ED after developing severe lower lumbar back pain, with associated left sided lower limb numbness and increasing difficulties mobilising over the last 5 days

You have developed weakness in your right leg over the last 5 days after having chronic back pain for approximately 10 years since a rugby accident. However, this 'feels' different.

The back pain originates in the lower back and radiates down into the thigh of your right leg. You have become concerned as you are having difficulties lifting your leg from the hip. You can kick out at the knee as normal and move your foot as normal but your right-sided hip movement is severely restricted and so is eversion of the ankle (the sole of the foot increasingly facing away from the other foot) .

You also have numbness around your right buttock and feel there is some weakness when you squeeze your bottom cheeks together. Your left leg feels normal. When they check reflexes of the right leg, they are absent at the ankle.

You are concerned that this is a serious spinal injury and that you will need surgery.

Case 20

You are a 48-year-old male businessman. You were working on the computer when you suddenly became very dizzy and started feeling nauseated and had some vomiting. You find that it is very difficult to walk and you are extremely unsteady on your feet. You needed assistance from your colleagues who took you downstairs and had to help you in and out of their car.

You are normally fit and well and you do not take any regular medications. You had a similar, much less severe episode 3 years ago that lasted for a few hours but resolved spontaneously. You do not have any pain anywhere. You smoke 20 cigarettes a day.

When you are asked to perform heel to shin movements you struggle, and you are unable to walk in a straight line. In fact, when you are standing you find you are swaying quite significantly.

Case 21

You are a 24-year-old man who has been brought to the Emergency department with a painful swollen knee. You report being tackled by another player whilst playing football yesterday - the others player's boot went into your left knee. Since then you have had pain on the inside of your left knee and are finding it difficult to walk. Today you woke up and your knee was more swollen so you have come to the emergency department.

You have already spoken to another doctor and given your history. Now the junior doctor in the emergency medicine team has been asked to examine the knee.

When examined, you can tell the candidate:

The knee is more swollen than usual. When they feel your knee, you can tell them it hurts on the inside of your left knee when it is touched.

When they move your knee, you can tell them it's too painful to straighten it and you can't do it. When they then try to move it you find that you can fully straighten your leg. When they test the ligaments of your knee, you can tell them that it hurts the inside of your knee.

When they test the sensation in your leg, you can report normal and full sensation in all areas.
When they test your knee power compared to the right side, it is slightly weaker.
When they test other joints, you find there are no tender areas and you have full range of movement.
On walking you are limping on your left leg due to knee pain.

Case 22

You are a 50-year-old woman who has self-presented to ED with pain in your left shoulder after falling off of your bicycle, landing onto your left outstretched arm. Since then you have been feeling pain that is worse when you move your arm.

The candidate should first look at both of your shoulders.

They should then palpate both shoulder joints. You should complain of pain as they press on the joint between your collarbone and your shoulder on the left side. You should also indicate to them that you feel that your left shoulder appears swollen and slightly deformed compared to the right side.

The candidate should then ask you to move your arms independently. You should complain of pain when you lift your arm in front of you, particularly once the arm is above shoulder level and when lifting your arm out to the side past your shoulder level.

The candidate will then move your arms themselves, similarly you should complain of pain when they lift your arm in front of you past shoulder level and to the side past shoulder level.

The candidate should perform a test where they hold your left arm across your body, putting pressure on the joint between your collar bone and your left shoulder. Please cry out in pain during this test and complain of a sharp pain between your collar bone and shoulder.

Finally the candidate will test the strength of various muscles around the shoulder. You complain of a sharp twinge in the area between the left collar bone and shoulder during these tests but have good strength.

Case 23

You are a final year medical student on a placement in the emergency department. You are shadowing a foundation doctor for the day in the resuscitation area. The team gets a priority call informing them that an unconscious female patient is being brought into the emergency department.

You are glad to have the opportunity to watch the foundation doctor manage this patient's airway as you are worried about having to do this once you have qualified and are on the wards. You ask the doctor to talk you through how they will manage the airway of the expected patient. You aren't confident about selecting equipment or your technique with manoeuvres and inserting airway adjuncts and devices. You are also concerned about how to respond if the airway remains compromised despite an intervention.

You have had a practical session in which you have been shown the different airway manoeuvres and pieces of airway equipment but you have never been able to practice this on a mannequin and you have never observed emergency airway management on a real patient. If the foundation doctor offers to demonstrate the equipment you are keen to be shown but you do not need to practice yourself.

Questions to ask if not already covered:

How do you know when you are achieving adequate ventilation?
Are there any situations that a nasopharyngeal airway shouldn't be used?
How can you tell which size of adjunct to use?

Respond well to: enthusiastic, encouraging approach with clear instructions and an opportunity to practice.

Case 24

You are a 67-year-old retired carpenter who has had trouble passing urine for about 6 months. You note that it has been very difficult to have a good stream when passing water, and you can never get a feeling of an empty bladder. You wake up a few times a night to pass water but it often takes a while to start.

You saw your GP about the symptoms a few weeks ago and you had a PSA test but you don't know the result. In the last few days you have been under the weather and have had some burning when passing water. You haven't been able to pass water at all today.

You have mild blood pressure and diet controlled diabetes. You are not currently on any medications. You are widowed and live alone but are feeling quite low mainly die to the worsening sleep you are getting due to waking in the night to pass urine.

The candidate will take a brief history from you, examine you and then recognise the need to insert a urinary catheter. They should explain the process to you, consent you and talk you through it as it happens.

Case 25

You are a 3rd year medical student attached to ED resus. A doctor has just received the results of an arterial blood gas. You will ask the doctor to explain the results to you.

You have read about ABG's and have seen one normal ABG before, but a doctor has never explained how to interpret and act on an abnormal ABG before. Throughout the teaching session you would like the following questions answered if not done so by the candidate:

How will the doctor act on the ABG findings or what will their management plan be?

What is base excess?

Is there much other information a typical ABG analysis/readout can give?

Obstetrics & Gynaecology

Case 1

Your name is Huda and you are a 26-year-old shop assistant. You have come to the Gynaecology outpatient clinic with a history of painful periods.

You periods started when you were 13 years old. They have always been regular – every 28 days, lasting 5-6 days with no bleeding or spotting between periods. You have not experienced any pain during sex and no bleeding after sex. You have no abnormal discharge. You have not noticed any pain when passing urine or opening your bowels. You have not experienced any rectal bleeding.

Your last period started 7 days ago. They used to be manageable, with heavy bleeding and mild cramping for the first 2 days. However, in the last 8 months, they have become very painful and have started to impact your work and social life. They are also heavier with clots and you now need to change your tampons every 3 hours on the first 2-3 days, although you have not experienced any leakage. You have been getting constant cramping lower abdominal pain radiating down your thighs, worse on days 2-3, occasionally so bad you have had to go home from work. You have tried taking Ibuprofen, which helps but wears off quickly.

You are otherwise fit and well with no other medical problems, and no recent weight loss. Your smears are up to date and have always been normal. You are in a long-term relationship and you use condoms and not tried any hormonal contraception. You have never had an STI. You have no allergies and do not take any other medication. You do not smoke and you drink 1-2 glasses of wine at weekends.

You work as a shop assistant and spend most of the day on your feet. Your boss has been understanding but struggles to find cover at short notice when you take time off. You are worried about the impact this will have on your career as you were hoping to be promoted to assistant manager this year.

You are anxious about what is causing the heavy, painful periods and you want to find a way to stop them impacting your personal and professional life.

Case 2

Your name is Celeste and you are a 34-year-old social worker. You have come to the Gynaecology outpatient clinic today with heavy periods.

For the last 10 months, you have noticed you periods are much heavier and more uncomfortable - still every 30 days, but now lasting 7-8 days instead of 4 days previously. You regularly pass clots, and have had some embarrassing experiences when you have leaked onto the bedding and through your clothes. You change your pads every 1-2 hours at times.

Your periods started when you were 12 years old. You have not experienced any bleeding between periods or after sex, and no pain during sex. You have no abnormal discharge. You have not experienced any excessive bruising, prolonged bleeding or nosebleeds. Your smears are up to date and have always been normal. You have never had as STI. You are married and use condoms with your husband. You had a miscarriage at seven weeks in 2013 and had 1 other pregnancy with a 5-year-old daughter but would like to have more.

You have no medical problems and no allergies. You have been feeling increasingly tired, especially around your periods. Your GP started you on Tranexamic Acid 2 months ago to which has been helpful but you are still having leaks. He also found you are anaemic and started you on iron supplements. You were not keen to start hormonal treatment as you were worried about how it would affect your body in the long run.

You do not smoke or drink alcohol. You moved to the UK from Ghana 15 years ago and you live with your husband and daughter and work as a social worker. Your mother also suffered with heavy periods but you are not sure why.

You are anxious to find out why you are bleeding so much and how to stop this, as you no longer socialise during your periods because you are scared of flooding. It is also causing problems with your husband as you are now having sex less often as your periods are longer.

Case 3

Your name is Martha, and you are a 24-year-old student doing your Masters in Journalism. You have presented to the Emergency Department with lower abdominal pain that started 4 days ago, and is now 6-7/10 in severity if asked. It is a constant dull ache and does not move anywhere, does not get better/worse throughout the day or with any positions although Ibuprofen has helped a little. You feel nauseous and sweaty, and you have no urinary or bowel symptoms.

You have not noticed any abnormal vaginal bleeding but have seen some yellowish/green frothy discharge. You have taken the COCP for contraception for the last 3 years, and have light, relatively painless bleeds for 5 days during the break. You have not noticed any bleeding after sex but occasionally do notice that it can be painful during penetration, which has been intermittent for the past 2-3 months, but you have not mentioned this to your GP.

Three months ago, you changed sexual partners and had an STI check where you were found to have chlamydia. The nurse practitioner at the clinic gave you given a week-long course of treatment, however you did not complete this as you were concerned it would interfere with the pill and you are worried about getting pregnant. You have not had any other sexual partners since then. If asked, you have had 3 male sexual partners in the last 6 months, and had a combination of oral, anal and vaginal sex, occasionally unprotected with all three. You have had 1 previous episode of chlamydia treated 2 years ago. You are not aware of any partners having HIV or Hepatitis or being IV drug users, and you have never used drugs. You had a negative HIV test at the clinic 3 months ago.

You have not been offered a smear test yet. You got pregnant once last year, which ended in a medical termination at 7 weeks, but you would like to have children in the future.

You are otherwise well with mild asthma managed with a salbutamol inhaler when required. You have no allergies. You live in a flat share while doing your Masters. You have no other relevant family history.

You are concerned this could all be because you did not complete the treatment from the STI clinic, and if the possibility of pelvic inflammatory disease is explained, you are very concerned that this may mean you will not be able to have children in the future.

Case 4

Your name is Ellie, and you are a 34-year-old teacher. You and your partner of 5 years, James, have been trying to conceive for the past 1 year. You try to have unprotected sex 3-4 times a week but you are both becoming quite stressed with work and with the lack of success in getting pregnant and so it is not always possible.

You have never been pregnant although James has 2 young children from a previous relationship. (Try to steer the candidate away from questions about your partner.)

You started having periods at age 13, and they were initially irregular but you now have a 30-day cycle and bleed for 5 days. This is always very heavy and very painful and has actually been getting worse. The pain can often start 1-2 days before your period actually starts. You have no pain during sex, after sex or between periods. Your smears are up to date and always normal and you have never had an STI.

You have no issues with your weight, and you do not have problems with excess hair growth, acne or nipple discharge.

You previously used the depot injection but stopped 2 years ago. You have no other medical issues aside from an appendectomy when you were 14 years old. You currently take folic acid in preparation for pregnancy. You have no other allergies. If asked about family history, you recall that your mother may have also had heavy, painful periods but she is now well into the menopause.

You are concerned that you will never be able to have children. James tries to reassure you but you are worried he will leave you and you keep pushing him away, which is causing friction in your relationship. You work as a teacher, which is also very stressful. Home and work has been so difficult that you reluctantly admit you have started smoking 5 cigarettes a day again after stopping 2 years ago.

Case 5

Your name is Natalie, and you are a 27-year-old lawyer. You have been referred by your GP to the General Obstetrics Clinic with uncontrollable itching. You are currently 30 weeks pregnant with your second baby.

You have experienced itching over the past two weeks and it is gradually getting worse. If asked specifically, it is affecting the palms and soles more than anywhere else, but is also noticeable on your tummy and legs. At first, you thought it would get better on its own and so you left it for a week and moisturised daily. However, as it became more intense, you went to your GP and he referred you here.

You have not noticed any yellowing of your skin or eyes. You have had no abdominal pain or change to your urine or stools. You feel well in yourself with no fevers, sweats or headaches and do not feel confused. You have not had a rash per se, but have redness from intense itching.

There has been no change in washing powder, soaps or creams. You have not started any new medications or taken anything over the counter. Nobody else you have been in contact with has experienced similar symptoms.

You have no significant past medical history. You take no regular medications and have no known allergies. You have no relevant family history. You live with your husband and two daughters aged 6 & 8 who are all fit and well. Both girls were normal vaginal deliveries at full term without complications. You have had no other pregnancies or gynaecological symptoms.

You are a non-smoker and used to drink 2-3 glasses of wine a week prior to getting pregnant.

Your main concern is finding out what is causing this intense itching as it is really impacting on your quality of life and you are worried it could be something serious. You are constantly thinking about it and your skin is starting to become sore from all the scratching. You would like to know if there are any medications that may help with the symptoms.

Case 6

Your name is Kiran, and you are a 27-year-old bank manager. You have presented to the Maternity Triage Unit with vaginal bleeding since yesterday. You are currently 32 weeks pregnant with your first baby.

Yesterday, you noticed some light spotting with fresh red blood. You tried not to panic as you had sexual intercourse the night before and thought it may be due to this. Today, the bleeding has been heavier and you noticed your pad was quite significantly stained today so decided to come to the hospital. You also noted a sharp 'twinge' in your lower belly this afternoon when you had heavier bleeding, although this has now settled. You have not noticed any vaginal discharge and have not had a rush or trickle of fluid. You felt the baby moving lots mainly in the morning but it has been quieter this afternoon, which you put down to the baby being asleep.

You have not had any episodes of bleeding in this pregnancy until now and it has otherwise been uneventful. If directly asked, your 20-week scan showed a 'low-lying placenta' but the sonographer advised you this was quite common.

Your first and only other pregnancy was 5yrs ago and you gave birth to a healthy girl. The pregnancy was normal but you had an emergency caesarean for failure to progress and fetal distress. You intend on having a vaginal birth (VBAC), which the midwives have been happy with.

You last had a smear 2 years ago and it was normal. You have never had an STI, and your husband is your only sexual partner. You are otherwise fit and well. You have no regular medications and no allergies.

You do not smoke or drink alcohol. You work in a bank, which can be quite stressful. You live with your husband and daughter. You are all very excited to have a new addition to the family and you feel well supported by your partner and family.

You are very concerned about the bleeding and worried that the baby is in danger or might be premature. You are very anxious that having sex may have harmed the baby and you blame yourself.

Case 7

Your name is Winona, and you are a 32-year-old optician, currently on maternity leave. You have presented to your GP feeling unwell for the past 24 hours with a fever. You noted your temperature was 38.3 at home this morning but did not want to take Paracetamol as you are breastfeeding.

You gave birth 5 days ago and you were discharged home after 1 day. You gave birth to a healthy baby girl called Sammie, who is your first child. You have had no other pregnancies. The pregnancy was uncomplicated with normal antenatal scans. You went into labour at 39^{+2} weeks when your waters spontaneously broke at home. You came into hospital and delivered normally on the midwife led unit after 16 hours of labour. You had a small tear during the labour that did not require stitching but has been a little sore. You are passing a small amount of fresh blood vaginally but this is now much less. You have not noticed any discharge or smell.

You have been breastfeeding Sammie. At first it was going well but the last 2 days your right breast in particular has become very tender and the nipple is cracked. The breast is redder and hotter than the left. You have not noticed any rashes elsewhere.
You have been eating and drinking well until yesterday when you started to feel unwell. You have no nausea or vomiting. You have had no pain when urinating, frequency or change in colour/smell. Your bowels are opening daily with no diarrhoea. You have no cough or coryzal symptoms.

You have no past medical history and no regular medications or allergies. You have never smoked and only drink alcohol occasionally, but that was before you were pregnant. You live with your husband and new baby and are currently enjoying your maternity leave.

You should specifically ask if taking medications such as Paracetamol and antibiotics will harm Sammie and if you can continue breastfeeding.

Case 8

Your name is Yee, and you are a 29-year-old pharmacist, currently on maternity leave. You have presented to your GP for your 6-week postnatal check. Your baby, Ella, has already had her 6-week check, which was normal.
You delivered 6 weeks ago at 37 weeks. You used gas and air during a normal vaginal delivery. It was quite traumatic for you as you had an episiotomy and had stitches; so sitting has been painful but has improved in the last few weeks. The health visitor reassured you it is healing well but you still have some discomfort when sitting for a long time. You are no longer experiencing any bleeding or discharge and have not noticed an offensive smell. You have not started your periods yet.

You are opening your bowels normally and passing urine but noticed you have small accidents when you laugh or cough. This is a concern as you do not want to continue wearing pads all the time, especially since the post-delivery discharge has now stopped.

You are currently fully breastfeeding and have no pain or problems with milk production. Ella has been gaining weight as expected and you are bonding well. You intend to fully breastfeed until at least 6 months. Your mood is generally quite good, apart from being very tired as you try to sleep train your baby (unsuccessfully). Your husband is very supportive but is about to start back at work full time so you will be on your own. You are anxious about this but have a good support network of friends and family nearby.

You plan to use condoms for contraception but have not had sex yet as you still feel a bit sore down below.
You have no other medical problems and are not on any medications and do not have any allergies. You do not smoke or drink alcohol. You currently live with your husband Simon and Ella.

Your main concern is the urinary incontinence when you are out and about, especially as you will be left on your own with the baby. As a result you have not made many trips out of the house, which is making you feel a bit isolated.

Case 9

Your name is Kyra, and you are 25-year-old postal worker. You have presented to the GP surgery after receiving a letter to attend for your smear test. You are quite nervous and so have booked a double appointment with the doctor. You would like to know what the procedure involves and why it is important. If it is described as a 'screening' programme, ask more about what this is.

You are currently not sexually active but have been in the past. Explain this to the candidate and ask if it is still necessary to have the examination.

Your last period was 14 days ago and you have not had any bleeding, discharge or pain. You have no known medical problems, you are not on any regular medications and you have no known allergies. You smoke 5 cigarettes a day.

You are quite nervous about the procedure as you have heard some horror stories from your friends. The doctor should be sensitive to these concerns and reassuring.

If asked for questions:
- What if there are abnormalities? Will that mean I have cancer?

Case 10

You are Frances, a 58-year-old writer and you have presented to the Gynaecology clinic. You have been experiencing intermittent vaginal bleeding for the past 2 months, and your GP referred you as a '2 week wait' referral to the Gynaecology team. You had an ultrasound scan last week that showed that the lining of your womb was thicker than expected, and so they have advised you to have a biopsy. You were quite upset when you found out the results of the ultrasound, as you are very afraid of it being cancer. The doctor advised you to come back in a few days to discuss the procedure to get a biopsy, which is why you are here today.

You went through the menopause over 5 years ago and have had no bleeding since you were 53 years old until now. Everything has happened quite quickly and you have not had time to process it, but the doctor advised that there are a few different options now in order to get the biopsy.

You are very anxious about having the procedure while awake and you would prefer to be asleep so you will not feel anything. You expect it is a bit like a smear test but worse, which you do find uncomfortable at the best of times.

You are otherwise well and on no medications. You have never had general anaesthetic or any surgical procedure, and you have not had any other gynaecological issues. You have no drug allergies. There is no family history of note.

Please steer the candidate away from asking a full history as you have been asked this before, and you are only here to find out about the procedure.

Case 11

You are Megan, one of the first year student midwives. Today is your first day in the community and you are meant to be shadowing the practice midwife at the GP surgery. Unfortunately, she has just called in sick and the clinic has been cancelled. The practice have kindly arranged for one of their Foundation Year doctors to give you a short talk on the mechanisms and stages of birth.

You are aware that there are three stages of labour, although you are not quite sure what happens in each stage. You have seen two births before but found it all quite emotional so cannot remember the details

The doctor will then talk you through this, and if they are using lots of jargon, ask questions to clarify.

If asked if you have any questions once they finish:

What usually causes prolonged first stage of labour?

Case 12

Your name is Sia and you are a 25-year-old PR manager. You have come in to the GP surgery today to have a vaginal examination and cervical smear. You have already consented to have the procedure and understand the risks and benefits.

Decline a chaperone if offered.

The candidate will perform a bimanual examination and cervical smear on a mannequin but should communicate with you as though you are being examined.

Case 13

Your name is Lucy and you are a 28-year-old fashion editor. You have come in to the General Obstetrics Clinic today for a routine check up at 28 weeks as you have been diagnosed with Gestational Diabetes (only give this information if asked). You feel well and have had no pain and your sugars are well controlled.

The candidate has been asked to examine your pregnant abdomen (for which they will use the mannequin provided). They should, however, communicate with you as though you are being examined.

If the candidate does not ask if you are in any pain before examining, please express your discomfort.

Case 14

You are Gina, a 35-year-old fashion editor. You have received a letter from your GP to come into the surgery to discuss the results from your recent smear. You are worried because you have not received such a letter before. All previous smears have shown no abnormalities.

You are otherwise fit and well and have had no symptoms. You are married with 2 young girls aged 2 and 4.

You searched online about what an abnormality could mean and have questions related to changes that could be present. You are worried that this means you have cancer, and you don't know how you would cope with such a diagnosis.

If asked for questions and not already covered:
What is HPV?
What does CIN mean?
What happens when I go for colposcopy?
What have I done to get this and is there anything that I can do to prevent it?
Is there anything I can do to reduce my risk of getting this?
Is it hereditary? Will my daughters be at risk?

Case 15

You are Celia, an 18-year-old university student. You have asked to speak to your GP today as you are thinking about starting the oral contraceptive pill.
You have been with your boyfriend for the past 6 months and have been sexually active for the last 4 months. Your boyfriend is 20 years old. You have only been using condoms until now, but you want to explore other forms of contraception. You spoke to your friends who suggested the 'combined' contraceptive pill. You are keen to start the combined pill, but you also wanted to know a little more about the progesterone-only pill as well.
Your boyfriend is your only current sexual partner. You have never had an STI, and your partner had a negative STI check prior to starting sexual intercourse. You have not noticed any vaginal discharge. Your menstrual cycle is regular occurring every 28 days and lasting for 5 days. You do not have very heavy menstruation or irregular bleeding. You have never been pregnant.
Your only significant past medical history includes mild asthma for which you use a salbutamol inhaler as required. You have no history of migraines. You have no other regular medications or allergies. You smoke 5 cigarettes a day. You do not regularly drink during the week, but may have 2-3 glasses of wine on a night out over the weekend. You are not overweight.
Your family history includes a mother who is hypertensive and a father who is diabetic and a smoker.
You have some specific questions about the use of the combined oral contraceptive pill:
What are you chances of getting pregnant while on the COCP?
What are the side effects?

Can you still contract a STI?

Is there an increasing risk of getting cancer?

What happens if I miss a pill?

Will the pill affect my long-term fertility once I come off of it?

Case 16

You are Marc, a 19-year-old choreographer. You have presented to the GUM clinic today after having unprotected sexual intercourse with a casual partner last week and wanted a routine STI check.

You are bisexual, but in the last 6 months, you have had 3 male partners. You are usually very careful with using condoms, but on this one occasion you were quite drunk and got carried away in the moment. You are concerned that you could have contracted HIV. You are currently only sleeping with this one casual partner for the last 3 months, prior to which you had a negative HIV and STI check, but you do not know about your partner. On this occasion, you had anal, oral and oro-anal sex – both reciprocal and penetrative.

You have not travelled abroad to any high-risk areas. You have not had any previous partners with known HIV or from high-risk areas. You have never used intravenous drugs and have never had any blood transfusions and you do not believe your partner has either. You have never paid anyone for sex.

You currently feel well with no penile or anal symptoms. About a week ago you had a flu-like illness but that has now settled. You have no other medical history aside from treated chlamydia 3 years ago.

If asked, you would like to know:

How the test will be taken

How long will I have to wait before the results come back and how will they be given

What is HIV? How is it transmitted? Is there treatment for it?

Are there any other ways to protect myself from contracting HIV?

If the HIV test returned with a positive result, you would be devastated. You have heard it is a 'death sentence' and you are scared that it would change all your future life plans. You would be worried about being able to have a long-term relationship if you had HIV. You have a very supportive family and so you have a good support network to help you if the test came back positive.

Case 17

You are David, a 27-year-old photographer. You have come back to the GUM clinic today to discuss your new diagnosis of HIV last week. You have been quite shell-shocked, as it was totally unexpected. You have not yet told your family but you told one of your oldest friends who has been reassuring and helpful to talk to.

Today you have written down a few questions about how this happened and what happens now.

You are otherwise well with no other medical, drug or family history. You have been sexually active since you were 15 years old and only ever in a heterosexual relationship. You have never done drugs and do not smoke. You drink only at the weekend, and tend to binge drink when out with friends.

Three months ago you went to Malia on a boy's holiday and had a few episodes of unprotected sex with 3 or 4 unfamiliar partners. You are currently not in a relationship.

You are quite concerned about informing your manager as they have made lots of cuts to staff because of 'budget cuts'. You are worried that they will use this as an excuse to fire you, because people might be scared that they may catch it.

Questions you would like to ask:

How long do I have to live?

Is it the same as AIDS?

Can I still have sex?

If so, can I still have children?

Do I need to tell my workplace occupational health team?

When do I need to start treatment?

How do I know if the disease is getting worse?

Case 18

You are Avanti, a 24-year-old singer/songwriter. You have come to speak with the GP today after noticing your period was two weeks late. You did a home pregnancy test yesterday and have discovered that you are pregnant. You are in a new relationship and use condoms with your boyfriend, but admit that there have been a few accidents. You are quite upset as you have a number of concerns. You do not think either of you are ready for a baby, and your career is just starting to take off and you cannot afford to put this on hold right now. You and your partner are not financially secure, and you would not have the support of your conservative and deeply religious family.

Whilst you do wish to have children one day, you do not feel it is the right time and you cannot continue with the pregnancy. You have not told your partner, but your best friend is very supportive and you can confide in her.

You wish to know what your options are for termination, and would like this done as soon as possible. You are worried that leaving it too late will mean it cannot be done or you will start to show.

You have not had an STI check but will accept one if offered.
Your last menstrual period was 6 weeks ago. You have had no discharge, bleeding or pain. You have never had an STI as far as you are aware. You are otherwise fit and well, and do not smoke. You drink 2-3 glasses of wine a week, but not since finding out about the pregnancy.

Case 19

You are Gloria, a 25-year-old typist. You have presented to the GP today to discuss your concerns about starting a family with your husband. You are both from Nigeria and you are aware that you are a sickle cell carrier, although your husband has never been tested. You are worried about having children because of the risk of passing on the disease, and are also worried about the effect this may have on your pregnancy.

Your mother has sickle cell disease and has suffered with severe pain and has had frequent admissions for pain relief. Both you and your sister are carriers. You have never had any complications as a result of being a carrier and you are otherwise well. You do not really know much about how sickle cell is inherited, or what causes the disease.

You have some specific concerns about sickle cell disease:
What is sickle cell disease? What is the difference between having the disease and being a carrier?
Will my child have sickle cell disease?
Does it affect my chances of becoming pregnant?
How can you test my baby for sickle cell disease?
What happens if my baby has sickle cell disease?

Case 20

You are Heidi, a 30-year-old lawyer. You are 19 weeks pregnant with your first child. You have come to see the GP today because you were told to book an appointment to have your whooping cough vaccine next week. You were fully up to date with your own childhood vaccinations and do not understand why you need to have another one now, especially while you are pregnant.

This is your second pregnancy, but your first ended in miscarriage at 6 weeks. Whilst no cause for the miscarriage was found, you are still concerned about this pregnancy and the risk of having another miscarriage, despite being reassured that it is unlikely. You have no other health problems and took folic acid until you were 12 weeks.

You do not know what whooping cough is, and want to know if the vaccine is a) necessary and b) safe in pregnancy. You are concerned that every few years new data emerges about different vaccines and are worried this may turn out to be dangerous. You have been careful not to take any other medication and having been eating well to optimise your health. You want to keep this pregnancy as natural as possible and don't want to feel pushed into having the vaccine without understanding the risks. You are also concerned that you may get the disease from the vaccination.

You have some questions you would like answered (if not already addressed):
Can I get the disease from the vaccine?
Can the vaccine harm the baby?
Does this mean the baby will not need their immunisations at 8 weeks for whooping cough?
If I decide not to have the vaccine, will this affect my follow up and interactions with the midwife?
At the end of the consultation, you are still not sure about your decision but would like to think about it and come back

Medicine

Case 1
You have been admitted with cellulitis that requires treatment with intravenous antibiotics. You have an allergy to penicillin. You have just been commenced on an infusion of intravenous flucloxacillin and have started to feel unwell. You noticed that the nurse was busy when they started the infusion, as they did not check your red wristband or allergy status. You feel as though your tongue and lips are swollen. You feel itchy and have noticed a bumpy rash over your chest. You are finding it difficult to breathe and your chest feels tight.
If the candidate correctly recognises anaphylaxis and administers IM adrenaline, oxygen and fluids you start to feel better and less wheezy.

Case 2
You have been bought the emergency department by your family who are concerned. You have been feeling generally unwell since yesterday after the district nurse changed your long-term catheter. You are shaky, feverish and not your normal self. You are disorientated to time and place but are not known to have any memory problems.
If the candidate correctly recognises that you have sepsis and administers oxygen, IV fluids and antibiotics you start to feel better.

Case 3
You are known to have scarring of the liver and have had bleeding from your gullet before that they have fixed with a camera and some "elastic bands". You started vomiting a large amount of fresh red blood today, and are passing thick, black tarry stools that smell. You are feeling unwell and dizzy. You do not have any abdominal pain.
On examination you are tachypnoeic and have blood around your mouth. You have generalised abdominal tenderness, but no guarding or peritonism. You have been incontinent and there is melena in the bed. You have bilateral palmar erythema, spider naevi over your upper chest and are jaundice.

Case 4
You are Jim a 75-year-old gentleman. You have been referred to the respiratory clinic as you have been experiencing increasing breathlessness on exertion and a dry tickly cough, over many months. You worked in a shipyard building ships from the age of 16 until 15 years ago when you retired.

You are not in any pain, and are happy to be examined.

Case 5
You are Sarah a 42-year-old female. You have a history of type 1 diabetes and end-stage renal failure. You have previously had haemodialysis via a radiocephalic fistula on your left arm. The fistula is still functioning but is not longer in use, and there are no evident needling marks or "button holes". You have had a successful renal transplantation. Your graft is located in the right iliac fossa and is non-tender.

You are not in any pain, and are happy to be examined.

Case 6
You are Mable an 80 year-old-female. You have attended the cardiology clinic for your yearly check up. You have a history of rheumatic fever as a child. You have been feeling well in yourself.

You have an irregularly irregular pulse at a rate of 85 bpm. You have a displaced apex beat and a pan-systolic murmur that is heard loudest in the mitral area and radiates into the axilla. You do not have any features suggestive of heart failure.

You are not in any pain, and are happy to be examined.

Case 7
You are a 45-year-old female who was diagnosed with multiple sclerosis 10 years ago. You have come to the emergency department as you feel like you have lost all sense of balance and have had several falls over the past 3 days.

On examination you have an unsteady (ataxic) gait, particularly on heel-toe walking. Romberg's Test is negative. You have a bilateral intention tremor and nystagmus on lateral gaze. Your speech also sounds slurred.

Case 8
You are a 45-year-old lady who has been experiencing tenderness in your hands for several months. It is limiting your ability to perform normal daily tasks. It has been getting worse, but you have not yet seen your GP about. Now you have been admitted with a chest infection so you decide to mention it to the doctors looking after you on their ward round. When you are not moving your hands, you feel very little pain - so if the candidate asks you whether you are in pain at the start of the examination, say "no".

When the candidate starts to palpate your joints, you feel pain and grimace, but don't make a noise. If the candidate does not take notice of your pain, keep grimacing throughout examination then say "ouch" when you are asked to do movements of your hands. If the candidate acknowledges your pain, the examiner will ask them to proceed as if you have been given painkillers and you should then appear settled.

You do not have any nail, skin changes or scars. You do have visible swelling over the MCP joints, PIP joints and wrists bilaterally. Temperature is increased over the swollen joints, and they are tender to palpation. Your pulses are intact. You can make the prayer signs, but are unable to fully complete the range of movement. Power and sensation are intact. You are able to perform functional tasks, but they can be painful. You have some nodules on your elbows.

Case 9
You are a 78-year-old gentleman who has presented to his GP with a tremor. The tremor started in your right hand several years ago, but it has now spread to affect the left side.

The junior doctor has been asked to examine you, please be cooperative. You have a walking stick with you. You are not in any pain. You have a quiet, monotonous voice.

ARMS: When the candidate moves your arms around you are very stiff, with increased tone and cog-wheeling. The power in your arms is good, but every movement takes you a long time. You have difficulty with functional tasks and struggle to undo/do a button due to your tremor.

HANDS: At rest you have a 'pill-rolling' tremor, which is worse when distracted (e.g counting). When asked to do hand movements you are very slow and they get smaller and slower each time you repeat the action.

WALKING: When asked to stand you have a stooped posture and lean forwards. You have difficulty initiating movement, walk in shuffling steps and are very slow to turn around (taking lots of small shuffling steps). You do not swing your arms when you walk.
Everything else is normal (reflexes, coordination, power)

Case 10
You are a 65 year old gentleman. You have presented to the emergency department with a 2 hour history of central crushing chest pain. An ECG and bloods have been taken. The candidate has been asked to interpret the ECG and explain their findings to you.

Case 11
You are a 42-year-old gentleman. One week ago you developed a cough, and you were bringing up yellow-green sputum. Four days ago, you started feeling short of breath while walking up the stairs and this has been getting worse. You have been feeling hot and sweaty at times.
Your wife was concerned so she took you to the local emergency department, where they have started you on antibiotics and given you a bag of fluids. You still feel uncomfortable breathing, and are waiting for the results of your chest x-ray that was taken an hour ago.
You are otherwise usually well and you don't take any regular medications. You work as a bank manager and smoke 10 cigarettes a day.

You listen carefully to the explanation given by the candidate. You may prompt with questions about the most likely cause and next steps if required. You are happy with the explanation given, and do not have any further questions for the candidate.

Case 12

You are a nurse and have just started on shift. You are looking after Joe a 60-year-old man with COPD who has become increasingly drowsy. You run the ABG for the foundation doctor on call and give him/her the print out. The patient is not on any oxygen. If candidate asks you about the patient's history, say, "I'm not sure, sorry" and do not provide any additional information.

Case 13

You are a 32-year-old banker working in the city. You have been under a lot of stress working on a busy project over the past 8 months. This has involved several late nights at work to meet your deadlines, usually followed by a few drinks at the local public house. Your current alcohol consumption is in excess, comprising of one or two glasses of wine at lunch or business meetings, and another three pints of beer/cider after every night after work and most weekends, totalling on average 70 units per week (guidelines state weekly intake should not exceed more than 14 units for men and women).

Over the past few weeks you have been getting worsening generalised abdominal pains, dull in nature, but constant at a severity of 6/10 with associated vomiting. You have noticed that you are a bit shaky in the mornings but feel much better after your first drink at lunchtime. You have not had an alcoholic drink for the past two days and have not been eating, as you cannot keep anything down.

You have had your appendix removed but otherwise have no other medical conditions and are not on any regular medications. You have no known drug allergies. You have no family history of alcoholism, but your father had bowel cancer, and is now in remission. You live alone in a flat in the city. You do not take any recreational drugs.

You last had your bloods taken at the age of 14 when your appendix was removed. You smoke 5 cigarettes a day for the past 10 years. You are aware that your alcohol intake is excessive and are willing to cut down. You are concerned that your boss will find out and that you will lose your job.

Case 14

You are a nurse working on the ward. The candidate has been asked to set up a syringe driver with the following prescription;

5mg diamorphine over 24 hours
10mls water for injection

The patient is no longer able to take oral medications, and has pain control issues. The patient already has a subcutaneous needle in-situ that is clean and within date and safe to use. Please assist the candidate by double checking drugs, fluids and calculations with them.

Case 15

You are an 85 year old retired painter who has been experiencing left sided calf pain which has been getting progressively worse over the last six months. Over the last month the pain is present at rest. It is now starting to affect your mobility. You are an ex-smoker with a 40 year pack history. You have T2DM, hypertension and previously had a CABG at aged 65 due to triple vessel disease. You are anxious that you will be told you need an operation.

Case 16

You are an experienced gastroenterology nurse who is competent in checking and administering blood products. Following the candidates lead you should check the patient's identity, prescription, and the blood unit label with them.

You have just performed observations on the patient. The patient's pulse rate is 90 beats per minute, blood pressure 110/81 mmHg, respiratory rate 19, and temperature 36.3 degrees centigrade. The patient's cannula is patent and working well.

The porters brought the blood unit to the ward (out of the blood bank fridge) 20 minutes ago. You would like to know what to do if the transfusion takes longer than the prescribed three hours as you are aware of guidance to complete transfusion within four hours of the blood product leaving controlled temperature storage.

Case 17

You are a patient on one of the medical wards. You have just spiked a temperature of 38.1°C. The candidate is a foundation doctor who has been called to take blood cultures.

You have had bloods taken before, and are happy to have these samples taken. You do not have any concerns about the procedure.

Case 18

You are a 75 year old retired school teacher. Over the last few weeks you have become increasingly short of breath particularly on doing any form of activity. You are only able to walk to the bathroom before getting short of breath. Six months ago you were able to the shops down the road without much difficulty. You do not feel breathless when resting. However sleeping has become increasingly difficult as you become very breathless when lying flat and wake up at least a few times a night gasping for breath. You have resorted to sleeping in your arm chair. On direct questioning you note that your ankles have become increasingly swollen over the last few weeks. You deny wheeze, chest pain, cough, fever, palpitations and weight loss. You have not travelled recently.

Your mother had a heart attack in her 60s. Your father died of lung cancer aged 82.

You had a large heart attack six months ago and required 2 stents. You have high blood pressure and high cholesterol.

You take aspirin, clopidogrel, atorvastatin, ramipril, bisoprolol, lansoprazole and GTN spray. You are allergic to penicillin and have previously developed a rash when taking it.

You smoked 15 a day for 20 years but gave up at the age of 40. You drink two glasses of wine/week.

You live in a house with stairs with your wife who has Alzheimer's dementia. You are her full time carer. You are adamant that you cannot be admitted to hospital as your wife struggled to cope when you were admitted six months ago.

Case 19

You are a 23-year-old man who has gone to your GP because of bloody diarrhoea. This started around 4 weeks ago. Initially you thought it was food poisoning from a recent holiday to Spain, but it hasn't gone away. You open your bowels between 5-6 times a day and it is often bloody. You often experience severe abdominal pain that is worse before you open your bowels. You often having urgency and on one occasion have not made it to the toilet. You have noticed around 3-4 kg weight loss since this started. You haven't had any mouth ulcers, eye or joint pain or rashes but are often tired.

You are normally well with other medical conditions and don't take any regular medications. You don't drink much but started smoking a few years ago. You have a family history of diabetes (type 2) and your grandma recently had a stroke. There is no family history of cancer.

You were reluctant to come to your GP and are very embarrassed about the diarrhoea. Since not making it to the toilet you have been worried about going out with friends, which has affected your social life. You work as a bus driver and have had to take time off work.

Case 20

You are a 71-year-old lady who has presented to the emergency department with collapse.

Before the event: You were sat watching TV and went to make a cup of tea. When you stood up you felt nauseous and light-headed. Your husband said you went as pale as a ghost. You did not have any chest pain, breathlessness or palpitations.

During: The next thing you remember is being on the floor in the middle of the living room. Your husband said you were only unconscious for a few seconds. You did not have any incontinence and did not bite your tongue or have any jerking movement of your limbs during this episode. You did not have any injury during the fall.

After: You felt a bit disorientated and confused for a few seconds but after that you felt ok. You feel well now. Your husband was concerned and made you come to the ED.

You have never collapsed before, although over the last few weeks you have had some dizziness. This dizziness occurs first thing in the morning when you get out of bed or when you stand up from a chair. In fact, last week you felt dizzy when doing the gardening and had to have a lie down. You just thought it was due to the hot weather and your age. You have been well in yourself otherwise with no other symptoms and no recent illness. If asked you don't drink much water because you don't really like the taste but you do drink a few cups of tea a day, which perhaps isn't enough during the summer.

PMH: You have very little past medical history apart from the fact that your blood pressure used to be high. However, this is now well controlled because they have recently increased your medication.

Medication: You were taking a pill for your blood pressure, but it made your ankles swollen which didn't look very nice in the summer when wearing a skirt. So about a month ago your lovely GP started you on a new tablet and you take one in the morning. You can't remember what it is called but you've got the packet with you: 'bendroflumethiazide 2.5mg'

Case 21
You have had a nine-month history of weight loss and are starting to get concerned as you have not been trying to lose weight. You have noticed that your clothes are loose. You have had some loose stool for six months with occasional periods of constipation in between. Prior to this, your bowel motions were regular. You have also noticed that you are eating less and sometimes you might skip lunch as you don't feel hungry. You have noticed that you can be irritable at times and have had intermittent palpitations.

You have no other medical conditions. Your brother and sister are diabetic.

You have no allergies and do not take any regular medications.

You have been feeling worried because your mother died of breast cancer in her 60s and she lost a lot of weight in her terminal phase. You have decided to come in to find out what the cause of your weight loss might be, and whether you also have cancer.

Case 22
You are a 43 year old lorry driver. The reason you are visiting the practice today is to have a consultation find out the results of some routine blood tests. You are unaware that the tests have shown that you have Type-2-Diabetes.

Five years ago you were diagnosed with high blood pressure and high cholesterol and you take amlodipine 5mg/day and atorvastatin 40mg/ON.

You are aware that you are overweight at the moment and have struggled with dieting as you are unsure of where to start. Your work involves long drives and you often stop for fried food at service stations en-route. You would be willing to get advice from a dietician. You rarely have time to exercise but do enjoy playing football with your work colleagues. You have smoked 20 cigarettes/day for 20 years and drink around 8 units of alcohol/week

You are very anxious about the diagnosis of T2DM as your father who died of a heart attack at the age of 75 also had the condition. He suffered badly with foot problems. You hate the idea of having to inject yourself with insulin as you have a severe needle phobia. You know that blood sugar control is very important with diabetes but you are not sure why.

Only volunteer information regarding your concerns if you are directly asked by the candidate.

Case 23

You are Patricia, are a 52-year old lady. You are attending a gastroenterology outpatient appointment at the hospital as you have had a 6-month history of troublesome acid reflux. You have tried over-the-counter medications, and are taking omeprazole and ranitidine from your GP, but these have not fully alleviated your symptoms. You have lost 5lb weight over the last six months. After doing some research online, you are very worried you might have cancer.

You recently received a letter in the post with an appointment for a gastroscopy to look at your food-pipe and stomach. You have never had a gastroscopy in the past, and are anxious about what it entails and whether it will be a painful procedure. You are adamant that you want sedation for the procedure.

Other than this, you have no medical conditions or known allergies.

After the procedure, you are planning to drive across the country in preparation for your son's graduation the following morning.

Case 24

Your father is currently an inpatient being treated for a chest infection. You phoned the ward this morning to ask for an update and were told by the nursing staff that he had fallen overnight. You were concerned whether he had hit his head or fallen from a height. Unfortunately the nursing staff were unable to give you details as the fall was not witnessed by staff. He was found by a healthcare assistant sitting on the floor. They tell you he appeared to have no injuries.

You cannot understand how your father has fallen. Each day when you have visited him there has been a staff member in the bay. You are concerned that overnight the staff have 'not been paying attention' and 'care more about reading magazines'. You are particularly concerned that your father may have hit his head. You want reassurance that he has not sustained a head injury and if this cannot be offered you want to know how this will be investigated.

Your mother sustained a hip fracture following a fall in hospital the previous year. You saw how long it took for your mother to regain her confidence following this. You are concerned that your father has sustained a hip fracture and again would like this investigated. You have previously made a complaint using the Patient Advice and Liaison Service (PALS) and would like to pursue this route again.

As the doctor addresses your concerns your anger subsides. Once they explain that your father's injuries will be investigated appropriately and the cause of fall will be explored you feel relieved. You would still like to go to PALS to make a formal complaint. This is your right.

Case 25

You are the daughter of Cara, a 72-year-old girl, with known allergy to penicillin. She has been suffering with a cough, occasionally bringing up green phlegm and shortness of breath for the past five days and was admitted for treatment for community acquired pneumonia.
You were called by a member of the nursing staff to come into hospital to discuss Cara's treatment with the doctor.

You are met by the doctor in a quiet room, with a nurse present. You are informed that earlier today, Cara was given an intravenous dose of Co-amoxiclav to which she had an anaphylactic reaction.

You are furious that your mother has been put through this. You cannot understand how the mistake was made when you had clearly stated that she was allergic to penicillin on admission.

You are adamant to know the name of the doctor who prescribed the medication as well as the nurse who gave the medication. You would like to speak with them and you are considering pressing charges against them for harming your mother. You would like to know how this issue will be dealt with and how it will be prevented in the future.

You settle with reassurance that, whilst this unacceptable mistake has been made, Cara is stable and being closely monitored on HDU. You would like to know whether you can see your mother on HDU.

Paediatrics

Case 1

You are the father of a 10 year boy, Paul, who you have brought to the Emergency Department after ringing an ambulance. You were making breakfast in the kitchen when you heard a thudding noise coming from upstairs. You ran upstairs to find Paul on the floor not responding to you and jerking all of his limbs. You also noted Paul has wet himself whilst you were ringing for an ambulance.

This kind of thing has never happened before and you didn't know what to do. The fit did not stop until the ambulance arrived and gave him some medication to make it stop. You think the whole episode lasted about 20 minutes. You don't know what they gave him but are worried he seems very sleepy and lethargic but is now responding to you.

You really want to know what tests need to be done and what can be done now. You are worried he could have epilepsy like his uncle. Paul usually lives with his mum but stays with you often. His mum dropped him off last night and was complaining he has been very clumsy recently especially in the morning when he is eating his cereal, but has not been unwell.

His immunisations are up to date and there are no developmental concerns. He has no known drug allergies and does not take any regular medication. He has not required any hospital admissions in the past. He was born at term by a normal delivery with no postnatal complications. He does not have any siblings and despite your separation you still get on well with his mother.

Case 2

Your 8 month old son, Sam, has been unwell for the last three days with a cough and runny nose. You live with your husband and three other children aged 3, 5 and 8, they are all usually fit and well. Your 3 year old has recently started nursery. He has had a cough and runny nose but has not had any difficulty in breathing like Sam.

Sam is much worse today as he is audibly wheezy. You noticed some slight in drawing of his ribs. He feels warm and has been very unsettled overnight. He usually sleeps very well. You are even more concerned as in triage the nurse commented that his oxygen levels were low at 94%. Sam has gone off his food but is drinking well and has not any diarrhoea or vomiting. He has no drug allergies, takes no regular medications, is passing urine and opening bowels normally with a normal number of wet and dirty nappies.

Your eldest son has asthma and you feel Sam needs inhalers to help him breathe. You feel he definitely needs to be admitted to be managed properly as he seems to be getting worse. It is only 3 weeks before Christmas and you want him to be well for his first Christmas. You feel antibiotics are the only thing that will make him better.

Sam was born at term by normal delivery. He had some breathing difficulties when he was first born. you remember he was breathing fast and needed antibiotics for 2 days but can't remember exactly why. His immunisations are up to date and there have never been any developmental concerns.

Case 3

You are the mother of a 3 year old girl, Freya. You rang an ambulance after she had an episode of being unresponsive and shaking all her limbs on the sofa. The whole episode lasted about 3-4 minutes in total. She was thrashing around abnormally, moving all four of her limbs. Her whole body seemed to be shaking like she was having a seizure. After she stopped shaking she was unresponsive and seemed a bit limp. She was still not herself when the paramedics arrived.

She was not at nursery today as she has had a fever for the last 3 days. She is off her food but drinking well. You are annoyed as you saw the GP yesterday who told you it was a viral throat infection that would settle.

Over the course of the day despite use of both Paracetamol and Ibuprofen her temperature was not coming down. She last had Paracetamol 4 hours ago and Ibuprofen 2 hours ago. She still had a temperature of 39°C at home just before the seizure happened. She has been miserable all day and is still hot. She is not her usual happy self in the Emergency Department.

Freya has a 6 year old brother who had a similar episode when he was 4 years old. You were told it was a febrile convulsion. You think your mother told you that you had a similar episode when you were a toddler. You know what a febrile convulsion is, but you are concerned as the shaking seemed much worse than it was in your son.

Freya does not take any regular medications, but has had 2 bouts of tonsillitis in the last year requiring antibiotics. Freya was born at term via elective C-section for breech position, but had no postnatal complications. She is developing well for her age with a good vocabulary and is dry by day. Freya does not have any known allergies, but does suffer from mild eczema.

Case 4

Your GP has referred your 14 month old daughter to the Paediatric Outpatient Clinic. The GP has been concerned that your daughter has not been growing very well. You first went to see your GP a few months ago because you were concerned that your daughter was smaller than your friend's child, who is two months younger.

Your daughter tends to get sick quite a lot. If anyone around her has a cold, she picks it up too. Her colds seem to go to her chest, and she has had a few courses of antibiotics for chest infections. She has been admitted to hospital three times with chest infections, needing antibiotics into the vein, and oxygen on one occasion. Even when she is well, she is a bit chesty. If specifically asks, she often has runny stool, which is quite foul smelling, and can be difficult to flush away.

She was exclusively breastfed until she was 6 months old, and then you started to introduce some solids. She is a fussy eater. She usually drinks a bottle of milk with breakfast, when she has some baby porridge. She has a snack in the morning with a bottle of milk, and then lunch – usually a little bit of meat, some vegetables and potato, although sometimes she doesn't want to finish her lunch. She has a bottle of milk in the afternoon, and usually has some of what you have for her dinner. She has another bottle of milk before bed.

She has had one admission to hospital with bronchiolitis. She needed oxygen for a couple of days. Otherwise, she has been well. She is up to date with her immunisations. There is no significant family history.

She is a quiet but content little girl. If asked, she sat without support at 11 months, but she cannot walk yet. She babbles and seems to know her name.

You live at home with your husband. She is your only child. Your husband's parents are around a lot and help you with childcare. Your husband smokes, but you do not. You are not known to social services.

Case 5

You have brought your four month old baby to the Emergency Department because he burned his arm two days ago. He was sitting on his changing mat, and reached across and knocked over your cup of tea from the dining table while you were out of the room. He cried a lot at the beginning, but settled with a cuddle. It did not look like a bad burn, so you did not ask anyone to see him. The burn is over the back of his hand. You brought him today because it seems to be bothering him more, and you think it might be infected. You have just come for some antibiotics, and want to get back home.

Your baby was born at term. He is your only child, and it was an unplanned pregnancy. He was well after he was born, and you were discharged on the same day. He was difficult to feed initially, and sometimes he still takes a long time to feed, which can be difficult. Your scans were normal, and he has been well since he was born. He is on no regular medications, and has no allergies that you know of. You have not managed to get around to making an appointment for his immunisations, but you plan to at some point.

There is no family history of note. You have no medical problems.

In terms of development, he can smile, and can support his head. His hearing and vision seem fine, and he passed his newborn hearing check.

It's just the two of you at home. The baby's father left during the pregnancy, and you have not heard from him since. If asked, before he left he would hit you occasionally, but you never reported him. Everything at home is fine. You were seen by the 'young mums' midwife because you are 18, but you are not otherwise known to social services. Your parents live in

Scotland, so are not around to help you, and you have been too busy to keep up with your friends since the baby was born. If probed, you are feeling isolated.

If the candidate summarises their history to you, you change your story, to say that the tea cup fell from a low table next to the changing mat.

You are unhappy to have to go through all of these details as you really just want antibiotics for your child. You become defensive if concerns are raised about the burn, and demand to leave once the antibiotics have been given. If challenged by security or the police you will concede and stay.

Case 6
You were seen at home by the community midwife for the 5 day postnatal check today. The midwife was concerned about your baby, because he has lost 12% of his birth weight. She told you to go to ED, and called ahead to say that you would be coming.

You have been exclusively breastfeeding your baby. He seems to be hungry a lot, and feeds all the time. It is difficult to settle him when he is off the breast. He feeds every hour, if not more often. He will fall asleep on the breast, but if moved, he wakes and starts to suck again.

He has passed urine twice in the last 24 hours, but has not opened his bowels. He has not been vomiting. You are concerned that he might be a bit more sleepy today. When he was awake yesterday, you thought that his eyes looked a bit yellow.

He was born at 39 weeks at this hospital following a normal delivery. He was fine after he was born, and went straight onto the breast. Your waters broke about 6 hours before he was born. You have been well in yourself, and have never heard of 'Group B Streptococcus'. You were discharged home the same day. He is your first baby. Your husband works during the day, but your mum is also around to help, and you feel well supported at home. You are not known to social services.

You have not given him formula, and you are very reluctant to do so. You have been told that formula can be harmful for babies. If questioned further, you become tearful, and say that you would feel like a failure as a mum if you were unable to provide enough milk for your baby. However, with clear and empathetic explanation, you would agree to give formula.

Case 7
Your teacher noticed the cuts on your arms earlier and told your Mum about it. You told your Mum that you cut your arms deliberately, so she brought you to the ED to have your arms looked at.

You've always been very healthy and have never even been to a hospital before. You are shy and quiet, have never had a boyfriend, and have a really good group of friends. You enjoy school, but are finding Year 8 stressful as the work is harder; you are worried you might start to get lower grades, like B's and C's, and then your teachers and parents will be disappointed.

You live with your Mum, Dad, and 8 year old brother. Recently, Mum and Dad have been arguing a lot about things like the washing up and the laundry; they never hit each other or say swear words, but they didn't used to argue like this and you're worried that they might get divorced like some of your friend's parents. Your parents are always loving towards you and your brother, but you wish they wouldn't argue so much. You used to be really happy but now you often cry at home, and don't sleep as well as you used to. You haven't talked to your friends about it because they're upset about their own parents splitting up, and you're worried you might upset them more.

You used some scissors from your art box to cut your arms last night – you didn't plan to do it and have never done anything like this before, but you were upset after hearing your parents argue and somehow it made you feel better. You didn't mean to hurt yourself by doing it. You find your Mum easy to talk to, but didn't tell her or anyone else because you didn't think it was a big deal. You didn't expect anyone to notice the cuts or be so worried about them, and are quite embarrassed to be here.

You have never thought about killing yourself, and have never made any plans to do so. You don't have any plans to cut yourself again, but you are worried how you will cope with Mum and Dad arguing, as well as the stress of schoolwork. If the candidate asks if you think you would like someone (e.g. CAMHS, school counsellor) to talk to regularly, you really like this idea.

You will be quiet, answer questions briefly and make little eye contact initially. If the candidate speaks to you softly, and is empathetic, then you will engage with them much more, making eye contact and answering their questions fully.

Case 8
You are Oscar's mother; he is you and your partner's first baby. You have rushed him to the ED because he had a floppy episode whilst feeding. You are shaken up, and on the verge of tears.

Your pregnancy was unremarkable, with normal scans and blood tests; this was a relief, after you and your partner suffered a miscarriage last year. He was born in hospital by normal vaginal delivery at 39 weeks. Your waters broke 6 hours before he was born, you had no temperature or IV antibiotics during labour, and you have never been told you have Group B Streptococcus. Oscar didn't require any resuscitation or neonatal unit care, and you were both discharged home the next day.

You have been breastfeeding Oscar since birth; his birth weight was 3.2kg, and he weighs 3.5kg now. He normally feeds on the breast every 2-3 hours, for 20 minutes. On this occasion Oscar had been feeding for around 15 minutes when you noticed he had stopped sucking – you looked down to see he was much floppier than normal. He seemed slightly pale, but you don't remember him looking blue; you picked him up, shouted for your partner, and blew in his face. He then vomited up a small amount of milk and gave a cry, before settling down as he normally would after a feed. The whole episode probably lasted 10-15 seconds, but felt much longer.

Oscar has been his normal self in the two hours since this happened, but you are now scared to feed him again – you want to know what you can do to stop this happening again, as at the time you and your partner both felt at the time that Oscar might die. Neither of you are happy to go home until you are certain this won't happen again. You and your partner are not related, and you are not married but live together; you both work as civil servants, and have no significant past medical history.

Other than today's floppy episode, Oscar has been a very healthy baby and has no current signs of illness. He has never had a floppy episode before, although vomits a small amount of milk after each feed which you were initially worried about; however, your health visitor reassured you that it was normal, particularly as he is gaining weight well.

Case 9
Examination findings are normal except for a soft systolic murmur heard at the upper right sternal edge. This does not radiate (if assessed), there is no heave or thrill (if assessed) and both femoral pulses are well felt. The baby is pink and not cyanosed.

If requested, tell the candidate that both pre and post ductal saturations are 98% in air and the mean four limb blood pressures are all within normal limits.

Case 10
You are a 9 year old boy, who has recurrent abdominal pain. Examination findings are entirely normal throughout.

Case 11
Cardiovascular examination reveals an ejection systolic murmur at the upper right sternal border which radiates to the interscapular area on the back. There is no heave or thrill palpable. Upper limb pulses are well felt. There is no radio-radial delay but radio femoral delay is present. Femoral pulses are more difficult to palpate but present.

If requested, four limb blood pressures are as follows:

RUL 135/70
LUL138/72

RLL 108/58
LLL 110/65

Case 12

You are a 15 year old boy with cystic fibrosis and are used to being examined by junior doctors for exams and in clinics. You are currently an inpatient for a planned course of antibiotics but are feeling well in yourself.

Respiratory examination reveals that he is short for his age, has clubbing of the fingernails and bibasal crackles, likely secondary to bronchiectasis. He also has an increased antero-posterior diameter of the chest.

Case 13

You are a 9 year old girl who has weakness in your arms. At rest both arms are kept across your body, flexed at the elbows and wrists. Your arms are stiff in all muscle groups with clasp-knife responses at both elbows. You have increased deep tendon reflexes in all areas bilaterally. Power in all areas in reduced, with flexor muscles being stronger than extensor muscles.

Case 14

You are an 8 year old boy who was born at 28 weeks gestation, who has a history of grade 3 IVH has been brought to clinic for his routine follow up. The child displays a circumducting gait consistent with a left hemiplegia. There is increased tone throughout the left leg. Power is reduced in the knee flexors, with increased deep tendon reflexes in all areas in the left leg. Right leg examination is entirely normal. The candidate will not be asked to test pain sensation or proprioception.

Case 15

You are Sarah, a 14-year-old girl who has been diagnosed with asthma. You have been told a little bit about what asthma is and understand that it is a condition where the airways in the lungs tighten, making it difficult to breathe. This causes you to have a cough and a tight feeling in your chest, as well as a wheeze. It is usually triggered when you exercise. You know you have to take inhalers but you are not really sure how long for. You are a bit worried about school and what you need to do if you feel unwell or need your inhalers at school.

You want to understand what asthma is, why you need your inhalers and when you need to talk to and adult about your condition, before you go home. If any medical language is used or there are words that you don't understand, you should ask the candidate to explain what is meant. You are on the ward with your Mum when the doctor comes to talk to you.

Case 16

Your son Ben is 18 months old and he has been admitted to the children's ward following a febrile convulsion. He had been unwell at home with a fever and runny nose for three days and then had a high fever of over 39°C at home. He became unresponsive and began shaking and jerking both his arms and legs. You were extremely worried and called an ambulance. The movements had stopped by the time the ambulance arrived and Ben did seem better in himself but he was still sleepy. Since you arrived at the hospital, he has been moved to the ward and although he is back to his usual self now, you still aren't quite sure what happened. You remember the ambulance crew mentioning something about a "fit" but were so worried at the time that you didn't really take much in. You have asked for someone to come and explain to you what happened.

You have a friend who has a little girl with epilepsy and she has seizures very frequently. You want to know that if Ben has also had a fit or seizure, then does he have epilepsy too and will he need to have medication or have fits again?

Case 17

You are the mother of Jack, who is 18 months old. You have asked to speak with a doctor.

You have brought Jack to the Paediatric Emergency Department as he has had a dry cough, runny nose and a high fever for 24 hours. The doctor who assessed Jack said that he had a viral infection and advised you to give paracetamol if needed. You are concerned that Jack has a chest infection and should have antibiotics. You have an older child who was admitted to hospital with a chest infection when he was a similar age to Jack. He received antibiotics and you want Jack to have the same treatment.

It is 2am and you have had very little sleep in the past 24 hours, as Jack has been miserable and coughing constantly. You want the antibiotics so that Jack will get better. You do not wish for him to need admission to hospital, as your older child did. If the doctor is unable to explain to you why Jack has not been given antibiotics, you become frustrated and ask to speak with a more senior doctor. If the explanation is satisfactory, you are reassured and willing to take Jack home.

Case 18
You are 25 weeks pregnant to your first baby and unexpectedly have developed contractions. The obstetric team have told you that the baby may be delivered in the next few hours and gave you an injection of steroids to help with the baby's lungs. You are extremely anxious and scared.

Prior to this, your pregnancy so far has been going very well with normal scans and blood tests. You had a water infection one week ago that was treated with antibiotics. Following meetings with your midwife you had made a plan for a natural home birth and you are very keen to exclusively breastfeed your baby. You wonder if you can still do this if the baby is born prematurely. You also want to know if there is anything to be done to prevent the baby from being delivered early.

Other question that cross your mind is whether the prematurity will affect the baby's brain and development. You become upset when the subject of death or disability is discussed. Your partner is currently in the United States on a business trip and you have been on your own at home. However, your parents live close by and you would like the doctor to come back and explain things again when they arrive.

Case 19
Your baby was born quite unwell a few hours ago totally unexpectedly. You had a normal pregnancy but the midwives told you that the baby's shoulder got stuck during delivery. Instead of giving the baby to you after birth he was taken away to the paediatricians and was admitted to the special baby unit where he is now breathing with the help of a machine. You visited the baby earlier and you were told that the baby was stable and hopefully the tube would be removed soon. You are shocked and upset when you hear that he has had seizures and needs to be moved to a different hospital.

You are very worried about the long term implications of what has happened and specifically if the baby has suffered brain damage. You are distressed about not having the baby with you and not being able to breastfeed. You are worried that he will be far away and you will not be able to see him. You are reassured when you are told that you may visit him at any time.

You hope that he recovers quickly and that you are able to take him home soon. However, you are happy to agree with any medical treatment that is considered best for him as long as it is properly explained.

Case 20
Your 7 month old baby has developed coughing and wheezing over the past 2 days that has been getting worse. His 3 year old brother has had similar symptoms. You brought the baby to the hospital because he refuses to feed and you are worried that his breathing is getting worse.

Prior to this your baby has been well and you have had no health concerns about him. He was born by natural delivery at term with no problems and he is gaining weight and developing well. He is fully immunised. His brother and father are healthy. You suffer from mild asthma and you wonder whether he is developing the same.

You are very keen to go back home since it is your first day back to work tomorrow morning.

Case 21
You are the parent of Iris who was admitted for the first time two days ago with viral wheeze following a cold. She has had similar episodes of wheeze on her chest before but has not previously been so severe. You are anxious about stopping the nebulisers and going home with just the inhalers and spacers.

The FY1 doctor has come to see you while Iris is spending time with the play specialist. You have seen them before on the ward round these last couple of days. You tell the doctor that you've seen the inhaler and spacer before at home but that your partner usually gives it to Iris if she needs it.

Case 22

You are a 37 year old woman on the postnatal ward and your baby boy Simon was born yesterday morning by normal vaginal delivery. He is your first child born at term. You had an uneventful pregnancy and as far as you know, both of your antenatal scans were normal. You did not have any additional tests during pregnancy to assess for Down's as you felt the risk was low despite your age. You have no past medical history and only take the vitamin supplements you were given during pregnancy. You are a non-smoker and a very occasional drinker but have not had any during pregnancy. Your husband is very supportive and has been very excited about the birth.

After Simon was born the midwife had some concerns about his appearance and asked the paediatrician to come and speak to you. The paediatrician agreed that Simon showed signs of Down Syndrome and asked permission to do a genetic test to confirm the diagnosis of which the results are now awaited.

You are feeling very guilty for not having more tests during pregnancy and are not sure how you and your husband will cope with this unexpected news. You are too scared to look on the internet to find out more about the condition but have heard of Down Syndrome and think it means Simon will be quite disabled. You've let your midwife know of your concerns and she has asked another paediatric doctor to come and speak to you.

You would like to know how Simon will be affected both now and in the long term. You would like to know what help there will be for Simon and most importantly when the results would be back.

Case 23

You are the mother of Benjy, an ex premature baby (32 weeks gestation) who is still in the Special Care Baby Unit but is now 8 weeks old. He is due his routine 8 week immunisations today.

You have no particular objections to your baby having immunisations but wonder if there are any oral formulations of the vaccines that he could have instead because he's had to endure so many needles so far. If the doctor mentions that he may be unwell with a fever after the vaccinations, you should ask whether that means he will need antibiotics as he has received three courses of intravenous antibiotics over the past 8 weeks for similar reasons.

You would like to know if there are any other likely complications as a result of these injections.

Case 24

Your 4 year old son has been admitted to the children's ward today with pneumonia after being unwell for the past 2 days with high fevers, cough and difficulty in breathing. He is being treated with intravenous antibiotics and facemask oxygen, which the nurses seem to keep turning up. He has only really had 2 cups of water in the past 2 days and he keeps vomiting, so the nurses are waiting for the doctor to come and prescribe some fluids.

You have been really worried about him for the past hour as he is becoming more drowsy. You just went out of the room for 1 minute and have come back and now he is not responding to you.

He was born at 29 weeks gestation, and has chronic lung disease, requiring home oxygen for the first year of life. He has been admitted to PICU at 9 months of age with bronchiolitis but not again since then. He has no history of cardiac defects or other medical problems and has only been admitted to hospital once in the past year for a chest infection. He has some mild motor developmental delay. He is attending nursery and is up to date with his immunisations.

Case 25

No actor required for this station.

General Practice

Case 1

You are a 60 year old gentleman Peter, who has recently signed up at the GP practice. You visited the practice nurse who noticed your blood pressure was high and has asked you to see the doctor.

ONLY OFFER INFORMATION IF SPECIFICALLY ASKED

You have had no obvious symptoms. You feel well in yourself. You have Type 2 Diabetes for which you are on Metformin and have no allergies. Your father died of a heart attack aged 60. You have smoked 20 cigarettes a day for 40 years. You drink a couple pints every weekend. Your diet consists of a 'fry-up' in the morning, some sandwiches for lunch and often a takeaway for dinner. You snack often. You have quite a lot of salt in your diet. You have been gaining weight slowly over the past few years and now weigh 90kg. You rarely exercise, but you are a builder and your work consists of manual labour and therefore feel it is enough.

The candidate will now have a discussion with the examiner. Following this they will take some time to address your ideas, concerns and expectations. You have some specific questions:

What does high blood pressure mean?
Your father had high blood pressure and he died of a heart attack will the same happen to you?
What food should you avoid?
Which medications will they start for high blood pressure and what are the side effects?

Case 2

You are a 50 year old lady Amanda, who has come to the GP as you are worried about the palpitations you have been having recently.

ONLY OFFER INFORMATION IF SPECIFICALLY ASKED

It feels uncomfortable because you become very aware of your own heartbeat and it seems really fast. They last about a few minutes and tend to disappear when you rest. They first started a year ago and seem to be getting worse. They come on often when you exercising and occasionally at rest. There is no prior warning.
There is occasional central chest tightness. This is a non-radiating, dull pain, 4/10 in severity and disappears as the palpitations do.
There is no shortness of breath or feeling faint. You haven't noticed any weight loss or change in appetite. You dress appropriately for the weather and you do not sweat over much. You do not suffer from headaches.
You have no other medical problems and are not on any medications and have no allergies.
You are a smoker (10 a day for 20 years) and drink in binges. You have the occasional coffee. You take no recreational drugs. You are a lawyer.
Your mother passed away of breast cancer when she was 65.
If asked about your ideas, concerns and expectations please offer the information below
You are concerned that these episodes will one day lead to a heart attack and you will die early.

Case 3

You are a 70 year old woman Diana, who has come to see the GP because you have been feeling more breathless and coughing more than usual in the past week or so.

ONLY OFFER INFORMATION IF SPECIFICALLY ASKED

Normally, you walk slowly and your breathing is not affected, but you get quite breathless going up stairs or hills. You cough early in the morning, often bringing up some white or clear phlegm.

For the past week you have been struggling to walk 100 meters, you have to stop due to your breathing and you have noticed a wheeze. You have been using your blue inhaler twice as often as usual. It has been a struggle to continue your everyday activities. During the day you have been coughing more but still bringing up white or clear mucus, no blood. You have not had fevers or night sweats. You have not lost any weight recently. You do not struggle with breathing when lying flat and you do not wake suddenly from sleep very short of breath.

You have had no pain or swelling in your legs. No recent foreign travel or long-haul flights and no recent contact with anyone with an infection.

You have COPD (diagnosed 10 years ago). You have had fairly frequent chest infections (2-3 per year) but you have only been admitted to hospital 2-3 times in total. You have never needed intensive care. You have no known heart problems and no history of previous clots. You take Seretide one puff twice a day, Spiriva one puff once a day, your blue salbutamol inhaler as and when you need it. You have been taking your medication as prescribed.

You had trouble with inhaler technique so you now use a spacer and have no problems with it. You do not have home oxygen or home nebulisers. You have the flu vaccine every year. You have no allergies.

You have a family history of high blood pressure. You are not aware of any lung cancer in the family. You were a secondary school teacher but retired 5 years ago. You live with your husband and you are both still independent and physically active. You are an ex-smoker (20 a day for 40 years) and you quit about 10 years ago. You do not drink. You do not have any pets.

If asked about your ideas, concerns and expectations please offer the information below
You're not sure what is causing your symptoms. When your symptoms have got worse like this in the past it is usually due to a chest infection. You are concerned that this is not just a transient worsening of your symptoms but the disease progressing.

Case 4
You are Jack a 60 year old retired missionary. You have had a dry cough for a long time and you have become concerned why it's not going away.
ONLY OFFER INFORMATION IF SPECIFICALLY ASKED
The cough started about 2 months ago and has been present every day since it started. The cough is normally non-productive but you sometimes bring up small amounts of red blood when you cough.

You have no chest pain or back pain. You now experience shortness of breath when walking up stairs. You do not feel more short of breath lying down and you do not wake suddenly from sleep gasping for breath. You have not noticed any swelling of your ankles nor any painful swelling of your calves.

You have lost your appetite and have lost a lot of weight but you are not sure how much. You have not had fevers or night sweats. You have high blood pressure. You have never been diagnosed with asthma, COPD, tuberculosis or HIV. You have never had a heart attack or a clot in your leg or lung. You take Losartan. You have no drug allergies. You have no family history of cancer.

You are now retired but worked for many years as a missionary in areas with a high prevalence of tuberculosis including India and Somalia. You may have been in contact with people with active tuberculosis but did not suffer any symptoms yourself. You had the recommended vaccinations prior to travel. You have never been exposed to asbestos. You smoked 10 cigarettes a day from your mid-teens until five years ago. You do not drink alcohol. You live with your wife of many years. Your wife has not been coughing.
If asked about your ideas, concerns and expectations please offer the information below

You think this might be cancer. Your wife is in the early stages of dementia and you are her main carer. You have no children and few local friends due to your itinerant lifestyle. You are concerned about who will look after your wife if this is something serious. You are expecting blood tests and scans but think this will take a long time on the NHS.

Case 5
You are a 33 year old woman, Bekah and you have come to the GP because you have been having headaches for 3 months.
ONLY OFFER INFORMATION IF SPECIFICALLY ASKED
They are usually only on the left side of your head and are throbbing in nature. They are 8/10 in severity at worst. You have about 2-4 headaches per week and they last 2-3 hours. You can generally tell when you are about to have a headache as

you have a strange visual sensation about 15 minutes beforehand. You have vomited a few times when you have had a headache and generally feel nauseous.

You think the headaches may be triggered by coffee or alcohol. Nothing particularly makes them worse but the pain does improve when lying down in a dark room. You take paracetamol every four hours during a headache. This helped initially but no longer has any effect.

You also have asthma which is generally well controlled with a blue inhaler if you get wheezy. You are also on the oral contraceptive pill for contraception.

Your mother suffers from tension headaches and you wonder if these are the same thing.

You work as a lawyer and live with your partner and your daughter. You have a very stressful case at the moment and are getting very little sleep.

If asked about your ideas, concerns and expectations please offer the information below

You are very worried as you have started to miss work because of your headaches and this is becoming very stressful. You would like some stronger pain relief and an explanation of what these headaches are and how they can be avoided.

Case 6
You are Colleen and have presented to the GP surgery, as you are worried about his progressing confusion. He is now 82 years old.
ONLY OFFER INFORMATION IF SPECIFICALLY ASKED

You are worried about your husband as he growing increasingly confused. You have come in today as he was recently aggressive towards you and you feel you cannot cope anymore. This has been going on for many years. You first noticed your husband's memory was awry 4 years ago when he began forgetting simple things like where he had put his keys. This has got worse and now he is beginning to forget friends and family.

He is often awake at night and often calls out during his sleep. He gets agitated very easily. He does not seem depressed or flat in his mood. His cognition does not seem to fluctuate through the day. He has no hallucinations.

This seems to be have been a slow progressive worsening rather than a sudden deterioration. There have been no recent signs of infection - no cough, no fevers, no urinary incontinence, no diarrhoea.

His mobility is fine and he is able to take himself to the toilet but there have been accidents recently. However you are his main carer and have to help him with washing and dressing. You prepare his food now, as there have been dangerous occurrences where he has left the gas on and recently you found him wandering outside alone with no good reason. This has changed your life as he no longer cooks for himself and this was a huge passion of his.

He has a past medical history of high blood pressure for which he is on Amlodipine. He has no drug allergies.

He is a retired lawyer and did not smoke or drink very much. You do not have any family around, as they have moved to Australia, and friends have their own problems that have come with age.

If asked about your ideas, concerns and expectations please offer the information below

You are worried about your husband's health and safety, as you can not leave him in the house alone anymore. You fear it may be dementia. In addition it has impacted your life greatly and at your age are finding it difficult to cope at home, especially with controlling his behaviour and aggression, but also just with washing and dressing him.

Case 7
You are Philippa, a 38 year old who has recently been diagnosed with Multiple sclerosis following two admissions to hospital. These admissions were prompted by an episode during which you experienced visual symptoms and an episode of right sided weakness, that has improved but remains, causing a slight limp.

ONLY OFFER INFORMATION IF SPECIFICALLY ASKED

You have come to the GP today because you have had a cough, runny nose and sore throat. You never really get unwell and you are worried this is related to your MS. You have not had a fever, your cough is non productive. You have not had any shortness of breath or chest pain. You have been taking lemsip which is helping. You have no other medical problems and no drug allergies. There is no family history of multiple sclerosis. You are a teacher and have been in contact with lots of 6-7year olds who have come down with the flu. You do not smoke or drink. You live with your fiance.

You have not felt fatigued or in pain recently. You are not experiencing any tingling or pins and needles. Your eye symptoms have resolved. You have no incontinence or urinary symptoms.

If asked about your ideas, concerns and expectations please offer the information below

When asked by your GP what you know about MS, confess that you are feeling quite overwhelmed by all the information you have been given and feeling quite confused. You are not sure about which symptoms could be due to MS. When the GP/candidate explains that this is unlikely related to your MS, ask which things you should look out for and what to do if you get these symptoms. Can the GP provide new medications?

You wonder if your leg is going to get any better at all as the limp is causing quite an inconvenience. Will all new symptoms continue to get worse?
Another big concern you have is your job. You are a teacher in a busy primary school and have to move classrooms to teach different classes, which is difficult with your leg. Will you have to quit your job?
Since your diagnosis you have been feeling very anxious and worried. You are struggling to sleep at night because you worry about the future- you don't want to have to use a wheelchair or have carers.

Case 8
You are a 45 year old gentleman Harry who has presented to the GP surgery as he would like to cut down on his alcohol intake.

ONLY OFFER INFORMATION IF SPECIFICALLY ASKED

You feel quite nervous about coming in to see the GP and are embarrassed that things have gotten this bad. Your girlfriend has recently given you an ultimatum that you must either seek help or she will leave.

You have always enjoyed a drink since you were younger and you feel 'you have always been a good laugh', but you have never had an alcohol problem in the past. You started drinking more about a year ago when you had a difficult time at work, following being suspended.

It used to start with having a glass of wine when you came home from work, and escalated to drinking a bottle of wine every day. However, in the past 3 months you have had to take many sick days as you felt too unwell to go in, and your boss has had several conversations with you about this, the most recent being last week where he told you that he has smelled alcohol on you and he was concerned so he has told you to take time off as leave.

You have found yourself having to have a drink in the morning to help you start your day. Usually this is a can of cider. You do not drink that much spirits. If asked to quantify exactly how much you drink you have 1 bottle of wine a day, and go through a 8-pack of cider in a week.

You deny any other drug use, but you smoke 20/day. You deny any other physical health problems or history of mental health. You have not had any problems with legal authorities.

You have no symptoms of gastritis, memory loss/confusion, no pins and needles in your hands and feet, and you do not experience palpitations.

If asked about your ideas, concerns and expectations please offer the information below
Your relationship with your girlfriend has become very difficult and you find you now mostly argue about your drinking, as she wants you to stop. She is upset as she is worried that you will lose your job and she will not be able to support you

both. You feel very guilty and ashamed that she feels this way, but you get annoyed because that is all she says to you now.

You are willing to seek help as you have realised you need to change.

Case 9
A 37 year old gentleman Sam, has presented to the GP surgery complaining of rectal bleeding.

ONLY OFFER INFORMATION IF SPECIFICALLY ASKED
This has been for the past month and happens intermittently. It is bright red blood and you notice it on wiping mostly, however recently you have noticed it in the toilet pan, which has made you more concerned. You do not think the blood is mixed in with stool. If asked about change in bowel habit, you cannot identify any obvious change. You have not had any diarrhoea. You have not been constipated but occasionally you do strain which is associated with pain followed by itching. You deny any black tarry stools, mucus in the stool, abdominal pain, or weight loss.
You report you eat a reasonably healthy diet. Only if asked directly, you do not eat enough fibre nor drink a lot of water.

You are a fit and healthy person. You have seasonal asthma and have inhalers blue and brown. You do not have any allergies. You are a non-smoker and drink very occasionally. You do a lot of exercise and work as a builder. You have no family history of bowel disease.

If asked about your ideas, concerns and expectations please offer the information below
You are worried about the bleeding and would like to know if it is something sinister and if there is anything you can do to manage it.

Case 10
You are a 50 year old woman Sarah, who has presented to the GP surgery after having found a lump in her breast.

ONLY OFFER INFORMATION IF SPECIFICALLY ASKED

You first noticed it about two months ago on the left upper side of the breast, whilst bathing. However, you did not think much of it at the time. It's not particularly painful but you think it's grown in size over the last two months, to about the size of a marble. It's quite hard in nature and it seems to be quite fixed. You've not noticed any discharge from the nipple, but you did notice a speck of blood on the inner surface of your bra the other day. The breast itself looks normal, with no skin or nipple changes. Your weight has been stable, you've not been in pain and as far as you know, you've not noticed any swellings elsewhere. You have not had any trauma to the area.

You've stopped having your periods about 18 months ago. You've not noticed any abnormal bleeding or discharge from down below. You're a mother of two children, aged 13 and 17, both of whom were born vaginally with no complications during pregnancy or childbirth. You don't have any medical problems, nor are you on any regular medications; though you've been experiencing some hot flushes recently and your GP believes this is down to the menopause, you've been reluctant to try HRT yet.

You don't smoke, but you do drink about 15 units of alcohol per week.

If asked about your ideas, concerns and expectations please offer the information below
However, your mother died of ovarian cancer in her 50s and you have read in the newspaper that there is a link between that and breast cancer—and you are worried that this may too be cancer.

Case 11
You are a 64 year old gentleman Winston who has presented to the GP surgery complaining of blood in his urine

ONLY OFFER INFORMATION IF SPECIFICALLY ASKED

It's bright red in colour, and painless. It's been troubling you for the past week, within which you've noticed it becoming more and more frequent. You've also noticed you've been having more of an urge to urinate recently. You haven't had any abdominal pain, no burning or stinging when you pass urine, no discharge from the penis, nor have you had any fever.

You've not had any falls or otherwise any trauma that might have otherwise explained the bleeding. However you have been feeling a bit run down recently, and you've been having to stop to catch your breath when climbing the stairs. You think you've lost a bit of weight, as your shirts do not fit as they once did.

You're otherwise well, you have high blood pressure which is controlled by tablets but have not had any major illnesses in the past. You have been a lifelong smoker (20 a day since childhood) and you've found it difficult to give up. You have the occasional pint.

You are a semi-retired decorator. Your family have all been well, but your father who used to run the decorating family business, had some bladder problems late in his life.
If asked about your ideas, concerns and expectations please offer the information below
You're worried about whether you're going to need a catheter because of the bleeding. You remember having had to care for your father who suffered from infections and blockages of the catheter and you think you would struggle to cope with one.

Case 12
A 55 year old woman Geeta has presented to the GP surgery complaining of feeling unwell.

ONLY OFFER INFORMATION IF SPECIFICALLY ASKED

When the consultation begins explain that you have just done a urine dip test with the nurse who has given you the following results to take to the doctor.

Nitrites moderate
Leucocytes moderate
Blood negative

For the last 3 days it has been painful when you pass urine, it is a burning sensation. I have been going to pass urine more often and have had to rush to get there on time. You have not had any incontinence. You have not noticed any blood in your urine. You have not had any fevers. You have also had some lower tummy pain that is a mild ache from time to time.
You have high blood pressure but no other past medical history. You have only had one previous urinary tract infection in your twenties. As far as you know you do not have any renal tract abnormalities and have normal functioning kidneys.
You live with your husband and are not sexually active. You have not had a recent sexual health screen but feel you are not at risk of a sexually transmitted infection. You have not had any abnormal vaginal discharge or bleeding. You do not smoke and do not drink. You are a housewife.
The candidate will now have a discussion with the examiner. Following this they will take some time to address your ideas, concerns and expectations. You have some specific questions:

Ask the doctor what your symptoms could be attributed to, as you thought it may be a urinary tract infection.

You have been doing some reading of your daughters medical textbooks, as she is studying medicine currently and you had some questions about your condition. Ask them to explain what a recurrent UTI is, and ask what the difference between a relapse and a reinfection. You are wondering if you fall into the category of recurrent UTI? Because you would like a kidney scan as you are worried.

The nurses always ask me to do a mid-stream urine, but no one has told me how to do this, could you explain.

Case 13
You are a 42 year old gentleman Praveen who has attended the GP surgery for a routine diabetic follow up but he is complaining of feeling funny in the last few weeks.

ONLY OFFER INFORMATION IF SPECIFICALLY ASKED

You were diagnosed with Type 2 diabetes 2 years ago and have been on Metformin and Gliclazide, which was added 8 months ago. Your past medical history includes asthma which is well controlled with Salbutamol inhalers alone. You smoke 10/day and drink 4-5 pints on the weekends with friends.

Every 3-4 months, you have a blood test done at the GP practice to check your diabetes control is satisfactory. The last test was within range so there were no changes to medication. You have annual checks for your eyes at the hospital. The GP also checks your blood pressure, feet, urine and blood test on regular intervals. You believe some of this for monitoring your heart, nerves and kidneys.

Unfortunately your diet has slipped lately due to being too busy to cook, so you have probably not had as great control as previously and you used to go on long walks and jogs, but due to work being more busy, you have been too tired.

Until the last 3 weeks, you were well but have recently noticed that you are increasingly having episodes where you feel faint and dizzy. This is accompanied with sweating and sometimes palpitations. You have not been worried much as eating seems to help these symptoms and so decided not to seek advice until today.

You were a builder but have recently been offered a job as an HGV driver which you intend to take up in the next few weeks. You do not drink alcohol and do not smoke.

Your family history includes both parents with diabetes. You have no allergies.

If asked about your ideas, concerns and expectations please offer the information below

You are quite happy with the current medications and do not want to make any changes to them. You are adamant they are fine, but if your doctor explains why it is dangerous for you to stay on Gliclazide as you are about to be an HGV driver and why the change in necessary, you understand and accept this. You then agree to try the new medication.

Case 14
You are a 38 year old gentleman Spencer who has presented to the GP surgery with a persistent red rash on both elbows for the last 6 years which has not grown in size.

ONLY OFFER INFORMATION IF SPECIFICALLY ASKED

You have noticed that the rash is quite thick, appears red although it is not painful, has not bled or oozed pus. There are no blisters and you don't have other rashes on the body. The rash sometimes reduces after you have worked in the summer when it's sunny. You think it often becomes worse when you are stressed.

You tried some moisturisers last year for this rash but they seemed to have hardly had any effect. You had left it then but now, as you will be attending your friend's wedding in 4 weeks, you want to get rid of it as it is extremely embarrassing.

You have had no fevers, joint pains, swellings, night sweats, weight loss or change in appetite. You have no ulcers in your mouth, have good bowel movement and no changes in your urinary habits.

You have previously had your appendix removed, but otherwise have been healthy. You have not been travelling in the last 3 years. You do not take any regular medications and you are only allergic to hazelnuts.

You have been a builder for the last 20 years, live with your wife and son aged 6, have no pets, smoke 15 a day and drink 2-3 pints of alcohol with friends every night after work.

You had an uncle who had a similar rash called psoriasis, but he had it more widespread and he always complained of pain in his joints. There is no other family history of rashes.

If asked about your ideas, concerns and expectations please offer the information below

A few weeks ago, you heard of a new drug called Methotrexate which you can take tablets of and is known to be very effective at controlling this type of rash. You are highly keen on taking it so that you can be free of it by the wedding. As it is a new drug, you believe it is also quite safe to take and want to try it.

You don't understand why the doctor is not happy to prescribe it – you ask if it is because it's expensive. It is only when they explain that it can potentially cause failure of production of blood and the immune system, cause lung and liver damage that you appreciate the risks and agree on trying a different treatment instead.

Case 15
You are Hugo a 59 year old who has presented to the GP with a small mole, which your wife noticed on your back 2 weeks ago

ONLY OFFER INFORMATION IF SPECIFICALLY ASKED

The mole started bleeding yesterday and she commented that it had doubled in size during this time. It does not hurt, but you find it is itchy sometimes.

You enjoy travelling, both as part of work and leisure and have spent a significant part of your life away from the country, largely in the Mediterranean countries, Southeast Asia and South America. During your trips, you often go to the beach or seek spots where you can sunbathe. You don't use sunbeds and have not really been consistent with using any suncreams. Your skin does burn sometimes.

Your past medical history includes Type 2 diabetes for which you take Metformin, but otherwise you have been well.

You are a landscape photographer so spend a lot of time outside. You smoke 20 cigarettes a day and drink 3-4 pints 2-3 times a week. You live with your wife and a pet dog. You do not have any allergies.

Your Dad had skin cancer when he was in his 60s but recovered from it after some procedure and your mother had breast cancer when she was in her 50s.

If asked about your ideas, concerns and expectations please offer the information below

You are not particularly worried that it is something bad– it just looks like a mole when you looked at it in the mirror but have come as your wife was worried about it. You would rather not bother the doctor with something like this and are not particularly keen on going to the hospital as you have never liked going to one, but if the doctor explains why he thinks you need to go see the hospital doctors, you understand his reasoning and agree to it.

Marksheets + Learning points

ENT	**190**
Anaesthetics & Critical Care	**210**
Orthopaedics & Rheumatology	**235**
Psychiatry	**260**
Surgery	**281**
Emergency medicine	**306**
Obstetrics & Gynaecology	**331**
Medicine	**351**
Paediatrics	**376**
General Practice	**401**

ENT

Case 1
History - muffled hearing

Task:	Achieved	Not Achieved
Introduces self & clarifies who they are speaking to and relationship to child		
Elicits history from parent/child in a concise manner		
Ascertains extent of hearing loss (whisper, soft words etc)		
Specifically asks about:		
Onset of symptoms		
Rate of onset (Insidious/rapid)		
Unilateral or bilateral symptoms		
Temperature/other skin changes		
Discharge (Color, smell, consistency)		
Associated pharyngitis		
Associated headaches		
Previous infections		
Deafness		
Dizziness/balance problems		
History of foreign bodies in bodily orifices		
Mastoid tenderness		
Asks about birth & past medical/surgical/drug history		
Checks allergy status		
Explores Ideas, concerns, and expectations		
Demonstrates good rapport and empathy with the patient throughout		
Relays a concise summary to the examiner		
Examiner's Global Mark	/5	
Actor / Helper's Global Mark	/5	
Total Station Mark	/30	

Learning points

The main differentials here include foreign body and an infection. These are the most common causes of ear presentations considering the age of the boy in this scenario.

It can be difficult getting a detailed history from children, so It is important to take time to elicit what information the child may be able to provide, to get a strong collateral history and then to ask direct questions.

It is also important to note the soft communication points (listening, rapport, empathy and question asking) are especially important in this station.

Case 2
History - discharge

Task:	Achieved	Not Achieved
Introduces self & clarifies who they are speaking to		
Specifically asks the following about the discharge:		
Color & Smell		
Consistency (thick, thin, serous, etc)		
Is it exacerbated by positioning?		
Timing (intermittent/constant)		
Unilateral or bilateral		
Does the discharge alleviate any headaches		
Screens for infective process:		
Pain/otalgia (ear, mastoid, peri-auricular area)		
Erythema (location and extent)/other skin changes		
Temperatures/rigors etc		
Previous infections		
Screens for symptoms associated with malignancy:		
Unintentional weight loss/loss of appetite		
Night sweats		
Lethargy/general malaise		
Associated nasal congestion		
Rhinorrhea, post nasal drip		
Asks about past medical/surgical/drug history & allergies		
Explores Ideas, concerns, and expectations		
Demonstrates good rapport and empathy with the patient throughout		
Relays a concise summary to the examiner		
Examiner's Global Mark	/5	
Actor / Helper's Global Mark	/5	
Total Station Mark	/30	

Learning points

Possible differentials for this station are acute otitis media, chronic suppurative otitis media, chronic otitis media, or in the context of trauma, CSF otorrhoea

Recognizing the relationship between nasopharyngeal malignancies and ear presentations is important re compression of the Eustachian tubes

Patients with significant family histories of malignancy can be very anxious about the possibility of them having the same. You will gain points in an OSCE and credibility in clinical life for being reassuring, confident and give an aura of a doctor that can be trusted by your patients

Case 3
History - bleeding ear

Task:	Achieved	Not Achieved
Introduces self & clarifies who they are speaking to		
Specifically asks the following about the discharge:		
Color		
Consistency (thick, thin, serous, etc)		
Events around onset of bleeding - trauma, foreign body (in a playground, swimming, fighting, etc)		
Timing (intermittent/constant)		
Screens for infective process:		
Pain/otalgia (ear, mastoid, peri-auricular area)		
Erythema (location and extent)/other skin changes		
Temperatures/rigors etc		
Previous infections		
Screens for other symptoms associated with bloody otorrhoea:		
Check for any palpable masses/lesions in the ear canal		
Hearing loss		
Tinnitus		
Dizziness and vertigo		
Facial palsy		
Checks for previous episodes of similar presentations		
Asks about past medical/surgical/drug history and allergies		
Checks the child's social circumstances, i.e. lives with siblings, no supervision at home, and generally checks that the child's home environment is safe		
Explores Ideas, concerns, and expectations		
Demonstrates good rapport and empathy with the patient throughout		
Relays a concise summary to the examiner		
Examiner's Global Mark	/5	
Actor / Helper's Global Mark	/5	
Total Station Mark	/30	

Learning points

Possible differentials for this station are foreign body, trauma, acute otitis media, chronic suppurative otitis media, chronic otitis media, Eustachian tube dysfunctions, or more rarely, the first presentation of a malignancy (ear canal squamous cell carcinomas, polyps, etc)

Most paediatric ear presentations that involve blood are either due to trauma or an infection. In the context of a young child in a playground, trauma (including foreign bodies) should be the top of the differential list. It is rare for patients in this age group to present with ear bleeding as a first sign of a pertinent malignancy.

In this particular scenario, there is a history of pre-existing contralateral hearing impairment. Dealing with the patient/parents has to be done in an exceptionally sensitive manner. When discussing the possibility of permanent damage to the left ear in this case, this should be done sympathetically and sensitively but ensuring there is no ambiguity in the message you convey.

Case 4
History - ' a lump'

Task:	Achieved	Not Achieved
Introduces self & clarifies who they are speaking to		
Briefly explains examination and obtains consent		
Asks about any hearing problems		
Asks about pain		
Assessment of lump		
Assessment of erythema and warmth		
Places lump between 2 fingers and attempts to mobilise it		
Assesses if fixed skin		
Assess if fixed to underlying structures		
Assess if compressible		
Checks if pulsatile		
Looks for punctum		
Tests for mastoid tenderness		
Repeats procedure on other ear		
Identifies abnormality		
Elects to use otoscope to check canal		
Checks contralateral ear first		
Ensures that lump does not extend into canal		
Asks to check for regional lymphadenopathy		
Demonstrates good rapport with the patient throughout		
Demonstrates empathy appropriately		
Relays a concise summary to the examiner		
Interpreters findings adequately		
Examiner's Global Mark	/5	
Actor / Helper's Global Mark	/5	
Total Station Mark	/30	

Learning points

All lumps should be assessed for adherence to underlying structures, a punctum, overlying skin changes, shape, consistency and colour.

All head and neck regional lymph nodes should be assessed, and the patient should be asked about any other swellings found in the axilla, groin or a sense of abdominal swelling that could indicate organomegaly

Must ask about pain BEFORE examining. Both in the OSCE and clinical practice, patients will cooperate and assist examinations far better if their pain is enquired about, acknowledged and dealt with as early as possible.

Case 5
History - Anosmia

Task:	Achieved	Not Achieved
Introduces self & clarifies who they are speaking to		
Elicits history from patient in a structured and concise manner		
Asks about onset of symptoms		
Asks about associated signs or symptoms such as pain, nasal discharge, blocked nose, difficulty breathing, snoring		
Asks about specific conditions such as sinusitis, rhinitis		
Asks about neurological signs/symptoms:		
Seizures		
Headaches		
Visual problems		
Asks about changes in mood, or personality		
Asks about changes on sense of taste		
Asks about facial trauma		
Asks about drug history/allergy status		
Asks about recreational drugs, namely snorting		
Family history		
Asks about smoking/alcohol history		
Asks about occupation		
Asks about past medical/surgical		
Explores Ideas, concerns, and expectations		
Demonstrates good rapport with the patient throughout		
Demonstrates empathy appropriately		
Relays a concise summary to the examiner		
Examiner's Global Mark	/5	
Actor / Helper's Global Mark	/5	
Total Station Mark	/30	

Learning points

Anosmia can be a subtle symptom and difficult to assess so often patients don't value it too much. However, its causes can be significant, and includes frequently missed pathologies such as head and neck/intracranial malignancies.

Note that head and neck malignancies have a high prevalence in patients of oriental origin

Following a thorough ENT examination, Investigations for anosmia include (and are not limited to) CT heads +/- contrast, CT sinuses, MRI head (including sinuses), Naso-endoscopy, etc.

Case 6
History & Examination - 'Red nose'

Task:	Achieved	Not Achieved
Introduces self & clarifies who they are speaking to		
History:		
Specifically asks for:		
Onset of symptoms and relation to returning from holiday (sun exposure)		
Any tenderness across the rash		
Any associated joint pain		
Asks about any past medical, drug history & allergy and family history		
Examination:		
Checks bedside clinical observations		
Inspection/		
Notes symmetrical appearance of rash		
Notes sparing of nasolabial folds		
Palpation/		
Notes that area is not tender		
Notes area is not raised		
Examine regional lymph nodes (no lymphadenopathy elicited)		
Examination – Joints		
If ascertained in history that has joint pain, offers to examine relevant joints (hands) – do not actually let candidate examine joints		
Examination – examination of nose		
Offers to examine both nostrils		
Explores Ideas, concerns, and expectations		
Demonstrates good rapport and empathy with the patient		
Relays a concise summary to the examiner		
Offers differential diagnoses		
Management plan (3 marks)		
Complete examination by looking for other skin changes elsewhere and joint examination		
FNE to look for malignancy		
Blood tests for auto antibodies and renal function		
Examiner's Global Mark	/5	
Actor / Helper's Global Mark	/5	
Total Station Mark	/30	

Learning points:

The patient has signs and symptoms suggestive of systemic lupus erythematosus (SLE). Other differentials include malignancy, sjogrens, sarcoidosis, dermatitis, sunburn, etc.

Recognize that it is a systemic condition and offer to examine for joint involvement (hand examination).

Recognize the need for further haemotological testing for auto antibodies, however can be a local reaction due to nasal pathology (malignancy), may require Fiber-optic Naso-endoscopy (FNE).

Case 7
Examination - Nose

Task:	Achieved	Not Achieved
Introduces self and clarifies role		
Briefly explains examination and obtains consent		
Asks about any breathing problems		
Asks about pain		
Assessment of nose		
Assessment of external nose – skin changes, deviation of bones		
Checks airflow by isolating nostrils		
Uses Thudicums appropriately		
Selects appropriate light source		
Looks in all accessible regions of the non-symptomatic side first		
Checks for discharge		
Checks for masses / FB		
Repeats procedure on other nostril		
Identifies abnormality (septal deviation)		
Proceeds to check oropharynx		
States would then examine the ears		
Checks regional lymph nodes		
Offers to use a Fiber-optic Naso-endoscope to assess the nasopharynx/posterior nasal cavity		
Demonstrates good rapport with the patient throughout		
Relays a concise summary to the examiner		
Interprets findings adequately		
Examiner's Global Mark	/5	
Actor / Helper's Global Mark	/5	
Total Station Mark	/30	

Learning points:

Air flow through both nostrils should be assessed first. Ask the patient to sequentially inhale and exhale sequentially through both nostrils. When examining the nasal cavity, open the nostrils using Thudicums (held using the thumb, fore and middle fingers). Ensure that you have an appropriate light source (either torch in other hand or headlamp) as you need to be able to visualize all areas of the nasal cavity

One of the least invasive ways of examining the nasopharynx thoroughly in a clinic setting is by using a Fiber-optic Naso-endoscope

As an examination of the nose/nasal cavity is incomplete without an oral exam, you should always offer to examine the oral cavity when faced with such a patient

Case 8
Examination - Nasal lump

Task:	Achieved	Not Achieved
Introduces self and clarifies role		
Briefly explains examination and obtains consent		
Asks about any breathing problems		
Assessment of nose		
Inspects for obvious nasal disfigurement		
Checks airflow by isolating nostrils		
Uses Thudicums and light source appropriately		
Assessment of nasal lump		
Assesses for erythema and warmth		
Assesses for a punctum or discharge		
Assesses if fixed to skin/underlying structures by placing the lump between 2 fingers and attempting to move it		
Assesses if compressible		
Assesses for overlying skin changes		
Repeats procedure on other nostril		
Identifies abnormality (lump fixed to skin)		
Proceeds to check oropharynx		
Offers to examine the ears		
Checks regional lymph nodes		
Offers to use a Fiber-optic Naso-endoscope to assess the nasopharynx/posterior nasal cavity		
Demonstrates good rapport with the patient throughout		
Relays a concise summary to the examiner		
Interprets findings adequately		
Examiner's Global Mark	/5	
Actor / Helper's Global Mark	/5	
Total Station Mark	/30	

Learning points:

When examining an abnormality in part of the body organ with laterality, always (or offer to) start with the normal side first; in this case, the normal nostril first
When inspecting the nasal cavity, open each nostril using the Thudicums held in thumb, middle and fore fingers. Offer to examine the oral cavity at the end of your exam, and also suggest using a Fiber-optic Naso-endoscope to assess the nasopharynx in more detail

In this age group, it is important to rule out malignancy, and as such, this should be top of your differential list. Other differentials for a lump on the nose include a polyp, sebaceous cyst, a post-traumatic lesion, or other rheumatological/autoimmune lesions such as SLE, sarcoidosis etc.

All lumps should be examined in a systematic manner in order to fully assess all aspects of the lump (size, shape, adherence to underlying structures including skin, overlying erythema/skin changes, compressibility, pulsatility, transluminence). In this case, remember to check the regional lymph nodes (in this case, around the neck and superior mediastinum)

Case 9
History & Examination - Nasal fracture

Task:	Achieved	Not Achieved
Introduces self & clarifies who they are speaking to		
Demonstrates an infection-control compliant approach: Bare below the elbow + washes hands at the start and at the end of the station		
Explains goal of encounter and seeks consent to proceed		
History:		
Takes a systematic pain history pain methodically (e.g. using "SOCRATES")		
Asks about time, date, and mechanism of injury		
Be specific and open regarding potential safeguarding issues (non-accidental injury, bullying etc.)		
Clarifies the onset and progress of nasal symptoms (bleeding, obstruction, anosmia, CSF leak)		
Asks about neurological and visual symptoms (headaches, nausea, diplopia etc)		
Ask about past and recent medical / surgical / medications history		
Checks social and family history		
Checks allergy status		
Examination:		
Checks (personally or ask for) basic observations: Temperature, HR, BP, SaO2 on air		
Considerately inspects and palpates the face for: Bleeding / bruising / deformity / tenderness / fractures		
Carries out nasal anterior examination for: Deformity / haematoma / bleeding / sniff test		
Carries out a brief neurological examination (cranial nerves, neck stiffness, pupils)		
Examine oral cavity for palate trauma / bleeding / teeth loosening		
Clarifies the patient's subjective feeling of facial deformity and explores the patient's and relatives' ideas, concerns, and expectations		
Demonstrates good rapport and empathy with the patient/relatives throughout		
Suggests a reasonable initial management plan		
Relays a concise summary of findings to the examiner		
Examiner's Global Mark	/5	
Actor / Helper's Global Mark	/5	
Total Station Mark	/30	

Learning points:

Nasal deformities affect the central aesthetic compartment of the face, and are therefore markedly noted and well appreciated by the patients and their relatives. The concern is usually significant and can lead to psychological impact that should be approached considerately.

The non-surgical management of nasal traumatic deformities is best achieved during the second week after the injury. During that period the swelling is usually regressed to allow precise appreciation of the bony deformity, and the fractured bones are still amenable to closed manipulation under GA.

A nasal septum haematoma, if untreated, can commonly become infected and turn into a septum abscess. This can cause complicated nasal deformities which are difficult and complex to treat. More importantly, such sepsis can spread into the orbit, sinuses, meninges, and cavernous sinus. Therefore, the early recognition and prompt treatment of a nasal septum haematoma in nasal trauma are crucial.

Case 10
Examination - Epistaxis

Task:	Achieved	Not Achieved
Introduces self & clarifies who they are speaking to		
Washes hands		
Permission obtained to perform examination		
Exposes and re-positions the patient appropriately		
Briefly checks vital signs & evidence of significant blood loss		
Recognizes/looks for obvious external abnormalities such as:		
Trauma		
Bruising to the periorbital region/mastoid process		
Lacerations		
Symmetry/deviation of the nose		
Swelling to the face		
Tenderness of the facial bones on palpation		
Assess for nasal discharge and notes features such as :		
Bright red blood		
Volume		
Mucus/CSF		
Palpates:		
The nose for tenderness/obvious fractures		
The facial bones for tenderness/obvious fractures		
Appropriately inserts a nasal speculum		
Notes presence/absence of foreign objects		
Relays a concise summary to the examiner		
Mentions further assessments/tests required		
Examiner's Global Mark	/5	
Actor / Helper's Global Mark	/5	
Total Station Mark	/30	

Learning points:

Epistaxis is commonly caused by trauma (including nose picking), iatrogenic (anticoagulants, surgery, cocaine), and bleeding disorders. The severity and onset of the haemorrhage define the most effective management (conservative, medical, or surgical). Therefore, thorough history taking is crucial in order to define the likely cause(s) and best management plan.

Epistaxis patients are commonly under significant stress due to pain and anxiety. This usually causes tachycardia, a rise in blood pressure and subsequently a higher risk of bleeding. Therefore the patient's anxiety and pain must be promptly assessed and addressed, preferably through a methodical manner (e.g. SOCRATES).

Although the cause can often be obvious such as in case of trauma, it is important to be methodical and look for cues and clues of other potential causes (eg: skin bruising can suggest anticoagulation use or coagulopathies)

Case 11
History - Dysphagia

Task:	Achieved	Not Achieved
Introduces self & clarifies who they are speaking to		
Specifically asks about:		
Onset of swallowing problem (gradual vs sudden)		
Difference between swallowing solids and liquids		
Associated pain		
Voice change		
Neck swellings		
Breathing difficulties		
Otalgia		
Halitosis		
Unintentional weight loss/Loss of appetite		
Night sweats		
General malaise/lethargy		
Asks about smoking/alcohol history and occupation		
Asks about past medical/surgical history		
Asks about Family history of malignancies		
Asks about drug history & compliance and allergy status		
Explores Ideas, concerns, and expectations		
Demonstrates good rapport and empathy with the patient throughout		
Relays a concise summary to the examiner		
Identifies the need to refer to secondary care via the 2 week wait suspected cancer pathway.		
Examiner's Global Mark	/5	
Actor / Helper's Global Mark	/5	
Total Station Mark	/30	

Learning points:

Main differentials to exclude are:

malignancy (malignant/benign), Zenker's diverticulum, GORD

In any head and neck malignancy station, asking about weight loss, tolerance of solids/liquids, family history and a quantified smoking & alcohol history are key

Remember to explore the non-malignancy differentials whilst taking a history. Singers are prone to having vocal cord polyps, and gastro-oesophageal reflux disease can also cause dysphagia

Case 12
History - Odynophagia

Task:	Achieved	Not Achieved
Introduces self & clarifies who they are speaking to		
Specifically asks about:		
Onset of swallowing problem (gradual vs sudden)		
Difference between swallowing solids and liquids		
Associated pain		
Voice change		
Neck swellings		
Breathing difficulties		
Otalgia		
Unintentional weight loss/loss of appetite		
Night sweats		
General malaise/lethargy		
Asks about smoking history and alcohol consumption		
Asks about past medical/surgical history		
Asks about Family history of malignancies		
Asks about drug history & compliance and allergy status		
Recent contact with someone with similar symptoms		
Explores Ideas, concerns, and expectations		
Demonstrates good rapport and empathy with the patient throughout		
Relays a concise summary to the examiner		
Identifies the likely underlying diagnosis of a peri-tonsillar abscess (quinsy)		
Examiner's Global Mark	/5	
Actor / Helper's Global Mark	/5	
Total Station Mark	/30	

Learning points:

Main differentials to exclude are: acute tonsillitis, peri-tonsillar abscess, pharyngitis, malignancy

In any head and neck malignancy station, asking about weight loss, tolerance of solids/liquids, family history and a quantifying smoking & alcohol history are key.

Remember to explore the non-malignancy differentials whilst taking a history. Younger patients are less likely to have malignancy, so an infection should be higher up the differential list

Case 13
History - 'Hoarse voice'

Task:	Achieved	Not Achieved
Introduces self		
Specifically asks about: Onset of symptoms – gradual/sudden		
Pattern of voice quality – fluctuating/constant		
Asks about voice use – work/recreation		
Asks about pain on phonation		
Enquires about difficulties breathing		
Enquires about difficulty swallowing		
Enquires about any neck lumps/swelling		
Enquires about indigestion/reflux		
Caffeine and water consumption		
Smoking history		
Alcohol consumption		
Occupation history		
Asks about past medical history		
Drug and allergy history		
Asks about previous surgery to the neck/mediastinum		
Explores Ideas, concerns, and expectations		
Demonstrates good rapport with the patient throughout		
Demonstrates empathy appropriately		
Relays a concise summary to the examiner		
Examiner's Global Mark	/5	
Actor / Helper's Global Mark	/5	
Total Station Mark	/30	

Learning points:

Hoarseness or dysphonia are terms used to describe a change in voice quality. A thorough history must include details surrounding the onset of hoarseness, any change in voice quality through the day (reflux laryngitis is commonly worse in the morning, nodules worsen with voice use through the day), associated upper respiratory tract infection and voice use habits including occupation and leisure activities.

A persistent hoarse voice for more than 2 weeks with no concurrent URTI in a patient over 45 years old meets criteria for a two week wait cancer pathway referral. Other red flags in the history include smoking, alcohol excess, a neck lump and associated stridor or dysphagia.

In addition to benign and malignant vocal cord lesions it is important to consider pathology that may affect the innervation of the larynx via the superior laryngeal nerve or the recurrent laryngeal nerve.

Case 14
History & Examination - Acute Stridor

Task:	Achieved	Not Achieved
Introduces self & clarifies who they are speaking to		
History:		
Specifically asks about: Allergy		
Previous medical history/drug history/drug chart		
Timing/type of last meal/drink		
Events leading to presentation		
Enquires about difficulties breathing		
Enquires about difficulty swallowing		
Enquires about any neck lumps/swelling		
Assessment:		
Assesses airway – comments on stridor and applies Oxygen		
Palpate neck – site of pain and check trachea is central		
Checks for cyanosis		
Assess chest expansion		
Notes use of accessory muscles		
Auscultates chest		
Calculates respiratory rate accurately (within 2 breaths per minute)		
Attaches pulse oximeter or asks for 02 Sats		
Explores Ideas, concerns, and expectations		
Demonstrates good rapport with the patient throughout		
Demonstrates empathy appropriately		
Relays a concise summary to the examiner		
Examiner's Global Mark	/5	
Actor / Helper's Global Mark	/5	
Total Station Mark	/30	

Learning points:

Stridor may be acute or chronic and can occur in childhood as well as adulthood. Stridor is distinct from stertor and may be inspiratory, expiratory or biphasic. Inspiratory stridor suggests a laryngeal obstruction, expiratory stridor suggests tracheobronchial obstruction and biphasic stridor suggests a glottic or subglottic obstruction.

In an emergency, take an A.M.P.L.E. history and perform examination in a structured A.B.C. manner. With experience you will be able to do both these tasks simultaneously.

AMPLE is primarily designed for trauma assessment but can be utilized in any emergent scenario where a concise history is required. AMPLE is Allergies, Medications, Previous medical/surgical history, Last meal time, Events surrounding injury/acute illness.

Case 15
Moulage - ATLS airway management

Task:	Achieved	Not Achieved
Introduces self & clarifies who they are speaking to		
Identify airway compromise as an emergency situation, and refers to the ALS/ATLS guidelines		
Call for senior help (Cons/anesthetist/crash team)		
Applies high flow oxygen (15L/min) via non re-breathe mask		
Attach monitoring for oxygen saturations and pulse rate		
Consider treatment for anaphylaxis		
Considers any neck pathology **before** extending and manipulating the cervical spine		
Performs chin lift and head tilt		
Describes use of an oropharyngeal airway		
Able to choose correct size – corner of mouth to ear lobe		
Describes use of a nasopharyngeal airway		
Able to choose correct size – patient's little finger		
Aware of contraindications to NPA (i.e.: skull base fracture)		
Consider supraglottic airway device such as a laryngeal mask airway		
Describes endotracheal intubation		
Mentions video laryngoscopy to improve the view of the laryngeal inlet (e.g. GlideScope)		
Mentions need for rapid sequence induction		
Mentions option for awake fibreoptic nasal intubation		
Describes temporary surgical airway – crico-thyroidotomy		
Describes definitive surgical airway – surgical tracheostomy		
Examiner's Global Mark	/5	
Actor / Helper's Global Mark	/5	
Total Station Mark	/30	

Learning points:

Airway compromise must be recognized as an emergency situation requiring senior assistance. Referring to guidelines such as ATLS is an excellent way to give your discussion structure.

Consider whether there are any contraindications to your actions, especially in the context of trauma. Skull base fractures can make nasopharyngeal airway placement hazardous and cervical spine injuries may impact on the ability to manipulate the neck.

A protected airway is defined as a cuffed tube inflated below the glottis. Although a supraglottic airway allows for positive pressure ventilation and obstructs the oesophagus it does not protect the airway from aspiration in the same way as a cuffed endotracheal tube. (ETT)

Case 16
History - 'lump in throat'

Task:	Achieved	Not Achieved
Introduces self & clarifies who they are speaking to		
Specifically asks about:		
Where is the lump in the throat sensation felt		
Onset of symptoms		
Ability to swallow fluids and solids		
Associated pain		
Voice change		
Breathing difficulties		
Weight loss		
Recurrent chest infections		
Description of neck swelling:		
Position		
Size		
Shape – smooth/irregular		
Surface – hard/soft		
Asks about smoking history and alcohol consumption		
Asks about past medical/surgical/drug history & allergy		
Explores Ideas, concerns, and expectations		
Demonstrates good rapport with the patient throughout		
Demonstrates empathy appropriately		
Relays a concise summary to the examiner		
Identifies the likely underlying diagnosis of a pharyngeal pouch		
Examiner's Global Mark	/5	
Actor / Helper's Global Mark	/5	
Total Station Mark	/30	

Learning points:

A feeling of a 'lump in the throat' is a common presenting complaint but is vague and can mean different things to different people. The medical term for this is globus pharyngeus but it is essential that any significant pathology is not missed.

This lady describes classical symptoms associated with a pharyngeal pouch (Zenker's diverticulum). Her lump is present when it fills with swallowed material. This can be confirmed with a barium contrast swallow and endoscopic stapling would be considered due to her recurrent aspiration pneumonia and weight loss.

Differentials in this case: Pharyngeal pouch, extrinsic esophageal compression (e.g. cervical osteophyte), benign stricture (e.g. Plummer-Vinson syndrome), malignant stricture, neuromuscular oesophageal dysmotility.

Case 17

History - 'neck mass'

Task:	Achieved	Not Achieved
Introduces self		
Explains goal of encounter and consent to proceed		
Asks if the patient wants a chaperone		
Clarifies if the patient has (and expresses willingness to address) any pain, discomfort, or needs methodically (e.g. "SOCRATES")		
Specifically asks about the following (one point each):		
The history of neck lump (onset, change in size, aggravating / relieving factors)		
Preceding events (trauma, travel, surgery, dental)		
Local symptoms (pain, tenderness, skin changes)		
Head and neck symptoms (dysphonia, dysphagia, odynophagia, sore throat, otalgia)		
Cardio-respiratory symptoms (chest pain, SOB, palpitations, cough, wheeze)		
General symptoms (weight, appetite, fevers)		
MSK symptoms: weakness in upper arms/thighs		
Neurological symptoms (headaches, vision, mood, dizziness)		
GU symptoms (urinary, periods, and ALWAYS LMP)		
Checks social / family history		
Checks past and recent medical / surgical history		
Checks drug history and allergy		
Elicits history in a concise and clear manner		
Explores the patient's and relative's ideas, concerns, and expectations		
Demonstrates good rapport and empathy with the patient and relatives throughout the encounter		
Relays a concise summary to the examiner		
Examiner's Global Mark	/5	
Actor / Helper's Global Mark	/5	
Total Station Mark	/30	

Learning points:

The differential diagnosis of a neck lump covers a wide range of conditions that can be classified into congenital, inflammatory, endocrine, and neoplastic. The associated systemic and local involvement can be significant, such as AF and extensive anxiety in this case. Therefore, a comprehensive history taking is crucial to identify the likely diagnoses and initiate a plan of action.

The systemic effects of endocrine neck masses can lead to significant cardiovascular and neurological duress. The patient's anxiety and pain must be promptly assessed and addressed, preferably through a methodical approach (e.g. SOCRATES).

A calm, confident, and reassuring approach by the doctor can play a key role in addressing the patient's anxiety. Good rapport with the patient and relatives also assists the doctor in establishing a clear coherent history and gaining the patient's trust (reflected here in higher points rewarded).

Case 18
Examination - 'neck mass'

Task:	Achieved	Not Achieved
Introduces self & clarifies who they are speaking to		
Explains the goal of the encounter and acquires consent to proceed		
Asks the patient for any painful / tender areas to be considerate towards these during examination		
Demonstrates an infection-control compliant approach		
Assesses for upper airway noises (stridor, stertor, gurgling, normal)		
Checks the patient's basic observations (temperature, BP, HR, RR, SaO2 on air)		
Carries out a general assessment of the patient (BMI, skin turgor, nail changes, peripheral oedema, bruising)		
Assesses the patient's voice quality (hoarse / breathy / strained / normal)		
Carries out a full inspection of the neck lump commenting on: scars, colour, symmetry or sinus		
Attempts to transilluminate the neck lump		
Carries out palpation of all neck regions (all 5 levels of the neck, thyroid gland, sub-clavicular, supra-clavicular, peri-auricular, TMJ's, occipital, and parotids), and systematically describes palpable masses (location, size, texture, mobility, tenderness, mobility)		
Carries out full oral cavity inspection (floor of mouth, buccal vestibules, gums, retro-molar areas, hard and soft palate, and oropharynx)		
Carries out a bimanual palpation of the floor of mouth (masses, stones), and massages the parotids while inspecting the parotid drainage points (opposite to upper second molars)		
Examines (or expresses will to) other lymph node regions (axillary, inguinal, popliteal)		
Demonstrates good rapport and empathy with the patient and relatives throughout the encounter		
Explains considerately and in lay-terms the examination findings and the needed further management steps to the patient and relatives		
Relays a concise summary of findings to the examiner		
Lists further clinical examinations that are required (FNE, FNAC)		
Lists required blood tests (blood film, FBC, LFT's, U&Es, LDH, infections serology, inflammatory markers, auto-antibodies)		
Suggests required imaging (USS / MRI / CT)		
Examiner's Global Mark	/5	
Actor / Helper's Global Mark	/5	
Total Station Mark	/30	

Learning points:

A neck node in an adult should be assessed comprehensively to rule out neoplasia. A full ENT and head and neck assessment is vital in order to exclude / diagnose a primary site of the suspected malignancy.

Vital diagnostic tests are available in outpatient settings (FNAC, FNE) and should be performed / requested to assist the diagnosis making process.

Patients who present with neck masses are commonly concerned regarding a possible malignancy. Clinicians should follow a professional and considerate approach in order to facilitate the clinical examination, gain trust and build rapport with the patient and his/her relatives.

Case 19

History - 'loss of vision'

Task:	Achieved	Not Achieved
Introduces self & clarifies who they are speaking to		
History of presenting complaint. Specifically:		
Monocular / binocular		
Onset of symptoms		
Redness of eye		
Pain/photophobia		
Current level of vision		
Associated ocular symptoms. Specifically:		
Double vision		
Preceding amaurosis		
Associated systemic symptoms:		
Fatigue		
Jaw claudication		
Scalp tenderness		
Headache history		
SOCRATES		
plus red flags 2 from (nausea, vomiting, postural variation, morning onset)		
Past ophthalmic history (including refraction – Short sighted)		
Past family/medical/drug history + allergy status		
Explores Ideas, concerns, and expectations		
Demonstrates good rapport and empathy with the patient		
Relays a concise summary to the examiner		
Suggests any 2 useful investigations from (1 mark only)		
ESR/CRP (inflammatory markers)		
Full blood count		
ECG		
Offers differential diagnosis (1 mark only)		
Giant cell arteritis / Temporal arteritis (arteritic ischaemic optic neuropathy		
Non arteritic anterior ischaemic optic neuropathy (i.e. embolic event)		
Examiner's Global Mark	/5	
Actor / Helper's Global Mark	/5	
Total Station Mark	/30	

Learning Points:

It is important to ask about specific symptoms e.g. photophobia, trauma, swelling, contact lens use as negatives can rule help rule out differentials.

Always ask about driving when taking an ophthalmology history. If you don't one day it will catch you out. Guidelines state that patients must have a visual acuity of 6/12 or better (with contact lenses or glasses if necessary) using both eyes together or in the only eye if monocular.

Asking about patients' ideas, concerns and expectations is especially important in ophthalmology. Sight is arguably the most important sense in humans, and the loss of vision can be a very debilitating disability, both physically and mentally. It is therefore important to demonstrate empathy towards patients' concerns, whilst and exploring their concerns and expectations.

Case 20
History & Examination - 'blurred vision'

Task:	Achieved	Not Achieved
Introduces self & clarifies who they are speaking to		
History:		
Checks if symptoms are uni/bilateral		
Asks the following about vision:		
Blurred/dimmed/distorted		
Diplopia		
Onset of visual loss (sudden/insidious)		
Timing of visual loss (transient/ongoing)		
Specifically asks about:		
Photophobia		
Pain - SOCRATES		
Examination:		
Using snellen chart assesses visual acuity		
With Pinhole		
Without Pinhole		
Tests colour vision with Ishihara plates		
Tests each eye separately		
Inspects pupils		
Tests accomodation		
Darkens room and asks patient to fix on distant object		
Tests direct and consensual pupillary reactions		
Performs swinging light test		
Indicates ideally patient's eyes should be dilated		
Tests red reflex using fundoscope		
Examines retina using fundoscope		
Demonstrates good rapport with the patient throughout		
Guides the patient through the examination		
Relays a concise summary to the examiner		
Examiner's Global Mark	/5	
Actor / Helper's Global Mark	/5	
Total Station Mark	/30	

Learning Points:
Differential Diagnoses
Inflammatory – Optic Neuritis, autoimmune disease, sarcoid
Ischemic – arteritic or non-arteritic ischaemic optic neuropathy
Nutritional – B12, folate, alcohol
Compressive – optic nerve, orbital or intracranial tumours
Systemic – severe hypertension, raised intracranial pressure

If a patient wears glasses, ensure that they wear them when checking visual acuity and colour vision. Don't forget to test each eye individually. If a patient cannot see any letters on a snellen chart check the vision in the following order: counting fingers, hand movements, perception of light. Learn and practice how to use a fundoscope prior to the exam. There is nothing worse than stressing and wasting time in the exam trying to turn it on!

The swinging light test is to check for a relative afferent pupillary defect. Shine the light in one eye for 3 seconds, then move the other for the same interval. Repeat as needed but do not spend longer on one eye than the other as this can bleach the retina and cause an artificial RAPD. If the right optic nerve is damaged, shining the light in the right eye will produce a normal efferent response in the left and right pupil. Moving to the right eye then causes a paradoxical dilation of both pupils as the stimulus is effectively diminished. A patient may tell you the light seems dimmer.

Anaesthetics & Critical Care

Case 1

Anaesthetic pre-assessment OSCE : Hernia repair

Task:	Achieved	Not Achieved
Introduces self & establishes rapport		
Clarifies planned procedure and indication		
Asks about previous anaesthetics		
Takes a medical history – cardiovascular/ respiratory/ systemic enquiry		
Asks about cardio-respiratory fitness/exercise tolerance		
Asks about acid reflux		
Asks about fasting status (solids & liquids)		
Takes a drug history including allergies		
Takes a social history (smoking/alcohol/illegal drugs)		
Takes a family history (including problems with general anaesthesia)		
Clarifies details of previous anaesthetic – was operation completed successfully, was patient woken up before surgery started, any awake fibreoptic intubation or tracheostomy, was he admitted to ICU?		
Seeks signs/symptoms suggestive of Obstructive Sleep Apnea – snoring, apneas, somnolence, obesity, hypertension.		
Performs a basic airway assessment (mouth opening/mallampati score/neck movement)		
Assesses dentition/asks about caps, crowns or implants		
Addresses patients concerns/answers questions		
Explains concerns about possible risks of general anaesthetic in understandable language		
Summarises case to examiner		
Identifies past history of difficult intubation		
Identifies need to discuss with senior and obtain previous anaesthetic chart		
Can suggest awake fibreoptic intubation and/or avoiding GA entirely by using a neuroaxial/regional technique.		
Examiner's Global Mark	/5	
Actor / Helper's Global Mark	/5	
Total Station Mark	/30	

Learning Points

The incidence of "failed intubation" is quoted as 1 in 1-2000 anaesthetics, and the more serious situation of "can't intubate can't ventilate" occurs in fewer than 1 in 5000 anaesthetics.

The ability to provide oxygen is far more important than being able to place an endotracheal tube, so an assessment of how easy it will be to ventilate the patient with a bag and mask is as important as assessing the likely ease of intubation.

If a patient is known to be a difficult intubation, the surgery could be performed, if appropriate, under spinal anaesthetic or regional nerve block. Alternatively, if an endotracheal tube is required it could be placed while the patient is still awake using a fibreoptic endoscope – Awake Fibreoptic Intubation.

Case 2

Anaesthetic pre-assessment OSCE - Patient with ischaemic heart disease presenting for elective surgery

Task:	Achieved	Not Achieved
Introduces self & establishes rapport		
Clarifies planned procedure		
Asks about previous anaesthetics		
Takes a medical history – cardiovascular/respiratory/systemic enquiry		
Elicits history of myocardial infarction and 2 coronary stents		
Asks about cardio-respiratory fitness/exercise tolerance		
Asks about recent follow up/investigations		
Asks about palpitations/loss of consciousness		
Asks about signs of cardiac failure		
Takes a drug history including allergies		
Takes a social history (smoking/alcohol)		
Performs a basic airway assessment (mouth opening/mallampati score/neck movement)		
Explains concerns about mildly elevated risks of general anaesthetic for patients with stable, optimised cardiac disease		
Addresses patients concerns/answers questions and offers a consultation with a senior anaesthetist		
Summarises case to examiner		
Identifies clinical picture of stable, optimised ischaemic heart disease		
Asks to see baseline observations		
Asks for a full blood count and U+E analysis		
Asks to see a recent ECG		
Knows that elective surgery should be postponed if patient has new/worsening angina		
Examiner's Global Mark	/5	
Actor / Helper's Global Mark	/5	
Total Station Mark	/30	

Learning Points

Ischaemic heart disease is a risk factor for complications during and after general anaesthesia. Cardiac conditions that are associated with the highest perioperative risk are:

Acute cardiac failure
Recent MI (<30 days ago)
Unstable angina
Arrhythmia
Symptomatic valvular disease

As well as patient factors, the perioperative risk is also related to the type of surgical procedure. High risk surgeries include supra-inguinal vascular, intra-thoracic and intra-abdominal procedures.

Asking about exercise tolerance is an extremely important screening tool. When trying to quantify a patient's perioperative risk, we usually express exercise tolerance in terms of 'metabolic equivalents' - or MET. 1 MET is defined as the oxygen consumption required to sit at rest in a chair. 4 MET is equivalent to climbing a flight of stairs and strenuous exercise is >10 MET. There is extensive evidence that an exercise tolerance of >4 MET indicates sufficient cardiorespiratory reserve to tolerate the physiological insult of undergoing general anaesthesia.

Case 3

Anaesthetic pre-assessment OSCE - Asthma with sensitivity to NSAIDs

Task:	Achieved	Not Achieved
Introduces self & establishes rapport		
Clarifies planned procedure and indication		
Asks about previous anaesthetics		
Takes a medical history – cardiovascular/respiratory/systemic enquiry		
Clarifies specific asthma history regarding emergency and critical care admissions		
Takes a drug history including allergies		
Elicits history of life-threatening reaction to diclofenac		
Asks about cardio-respiratory fitness/exercise tolerance		
Asks about acid reflux		
Asks about fasting status (solids & liquids)		
Takes a social history (smoking/alcohol/illegal drugs)		
Takes a family history (including problems with general anaesthesia)		
Performs a basic airway assessment (mouth opening/mallampati score/neck movement)		
Assesses dentition/asks about caps, crowns or implants		
Addresses patients concerns/answers questions		
Able to reassure patient NSAIDs are recorded as an allergy on the patient record		
Explains concerns about possible risks of general anaesthetic in understandable language		
Summarises case to examiner		
Can identify other NSAID agents (e.g., ibuprofen, parecoxib) as potential triggers		
Mentions use of peak flow measurement, pulse oximetry and chest radiograph as potential investigations		
Examiner's Global Mark	/5	
Actor / Helper's Global Mark	/5	
Total Station Mark	/30	

Learning Points

Up to 25% of individuals with asthma may suffer from NSAID-induced wheeze, it is essential to specifically enquire about previous NSAID usage in asthmatics.

The British Thoracic Society produces guidelines for the step-wise pharmacological treatment for asthma. Treatment with oral bronchodilator agents (leukotriene antagonists such as montelukast or methylxanthines such as aminophylline) should alert you to those patients with more 'brittle' asthma.

Multiple inhalers exist for patients with asthma and chronic obstructive pulmonary disease (COPD). It is helpful to learn which colour inhaler matches which therapy to aid you taking a drug history.

Case 4
Data interpretation OSCE – Waveform Capnography Analysis

Task	Achieved	Not Achieved
Introduces self.		
Establishes student ODP's baseline knowledge.		
Explains that capnography demonstrates how CO2 partial pressure changes over the respiratory cycle. Demonstrates inspiration and expiration on graph.		
Used to confirm correct placement of endo-tracheal tube.		
Used to demonstrate the adequacy of ventilation		
Used in cardiac arrest to assess adequacy of cardiopulmonary resuscitation or return of spontaneous circulation.		
Waveform One – identifies normal waveform.		
Waveform Two – identifies obstructive waveform.		
Waveform Two – suggests causes include equipment problems e.g. kinking or blockage of ETT/Airway Device and pathological causes e.g. COPD, bronchospasm, laryngospasm.		
Waveform Two – actions include checking patency of airway device and circuit, and examining patient for signs of upper and lower airway obstruction.		
Waveform Three – identifies sudden loss of cardiac output		
Waveform Three – suggests cause is cardiac arrest, or massive PE.		
Waveform Three – actions include looking for signs of life, instituting resuscitation, identifying and correcting reversible causes.		
Waveform Four – identifies spontaneous respiratory effort against ventilator.		
Waveform Four – causes include insufficient neuromuscular blockade, increased painful stimuli, insufficient depth of anaesthesia.		
Waveform Four – actions include administering further neuromuscular blockade/analgesia/anaesthetic, or assessing if appropriate to allow spontaneous breathing.		
Waveform Five – identifies likely disconnection in breathing circuit or capnography line.		
Waveform Five – check that airway device still in-situ, look for and correct disconnection in circuit or monitoring.		
Presents information in structured manner.		
Checks student's understanding, allows opportunity for questions.		
Examiner's global mark	/5	
Actor's global mark	/5	
Total station mark	/30	

Learning Points

End-tidal CO2 monitoring, or Capnography, is essential to anaesthetic practice; it confirms correct placement of an endotracheal tube, and allows us to assess the adequacy of ventilation.

End-tidal CO2 monitoring also gives information about the adequacy of cardiac output, and can detect low output states or sudden events such as a PE or Cardiac Arrest.

Abnormalities in the capnography trace can arise from a clinical problem, e.g. COPD or bronchospasm, or from an equipment issue i.e. kinking of the endotracheal tube. A systematic review of both patient and breathing circuit is required to identify and correct the problem.

Case 5
Data interpretation OSCE - Arterial blood gas analysis

Task:	Achieved	Not Achieved
Verifies this is a arterial blood gas from the correct patient at the correct time		
Identifies acidaemia		
Identifies hypoxia		
Identifies hypocapnia		
Identifies a metabolic/lactic acidosis		
Identifies normal sodium and chloride level		
Identifies mildly elevated haemoglobin level		
Identifies raised A-a gradient		
Identifies Type 1 respiratory failure		
Identifies concurrent metabolic acidosis with partial respiratory compensation		
Gives sensible differential diagnoses (e.g. infection, bronchospasm, PE, pneumothorax)		
States they would take a history and examine the patient		
States they would obtain baseline physiological observations		
States they would titrate oxygen to obtain a SpO$_2$ of ≥94%		
Would order tests directed towards their differential diagnoses (Accept any 2 of: CXR, CT-PA, urinary pneumococcal antigen, atypical screen, HIV test, baseline biochemistry, sputum and blood cultures)		
Recognises that the patient is unwell and asks for senior help		
Treats consolidation with antibiotics and can name an appropriate antibiotic regimen e.g. co-amoxiclav and clarithromycin. Stating 'I would check the hospital guidelines for community acquired pneumonia is acceptable'.		
States that the pCO$_2$ would rise and the pH would fall if the patient was tiring		
States that lactic acidosis is treated with a fluid bolus		
States expected PO2 50kPa (accept 45-52 kPa)		
Examiner's Global Mark	/5	
Actor / Helper's Global Mark	/5	
Total station mark	/30	

Learning Points

Although blood gas analysis is important, it should never supplant taking a history and performing a thorough examination.

Have a systematic approach to interpretation of blood gases

> Is the pH normal?
> Is the pO$_2$ adequate?
> Determine the respiratory component (pCO$_2$)
> Determine the metabolic component (HCO$_3$, Base excess)

In a young, otherwise healthy individual, a normal pO$_2$ on air is 13.6 kPa. A low pO$_2$ (e.g. the 10kPa seen in this case) despite supplementary oxygen is concerning and indicates a raised alveolar-arterial (A-a) gradient, the commonest cause of which is V:Q mismatch. As a simple rule of thumb, the arterial pO2 should be about 10 less than the inspired oxygen concentration. This difference is physiological and represents the addition of water vapour (humidification) and mixing with alveolar CO2.

Case 6
Data interpretation OSCE – ABG Analysis

Task	Achieved	Not Achieved
Introduces self		
Confirms patient details		
Confirms date and time of sample		
Comments on the pH and level of acidity		
Comments on oxygenation		
Determines any respiratory component		
Determines the metabolic component		
Comments on hyperglycaemia		
Outlines primary disturbance – severe metabolic acidosis		
States the presence of partial respiratory compensation		
Suggests diagnosis – Diabetic ketoacidosis		
Mentions other investigations – blood or urinary ketones, tests for possible precipitating cause		
Mentions A-E approach in initial resuscitation of patient		
Suggests initial management plan – fluid replacement and insulin,		
Outlines importance of regular blood glucose and pH monitoring		
Discusses potassium replacement		
Suggests definitive management – diabetes control, treatment of any underlying conditions		
States other causes of metabolic acidosis		
Presents data in structured manner		
Sensible approach to management of DKA		
Examiner's global mark	/5	
Actor's global mark	/5	
Total station mark	/30	

Learning Points

Having a clear structure when analysing data is important in helping process relevant information, especially in high-pressure situations. However obvious the abnormalities on a piece of data may seem, always stick to your chosen system to ensure you don't miss other concurrent issues.

Arterial blood gases are invaluable in providing essential information about patient physiology in emergency circumstances as well as useful monitoring tools. Becoming familiar with interpreting them will greatly improve clinical practice.

Metabolic acidosis is usually a medical emergency. The A-E approach in managing patients is critical but also be aware of the common causes and treatments.

Case 7
Critical care OSCE – Bleeding oesophageal varices

Task:	Achieved	Not Achieved
Introduces self to patient and seeks permission to perform assessment		
Takes focused history of acute problem – offensive black stools, asks about haematemesis		
Brief past medical and drug history including allergy status		
Social history, identifies excessive alcohol consumption		
Performs A to E assessment		
Picks up on clinical signs of hypovolaemia		
Recognises Upper GI Bleed as cause		
Calls for appropriate help – e.g. 2222/Major Haemorrhage call, senior doctor, ICU		
Gives 10-15L of Oxygen using non-rebreathe mask		
Establishes IV access, recognizes need for multiple sites/wide bore access		
Sends relevant blood tests including Crossmatch sample, FBC, Coag/INR, U&Es, LFTs		
Gives IV fluid bolus		
Gives O-negative blood		
Repeats A to E assessment following fluid/blood transfusion		
Requests other blood products – FFP, Platelets		
Requests IV Antibiotics and knows rationale for this		
Requests terlipressin and knows rationale for this		
Aware of need for urgent OGD		
Summarises case to examiner		
Remains calm and methodical throughout		
Examiner's Global Mark	/5	
Actor / Helper's Global Mark	/5	
Total Station Mark	/30	

Learning Points

Oesophageal varices are dilated veins, vulnerable to bleeding, which occur in patients with portal hypertension. They can be a cause of major haemorrhage.

An OGD is required to identify and treat the bleeding, which may include banding or sclerotherapy. As a last resort compression of the varices with a Sengstaken-Blakemore tube may be required but this will only be performed by senior doctors in parallel with intubation.

NICE Guidelines recommend giving terlipressin and IV Antibiotics in the acute treatment of variceal Bleeding. The former aims to reduce portal hypertension and reduce the pressure in the varices, while the latter reduces the incidence of hepatic-encephalopathy.

Case 8

Communication OSCE – Unconscious patient

Task	Achieved	Not Achieved
Ensures safe to approach, wears gloves		
Confirms patient identity and asks for background information		
Requests appropriate help (e.g. periarrest team/Medical Emergency Team call)		
Checks for signs of life - rules out cardiac arrest		
Checks physiological observations/attaches monitoring		
Airway assessment – confirms airway patency by looking, listening and feeling		
Breathing assessment – including application of high flow oxygen		
Circulation assessment – including intravenous access and blood tests		
Disability assessment – checks consciousness level and blood glucose		
Immediately treats hypoglycaemia using intravenous Dextrose (e.g. 100ml 20% dextrose then reassesses patient)		
Exposure - looking for rashes, injuries etc		
States will continually reassess conscious level and recheck capillary glucose after treatment		
Reviews patient notes and charts for further history – states medications to be reviewed		
Discusses with appropriate seniors – states will consider ITU if remains unconscious		
Identifies oral glucose gel & IM glucagon as additional treatments of hypoglycaemia		
States capillary glucose range of 6-10mmol/l for critically ill patients		
Gives concise and accurate summary		
Suggests definitive management for hypoglycaemia including regular blood sugar monitoring		
Systematic assessment of patient		
Professional approach to managing patient		
Examiner's global mark	/5	
Actor's global mark	/5	
Total station mark	/30	

Learning Points

The causes of a depressed conscious level are numerous - a structured A-E approach is essential to ensure that no reversible causes are missed! Remember 'DEFG' stands for 'Don't Ever Forget Glucose'!

Identification and immediate correction of abnormal physiology is a core part of the A-E assessment. Early reassessment after initiating an intervention is essential in both the OSCE and real life clinical scenarios.

Abnormalities of plasma blood glucose levels commonly accompany critical illness. The 'stress response' is associated with insulin resistance and hyperglycaemia, but the patient may also become hypoglycaemic if they receive hypoglycaemic agents when they are not eating properly. A variable rate intravenous insulin infusion ('sliding-scale') will ensure that the patient has their blood sugar checked regularly and that their insulin doses match their requirements.

Case 9
Critical care OSCE – Amitriptyline Overdose

Task:	Achieved	Not Achieved
Introduces self to patient/assistant and seeks permission to perform assessment		
Seeks further history, recognizes potential for amitriptyline overdose		
Performs A to E assessment		
Recognises partial airway obstruction		
Correctly performs simple airway manoeuvres		
Correctly sizes and inserts an oropharyngeal or nasopharyngeal airway		
Requests assistance i.e. anaesthetics/ICU to manage airway		
Gives 10-15L of Oxygen using non-rebreathe mask		
Establishes IV access		
Requests appropriate blood tests including paracetamol/salicylate levels		
Administers IV Fluids		
Requests and correctly interprets ABG		
Requests and correctly interprets 12 Lead ECG		
Seeks further information regarding tricyclic poisoning from poisons advice service (eg NPIS/Toxbase)		
Requests Sodium Bicarbonate infusion, or aware that this may be appropriate		
States need for ICU admission		
Reassesses after interventions		
Summarises case to examiner		
Can describe the signs and symptoms associated with tricyclic overdose		
Remains calm and methodical throughout		
Examiner's Global Mark	/5	
Actor / Helper's Global Mark	/5	
Total Station Mark	/30	

Learning Points

Tricyclic antidepressants such as Amitriptyline are dangerous in overdose. Their anticholinergic effects lead to tachycardia, pupillary dilatation, urinary retention, dry mouth and sedation; sodium and calcium channel blockade causes myocardial toxicity, with conduction delays producing broad QRS complexes and ventricular arrhythmias; alpha-receptor blockade causes hypotension.

Management of tricyclic overdose is largely supportive, but the administration of Sodium Bicarbonate can be useful, as it reverses the metabolic acidosis. A more alkaline pH increases the amount of amitriptyline bound to plasma proteins and hence reduces the amount of free drug available to exert its effects. It may also reverse the direct myocardial effects.

In any suspected poisoning, the National Poisons Information Service can provide useful information via their Toxbase website or telephone line. Toxicology is rarely a service that hospitals have on site so it is essential to utilise their online resources and print out the recommendations to remain in the patient notes.

Case 10
Critical care OSCE – Status epilepticus

Task:	Achieved	Not Achieved
Identifies self to team		
Mentions initial assessment of ABCDE		
States would attempt airway manoeuvres (head-tilt, chin-lift)		
Requests airway adjunct (e.g., nasopharyngeal airway)		
Requests suction		
Ensures high flow oxygen administration		
Mentions measurement of blood glucose		
Ensures adequate intravenous access		
Clarifies timing of onset of seizures		
Clarifies customary anti-epileptic drugs and treatment initiated so far		
Checks allergy status		
Requests administration of IV lorazepam		
Offers dosage of IV lorazepam (0.1mg/kg, up to 4mg)		
Requests intravenous loading dose of phenytoin (dosage of phenytoin not required to be known (15 – 18 mg/kg)		
Declares diagnosis of status epilepticus		
Able to name subsequent pharmacological agents for persistent seizures (phenobarbitaone, thiopentone)		
Calls for senior help / medical emergency team		
Summarises finding back to examiner		
Indicates potential need for escalation - general anaesthetic / intensive care		
Able to identify potential causes for seizure onset (e.g., infection, antibiotic interaction)		
Examiner's Global Mark	/5	
Actor / Helper's Global Mark	/5	
Total Station Mark	/30	

Learning Points

Patients with epilepsy frequently present to hospital with acute illnesses, often unrelated to their disease. Common triggers for seizures include missed anti-epileptic drug doses, poor compliance with medication, alcohol use, infection, and drug interactions. It is particularly important to check for interactions when prescribing acutely as certain medications can reduce seizure threshold (in this case, a quinolone).

The definition of status epilepticus traditionally required seizures to persist for longer than 20-30 minutes or for patients to have further seizures without returning to full consciousness in between fits. This is now evolving to recognise that most seizure episodes will terminate spontaneously within 2 – 3 minutes. Therefore, generalised tonic-clonic seizures lasting beyond 5 minutes may represent status epilepticus and require early proactive treatment.

The majority of hospitals will adhere to advanced life support seizure algorithms, however As epilepsy pharmacotherapy advances, newer agents (for example, levetiracetam) are likely to be incorporated into these treatment algorithms in place of older drugs (that are associated with significant side effects). It is important to remain up to date with current specialist guidance. Known epileptics may also have bespoke management plans in place.

Case 11
Critical care OSCE – Septic shock

Task:	Achieved	Not Achieved
Introduces self		
Briefly clarifies presenting history		
Briefly clarifies past medical history		
Assesses patient using an ABCDE approach		
Requests high flow oxygen administration		
Requests current vital observations (PR, RR, BP, SpO2)		
Requests blood glucose level		
Requests serum lactate level		
Requests further IV fluid bolus (up to 30ml/kg) to assess BP response		
Requests urinary catheterisation and monitoring of fluid balance		
Requests peripheral blood culture samples		
Indicates requirement for urgent administration of broad spectrum IV antibiotics		
Specifically checks patient allergy status prior to commencing IV antibiotics		
Clear communication style		
States would seek for senior help		
Able to name 'Sepsis Six' initiative		
Summarises findings and likely diagnosis back to examiner		
Able to name investigations associated with Sepsis Six (lactate, BP & MAP, blood cultures)		
Able to name therapies associated with Sepsis Six (fluid boluses, IV antibiotics, vasopressors)		
Aware of requirement for critical care for patients with septic shock		
Examiner's Global Mark	/5	
Actor / Helper's Global Mark	/5	
Total Station Mark	/30	

Learning Points

Sepsis is a potentially life-threatening syndrome resulting from the body's maladaptive response to infection. Alterations in microvasculature and perfusion result in shock and can progress to multi-organ failure if not recognized and treated early. In the UK around 40 000 deaths annually are attributable to sepsis.

In the UK the Surviving Sepsis Campaign, the UK sepsis Trust and the NICE sepsis guidelines have devised sepsis algorithms based on early warning scores. 'Care bundle' exist of the six evidence-based interventions that need to be completed in a finite time window from presentation, with the aim of preventing progression of the condition.

Early Warning Score systems to track unwell patients help to identify those at risk of developing sepsis. These may well include a 'trigger' for in-hospital referral to critical care services to achieve appropriate higher level care, such as vasopressor drugs and invasive monitoring.

Case 12
Critical care OSCE - Anaphylaxis

Task:	Achieved	Not Achieved
Introduces self to patient		
Briefly clarifies history of acute problem		
Briefly clarifies past medical and drug history		
Enquires about allergy status		
Performs ABCDE assessment		
Picks up on clinical signs - lip swelling, wheeze, hypotension, tachycardia, flushing/rash		
Recognises and verbalises diagnosis of anaphylaxis		
Escalates early and calls for appropriate help eg 2222 , senior doctor/ anaesthetist		
Administers IM adrenaline 500mcg		
Gives 10-15L of Oxygen using non-rebreathe mask		
Seeks precipitants - asks patient, nursing staff, looks at drug chart		
Stops IV Flucloxacillin immediately		
Gives 500-1000ml Crystalloid bolus		
Requests 200mg IV Hydrocortisone		
Requests 10mg IV Chlorphenamine		
Recognises deterioration and repeats ABCDE assessment		
States the need to repeat IM adrenaline after 5 minutes		
Summarises case to examiner		
Aware of need for ongoing treatment on ICU		
Aware of need for drug error incident reporting		
Examiner's Global Mark	/5	
Actor / Helper's Global Mark	/5	
Total Station Mark	/30	

Learning Points

Anaphylaxis is a severe, life-threatening, systemic hypersensitivity reaction. It causes a rapidly evolving compromise of the airway, breathing and circulation. Skin changes, e.g. urticarial rash, flushing or mucosal swelling, are absent in 20% of cases.

The most important treatment is adrenaline, which treats vasodilatation and bronchoconstriction, and also stabilises mast cells. The correct adult dose is 0.5ml of 1:1000 (500mcg) administered IM. The ideal site of administration is the middle third of the thigh, along the anterolateral border.

Mast Cell Tryptase levels confirm a diagnosis of anaphylaxis. Ideally 3 samples should be taken: during resuscitation; 1-2 hours after the onset of symptoms; and 24 hours later.

Case 13
Critical care OSCE - Severe hyponatraemia

Task:	Achieved	Not Achieved
Introduces self to patient + daughter and establishes rapport		
Briefly clarifies history from daughter and patient		
Assesses airway		
Assesses breathing (RR/inspection/palpation/ percussion/auscultation/SpO$_2$)		
Assesses circulation (HR/BP/CRT/3 lead ECG monitoring)		
Assesses conscious level- GCS or AVPU - notes V on AVPU		
Checks for external signs of head trauma		
Checks blood glucose		
Notes that all 4 limbs are moving		
Checks peripheral reflexes including plantar response		
Checks for neck stiffness		
Checks pupillary light reflexes		
Checks temperature		
Identifies hyponatraemia on venous blood gas		
Re Clarifies a medication history		
Explains problem of hyponatraemia		
Deals compassionately with patient and her daughter		
Escalates early to senior colleague		
Summarises case to examiner and presents a differential diagnosis (including SIADH and diuretic induced)		
Outlines treatment plan (correction of hyponatraemia with hypertonic saline in monitored environment)		
Examiner's Global Mark	/5	
Actor / Helper's Global Mark	/5	
Total Station Mark	/30	

Learning Points

A systematic approach is essential when assessing a patient with an abnormal conscious level - there are numerous potential causes especially in patients with multiple comorbidities and many of which are easily overlooked!

Hyponatraemia usually has multiple causes with SIADH and drug induced (especially diuretics) the commonest. It is important to know a list of potential causes based upon the patient's fluid status, serum and urinary osmolarities and urinary sodium levels.

In severe, symptomatic hyponatraemia (as in this case), raising the serum sodium by 4 to 6 mmol/L with hypertonic saline (e.g. 2.7% NaCl, 2ml/kg) should generally reduce symptoms and prevent cerebral herniation. Correction to a 'normal' level can then take place slowly over the next couple of days. Needless to say, senior help is essential!

Case 14
Critical care OSCE - choking

Task:	Achieved	Not Achieved
Introduces self		
Assesses airway by talking to the patient		
Correctly identifies patient has partial airway obstruction with an effective cough		
Encourages cough		
Recognises complete airway obstruction signified by silent cough		
Identifies patient is deteriorating and acts swiftly		
Calls for help / cardiac arrest call initiated		
Administers back blow before abdominal thrust		
Correctly administers 5 back blows		
Reassesses to see if back blow have cleared airway obstruction		
Recognises need for further treatment when airway obstruction persists		
Correctly administers 5 abdominal thrusts		
Reassesses to see if abdominal thrusts have cleared airway obstruction		
Repeats cycle of back blows and abdominal thrusts while patient remains conscious		
Checks for signs of life when patient appears to lose consciousness		
Diagnoses cardiac arrest and calls arrest team/2222		
Performs CPR 30:2 with help from nurse		
Proceeds through algorithm swiftly and calmly		
Question 1 - knows that foreign body should only be removed under direct vision/laryngoscopy by appropriately trained person		
Question 2 - knows that a surgical airway is a technique to restore oxygenation in this situation		
Examiner's Global Mark	/5	
Actor / Helper's Global Mark	/5	
Total Station Mark	/30	

Learning Points

Recognising signs of airway obstruction is a crucial skill. Remember, a partially obstructed airway is noisy. This noise is caused by turbulent air flowing past the obstruction e.g. stridor. Most concerning is if the patient with airway obstruction is silent - this means no air is moving and the patient has total airway obstruction. This must be relieved immediately or the patient will quickly go on to have a hypoxic cardiac arrest.

Never try to manually remove a foreign body in a patient who is choking. An appropriately skilled individual may be able to retrieve the object with suction or forceps under direct vision using a laryngoscope. To do this safely, the patient must be either anaesthetised or unconscious.

In situations where an airway cannot be established via the mouth or nose, Anaesthetists are trained to access the airway surgically by performing a cricothyroidotomy.

Case 15
Critical care OSCE: Cardiac Arrest

Task:	Achieved	Not Achieved
Looks for danger		
Checks patient for response		
Look, listens and feels for breathing for <10 sec		
Simultaneously feels carotid <10 sec		
Confirms cardiac arrest and calls for resuscitation team (2222)		
Starts chest compressions at 100-120/min at depth of 5-6cm		
Asks nurse to attach defibrillator pads whilst continuing CPR		
Asks nurse to ventilate patient with a bag valve mask (30:2)		
Pauses CPR to assess rhythm briefly		
Correctly identifies VF		
Charges defibrillator		
Clear command to stand clear and remove oxygen		
Delivers shock safely		
Resume CPR immediately for 2 mins then reassess		
Identifies PEA and administers adrenaline 1mg IV/IO immediately		
Continues CPR for 2 mins then reassess		
Identifies sinus rhythm Checks for pulse to confirm ROSC		
Summarises findings to examiner		
Identifies reversible causes with 'thrombus' most likely		
Examiner's Global Mark	/5	
Actor / Helper's Global Mark	/5	
Total Station Mark	/30	

Learning Points:

It is important to be able to deliver high quality chest compressions with minimal interruptions as this can significantly influence outcome. Performing compressions is tiring so no one person should ever do more than one cycle in a row where personnel allow for regular rotation. A key time to remember this is once the rhythm has been confirmed as shockable chest compressions should be restarted and continue while the defibrillator is charging.

Look for reversible causes and treat early – remember 4H's and 4T's of Hypoxia, Hypovolaemia, Hypo/Hyper electrolytaemia, hypothermia and Tension pneumothorax, tamponade, Toxins and Thrombus. Each cause should be considered and excluded fully.

Use an ABCDE approach immediately following ROSC and ensure necessary investigations are carried out to identify and treat precipitating causes. High quality of care must be sustained before safe transfer to critical care facility.

Case 16
Critical care OSCE - Spinal cord injury

Task:	Achieved	Not Achieved
Introduces self & establishes rapport		
Briefly clarifies history		
Feels hands and pulse		
Asks for pulse rate and blood pressure		
Checks conscious level		
Asks about pain		
Checks pupils		
Assesses limb tone		
Assesses sensation of limbs and torso - identifies sensory level at T4		
Assesses limb motor function		
Assesses limb reflexes		
Examines abdomen		
Visually inspects long bones/pelvis		
Asks for temperature/glucose		
Responds to patient's concerns appropriately		
Gives patient honest explanation without colluding		
Summarises case to examiner		
States would log roll and assess back/neck/sphincter tone		
Suggests CT or MRI for further investigation		
Can outline pathophysiology of spinal cord injury		
Examiner's Global Mark	/5	
Actor / Helper's Global Mark	/5	
Total Station Mark	/30	

Learning Points

An injury to the spinal cord above T6 may lead to interruption of the sympathetic chain and gives the characteristic cardiovascular picture of bradycardia and hypotension known as neurogenic shock. Paralysis of the intercostal muscles leads to a diaphragmatic breathing pattern. It is important not to mix this diagnosis up with the term 'spinal shock'.

After completion of the primary survey, urgent imaging is required to identify the lesion and, if appropriate, direct surgical intervention.

Decreased organ perfusion may lead to organ failure so early recognition and treatment is essential. Judicious fluids, atropine and vasopressor therapy may all be indicated.

Case 17
Communication OSCE – Analgesia for labour

Task:	Achieved	Not Achieved
Introduces self and establishes rapport		
Starts with open questions and allows the patient to talk		
Listens actively and shows empathy		
Clarifies patient's specific concerns about childbirth		
Explores patient's understanding of pain relief available for labour		
Elicits patient's particular concerns about epidurals		
Explains that there are several options available for pain relief – tailored to each patient's needs		
Mentions simple analgesia (paracetamol)		
Mentions gas and air/entonox		
Mentions other pain relief like TENS and water birthing		
Addresses patient's specific concerns about epidural analgesia		
States that epidurals are a very safe technique but acknowledges possible risks		
States that epidural analgesia is the most effective pain relief for labour		
States that epidurals do not increase the risk of caesarian section		
Explains that serious complications of epidurals are very rare		
Offers information leaflet about pain relief during labour		
Offers to refer to a senior anaesthetist if she would like further discussion		
Answers patient's questions in simple language		
Asks about birthing partner and family support		
Summarises findings and options to the examiner		
Examiner's Global Mark	/5	
Actor / Helper's Global Mark	/5	
Total Station Mark	/30	

Learning Points

There are numerous ways to provide analgesia for labour, ranging from breathing exercises, massage and family support, to epidurals. No single method is right for every woman and all labour experiences are unique. As healthcare professionals, our job is to provide accurate information that allows our patient's to make informed decisions.

There remains controversy about epidurals for labour and misinformation about the potential risks is often found online or through child birthing groups. It is a difficult subject in which to design clinical trials and so data is limited, however, what data are available suggest that there is no increased risk of caesarian section after epidurals, though the rate of instrumental delivery may be slightly higher.

The Obstetric Anaesthetist's association (OAA) provide excellent information leaflets for pregnant women and healthcare professionals which are freely available online (www.labourpains.com).

Case 18
Communication OSCE - Explaining anaesthetics drugs

Task:	Achieved	Not Achieved
Introduces self & establishes rapport		
Identifies learning needs of student		
Correctly identifies propofol & thiopental as 'hypnotics'/'induction agents'		
Correctly identifies morphine & fentanyl as 'opiates'		
Explains that morphine is longer acting than fentanyl		
Explains that fentanyl is more potent/stronger than morphine		
Identifies suxamethonium & rocuronium as muscle relaxants		
Explains briefly the difference between depolarizing and non-depolarizing agents		
Identifies ondansatron & cyclizine as antiemetics		
Identifies metaraminol & ephedrine as sympathomemmetics (accept 'drugs that increase the blood pressure)		
Explains that metaraminal & ephedrine act on alpha and beta receptors to have their effect		
Identifies atropine & glycopyrollate as vagolytics/drugs to increase heart rate		
Explains that these drugs block the action of the vagus nerve		
Identifies lidocaine & laevobupivicaine as local anaesthetics		
Explains that these drugs block nerve transmission by blocking sodium channels		
Specifies that local anaesthetics are given by subcutaneous injection or deposited around nerves		
Gives correct definition of 'balanced anaesthesia' (including anaesthesia/analgesia/muscle relaxation)		
Corrects misconception - explains use of volatile/intravenous agents to maintain anaesthesia		
Information pitched and paced appropriately		
Answers students questions clearly		
Examiner's Global Mark	/5	
Actor/Helper's Global Mark	/5	
Total Station Mark	/30	

Learning points:

A working knowledge of the drugs used in Anaesthesia is useful for all clinicians, especially if you are called upon to assist with the Anaesthetic care of a critically ill patient on the ward or in the Emergency Department - the Anaesthetist is bound to be very grateful for the extra help and it is important for you to known and understand what drugs your patient is having and the ongoing effects they will have on them.

Induction of general anaesthesia usually involves administration of an intravenous induction agent in combination with a short acting opiate like fentanyl. This combination produces rapid loss of consciousness and obtunds the laryngeal reflexes sufficiently to allow instrumentation of the airway. Muscle relaxants are typically added in order to facilitate endotracheal intubation.

Before conducting any anaesthetic the Anaesthetist will always prepare their emergency drugs, which must always be readily to hand in order to manage life threatening complications like hypotension, bradycardia or airway obstruction.

Case 19
Communication OSCE – Explaining conscious sedation

Task	Achieved	Not Achieved
Introduces self		
Confirms patient's name and date of birth		
Asks about prior knowledge		
Identifies and addresses patient's concerns		
Explains conscious sedation – informing patient that he will not be intentionally put to sleep but may be drowsy and responsive		
Explains indication for conscious sedation – relaxant and analgesic effect		
Informs patient about fasting		
Asks about medical history, drugs and allergies		
States medication may be given intravenously or intramuscularly		
Explains drugs used are quick-acting and last for short time after procedure		
Discusses risks of conscious sedation – allergic reaction, respiratory depression, hypotension		
Explains patient will be monitored whilst sedated and during recovery		
Briefly discusses process of OGD		
Explains patient should be able to go home soon afterwards		
States patient may return to normal activities the next day		
Ensures patient understands explanation		
Informs patient not to drive or engage in high risk activities for at least 24 hours		
Uses clear sentences, avoiding medical jargon		
Summarises discussion to the examiner		
Answers examiner's question		
Examiner's global mark	/5	
Actor's global mark	/5	
Total station mark	/30	

Learning Points

It is essential to have good knowledge of common procedures in medicine as well as how to explain them simply but thoroughly to patients. Practicing speaking without the use of medical jargon can go a long way in effectively communicating with patients. In particular be careful with the use of abbreviations that seem second nature to you but may cause confusion to the patient.

Post procedure instructions should not be neglected as they are often relevant, particularly so in this case where the patient must be advised against driving till the next day. Verbal instructions can often be forgotten so giving written instruction advice is often a recommended adjunct to your discussions.

Identifying the ideas, concerns and expectations of patients is important in directing the consultation, as information needed may not be what is assumed.

Case 20
Communication OSCE – Teaching midwife about spinal anaesthetic

Task:	Achieved	Not Achieved
Introduces self & establishes rapport		
Clarifies identity of midwifery student		
Explains rationale for spinal anaesthetic		
Describes process of siting spinal anaesthetic (positioning, identify level)		
Outlines common drugs used in spinal anaesthetic (local anaesthetic and opiate/strong pain killer)		
Outlines potential problems of GA for LSCS (fetal benefits, aspiration risk)		
Outlines benefits of spinal anaesthetic for elective LSCS (awake patient, partner presence, DVT)		
Explains some differences between spinal and epidural block (needle choice, catheter)		
Acknowledges importance of patient choice and consent for anaesthetic technique		
Indicates requirement for IV cannula		
Indicates requirement for monitoring (ECG, BP, SpO2)		
Indicates requirement for sterility of procedure		
Indicates requirement for presence of a trained assistant		
Indicates requirement for checking blood results (platelets, clotting) prior to commencing		
Indicates requirement to check patient allergy status prior to commencing		
States would ask for senior help in an emergency		
Uses clear language and terminology appropriate for seniority of student		
Clarifies understanding at intervals and doesn't get frustrated at questions from student		
Summarises back to examiner		
Answers questions from examiner in an orderly manner		
Examiner's Global Mark	/5	
Actor / Helper's Global Mark	/5	
Total Station Mark	/30	

Learning Points

Spinal anesthesia is a standard technique in obstetric anaesthesia, and is commonly used for a range of procedures on labour ward. It reduces the risk of DVT and blood loss compared to general anaesthetic, and when used for Caesarean section allows the mother to be conscious and partner to be present at the moment of delivery.

As doctors we frequently encounter different members of the multidisciplinary team, covering a range of specialties and seniority. Remember that communication skills between professionals are just as important as those with patients. Miscommunication is a common source of error.

Using the format of "chunks and checks" can be a helpful tool to ensure effective communication when teaching colleagues or describing procedures to patients. Split up the information into sections and confirm understanding before moving on. Remember you don't have to teach everything in one go and setting realistic and achievable learning objectives for the session will lead to a more enjoyable experience for both teacher and learner.

Case 21
Clinical skills OSCE: Oxygen delivery devices

Task:	Achieved	Not Achieved
Introduces self and establishes learning environment		
1) Can define atmospheric O_2 concentration (21%)		
2) Correctly identifies nasal cannulae		
3) States delivers ~ 28% O_2 at 2 L/min		
4) States delivers ~ 38% O_2 at 6 L/min		
5) Correctly identifies Hudson mask		
6) States delivers ~50% O_2 at 6 L/min		
7) Correctly identifies reservoir / non-rebreathe mask		
8) States delivers ~ 90% O_2 at 15 L/min		
9) States valve held down to inflate reservoir before applying to the patient		
10) Correctly identifies Venturi mask		
11) States FiO_2 delivery of Venturi attachments		
12) States specific oxygen flow rate determines FiO_2		
13) States Venturi flow rate can be found on collar of adapter (also accept: packaging)		
14) Fixed performance device: Venturi mask only		
Elaborates advantages / disadvantages for devices		
Scenario 1: Nasal cannulae selected		
Scenario 2: Venturi mask selected		
Scenario 3: Reservoir mask selected		
Scenario 4: Hudson face mask selected		
Examiner's Global Mark	/5	
Actor / Helper's Mark	/5	
Total Station Mark	/30	

Learning Points

The amount of oxygen a patient receives using any device is dependent on a range of patient factors. Variables such as the pattern of breathing, respiratory rate, route (nasal or mouth breathing) and device tolerance can lead to wide variations in actual inspired oxygen concentrations.

As with any device or piece of medical equipment, it is important to be aware of the correct usage of oxygen delivery devices and the need to prescribe oxygen. It is also useful to be aware of their limitations. Oxygen is too important to get wrong!

The normal peak inspiratory flow rate for an adult is around 30 L/min. Most oxygen supplies (wall and cylinder) have a maximum flow rate of 15 L/min. To allow concentrations of close to 100% to be delivered to the patient, the reservoir mask supplements the shortfall from the supply. For this reason, the reservoir must be inflated before it is applied to the patient.

Case 22

Clinical skills OSCE - Management of acute post operative pain

Task:	Achieved	Not Achieved
Introduces self		
Confirms patient is in pain		
Assesses severity of pain		
Asks for/says they would check patient's observations (HR/BP/SpO2)		
Checks past medical history		
Checks drug history		
Confirms allergies		
Documents allergies on chart		
Prescribes regular paracetamol 1g QDS		
Does not prescribe an NSAID		
Prescribes appropriate regular weak opiate		
Appropriate regular dose and interval of weak opiate		
Prescribes PRN strong opiate for breakthrough pain		
Appropriate PRN dose and interval for strong opiate		
Prescribes PRN antiemetic		
Prescribes 2 different classes of antiemetic		
Prescribes Naloxone		
Prescribes PRN laxative		
Writes legibly		
Prescription signed and dated		
Examiner's Global Mark	/5	
Actor / Helper's Global Mark	/5	
Total Station Mark	/30	

Learning Points

The WHO analgesic ladder is an excellent framework for managing acute pain and is core knowledge for any new Doctor starting on the wards - go and learn it if you haven't already!

'Multi-modal analgesia' is the term we use to describe an analgesic strategy that combines multiple drugs of different classes. In combination these drugs are more effective than they would be in isolation - in this regard they are said to act 'synergistically'.

Non steroidal anti-inflammatory drugs (NSAIDs) can be extremely effective additions to your multimodal analgesic strategy. However, they are not benign substances and some of the side-effects are potentially serious. Renal impairment is a particular concern in the elderly, or in those patients with other risk factors for acute kidney injury (AKI) in whom NSAIDs are to be avoided.

Case 23
Clinical skills OSCE - Opioid Conversion

Task:	Achieved	Not Achieved
Introduces self & establishes rapport		
Verifies identity of the patient and that the drug chart is for the correct patient		
Takes a focused pain history		
Attempts to assess pain severity		
Elicits history of constipation		
Elicits history of mild nausea		
Asks about allergies		
Asks about other co-morbidities		
Asks about oral intake		
Asks about history of taking oral analgesics		
States would complete allergy section of drug chart		
Prescribes appropriate dose of modified release morphine tablets (accept 20mg – 30mg bd of MST)		
Prescribes appropriate dose of immediate release morphine for breakthrough pain (e.g. oramorph or sevredol 10-20mg 2-4 hourly).		
Explains analgesic plan to the patient		
Suggests the addition of laxatives		
Suggests the addition of antiemetics		
Highlights the potential for other analgesics to be used e.g. short term ibuprofen		
Suggests the addition of naloxone as an emergency drug		
Explains the importance of good analgesia and that regular review will be undertaken		
Summarises case to examiner and answers questions		
Examiner's Global Mark	/5	
Actor / Helper's Global Mark	/5	
Total Station Mark	/30	

Learning Points

Effective postoperative analgesia is crucial in postoperative mobilization and recovery. The responsibility for this lies not only with the anaesthetists but with the doctors looking after the patient post operatively on the ward.

Intravenous morphine can be converted to oral morphine at a ratio of 1:2-3, so that 10mg of IV morphine is equivalent to 20-30mg of oral morphine. As well as a 'maintenance' dose, a breakthrough prescription should also be completed (for adults, 10-20mg of immediate release morphine is a good starting point).

Opioids can have troublesome side effects including constipation and nausea that may themselves hinder recovery, so it's often a good idea to make sure that concurrent antimetics and laxatives are also prescribed and that the patient is warned to look out for these adverse side effects.

Case 24
Clinical skills OSCE – Checking and administering a blood transfusion

Task:	Achieved	Not Achieved
Introduces self		
Clarifies Identity of patient : Name		
Clarifies Identity of patient : Date of Birth		
Clarifies Identity of patient : Patient Number		
Cross-checks 3-point identity with prescription chart		
Cross-checks identity with blood product label		
Checks group of blood unit		
Checks expiry date of blood unit		
Performs two-person checks		
Reviews appropriate duration of administration		
Ensures suitable cannula in situ and functioning		
Ensures appropriate blood giving set available (filter giving set)		
Enquires about consent for receiving blood transfusion		
Checks for any allergies		
Visually inspects unit for damage / precipitants		
Requests / asks to review pre-transfusion observations (pulse rate, blood pressure, respiratory rate, temperature)		
Advises set of observations 15 minutes after start of transfusion		
Advises set of observations 60 minutes post-transfusion		
Aware of maximum time for blood to be out of fridge before return to blood bank when asked		
Summarises case to examiner and answers questions		
Examiner's Global Mark	/5	
Actor / Helper's Global Mark	/5	
Total Station Mark	/30	

Learning Points

Serious complications of blood transfusion are rare. Most incidents of wrong-product transfusion are related to human error; therefore, most centres employ 2-person checks of the patient identity and blood product prior to administration. Positive patient identification requires "3-point verification". This is usually full name, date of birth, and a unique identifier number.

Blood banks keep packed red cells in temperature controlled storage until they are ready to be transfused. Once units have left the blood bank they must be kept in an insulated storage box to maintain a safe temperature and have completed transfusion within a 4-hour limit. They can be returned to controlled temperature storage within 30 minutes if no longer required.

A failsafe way to avoid transfusion complications is to avoid unnecessary transfusions altogether – most hospital blood banks will produce guidelines regarding appropriate use of blood transfusion.

Case 25
Clinical skills OSCE – Airway Manoeuvres

Task:	Achieved	Not Achieved
Checks safe to approach and tries to rouse patient using shake and shout		
Calls for help – senior doctor/fast bleep anaesthetist/2222 crash call		
Correctly demonstrates head tilt/chin lift (no history of C-spine trauma)		
Correctly demonstrates jaw thrust		
Selects correct size of nasopharyngeal airway for mannequin (Size 6 or 7 most women, Size 7 or 8 most men)		
Correctly inserts nasopharyngeal airway, after applying lubricant		
Demonstrates how to size an oropharyngeal airway – flange level with incisors, tip to angle of jaw		
Selects appropriate size of oropharyngeal airway for mannequin		
Demonstrates correct insertion technique for oropharyngeal airway – careful placement, upside down until encounters resistance from hard palate, rotates 180 degrees		
Requests and applies 15L O2 with non-rebreath mask. Does not use self-inflating bag to provide oxygen while patient spontaneously breathing		
States how would assess for improvement – no more snoring, synchrony of chest and abdominal wall movements, look, listen and feel for effective breathing		
Correctly applies face mask – chin to bridge of nose covered, no pressure on eyes, correct placement of hand(s) to hold mask – C-shape with around mask, lifting mandible forward with free fingers		
Successfully uses self-inflating bag to demonstrate chest rise – can ask assistant to squeeze bag if 2 hands needed to hold mask		
Requests the self-inflating bag be connected to 15L of O2		
Demonstrates appropriate rate of ventilation – 12-16 breaths/minute		
Selects appropriate size of iGel SAD, 4 for most patients as suggested by weight range written on device		
Demonstrates correct insertion technique – opens mouth, SAD correct way up, careful insertion into mouth, firm pressure until device comes to natural stop (May ask for jaw thrust from assistant)		
Correctly attaches self-inflating bag to SAD and demonstrates adequate chest rise		
Requests appropriate monitoring – minimum SpO2 probe, others could include ECG, NIBP, End Tidal CO2		
Suggests further management options – one or more of antagonists (naloxone, flumazenil) definitive airway management by anaesthetist, HDU/ICU admission		
Examiner's Global Mark	/5	
Actor / Helper's Global Mark	/5	
Total Station Mark	/30	

Learning Points

Airway obstruction and respiratory depression can occur following sedation

A self-inflating bag contains a one-way valve, which causes high resistance to breathing and makes it unsuitable for spontaneously ventilating patients.

Supraglottic Airway Devices form a seal above the larynx, reducing gastric distension from ventilation attempts with the self-inflating bag. The second generation devices such as the iGel also allow passage of a gastric tube, allowing the emptying of stomach contents.

Orthopaedics & Rheumatology

Case 1
History taking: Shoulder – instability and dislocation

Task:	Achieved	Not Achieved
Introduces him/herself		
Clarifies who they are speaking to, establishes age		
Checks occupation		
Positions themselves at appropriate distance from patient and maintains eye contact		
Uses open questions to begin the history		
Elicits history any pain shoulder joint		
Asks about episodes of dislocation, number, mechanism of injury and method of reduction		
Asks about current neurovascular symptoms		
Asks about current ability to use the shoulder		
Enquires about exacerbating factors such as weight, overhead activity or matches		
Enquires specifically about impact on daily activities and function, including employment		
Asks about previous shoulder injuries and elicits long term problem		
Asks about past medical history		
Asks about drug history and allergies		
Asks about relevant family history		
Asks about smoking, alcohol and recreational drug use		
Elicits patient's concerns		
Summarises clinical history		
Offers diagnosis and relevant differential diagnoses		
Suggests appropriate initial investigations including blood tests and XR AP and Lateral of the shoulder, and MRI scan		
Examiner's Global Mark	/5	
Actor's Global Mark	/5	
Total Station Mark	/30	

Learning Points

Anterior shoulder dislocations are a relatively common presentation in the emergency department and it is important to ask questions which help establish whether there has been any neurovascular injury. The classical area of numbness over the lateral aspect of the deltoid is referred to as the 'Regimental badge' sign and occurs following dislocation due to stretch of the circumflex humeral nerves.

It is important to ascertain the age of the patient, the mechanism of injury and whether there have been previous episodes. After a single episode of traumatic anterior shoulder dislocation there is around 50% chance of another dislocation.

Treatment options vary and evidence is controversial. It is common practice to treat first dislocation episodes with a brief period of immobilisation in a polysling following reduction. However, some advocate further investigation with MRI scan due to the association with Bankart injuries to the labrum.

Case 2
History taking: Hip – Osteoarthritis

Task:	Achieved	Not Achieved
Introduces him/herself		
Clarifies who they are speaking to and establishes age		
Checks occupation		
Positions themselves at appropriate distance from patient and maintains eye contact		
Uses open questions to begin the history		
Elicits history of pain		
Asks about distribution		
Asks about chronology of symptoms		
Enquires about alleviating and exacerbating factors		
Enquires specifically about impact on daily activities and function, including employment		
Asks about symptoms at night		
Asks about constitutional upset (e.g. anorexia, weight loss and fevers)		
Asks about past medical history		
Asks about drug history and allergies		
Asks about relevant family history		
Asks about smoking, alcohol and recreational drug use		
Elicits patient's concerns		
Summarises clinical history		
Offers diagnosis and relevant differential diagnoses		
Suggests appropriate initial investigations including blood tests and XR AP and Lateral of the hips/ pelvis		
Examiner's Global Mark	/5	
Actor's Global Mark	/5	
Total Station Mark	/30	

Learning Points

Osteoarthritis of the hip is a common condition which has a significant impact on patient's activities of daily living and this should be reflected in your history taking. It is important to ask about independent mobility, walking aids and walking distance to understand the impact the condition has on the patient.

Osteoarthritis of the hip may occur due to secondary causes so consider asking about developmental history, previous injuries or operations or family history of hip problems. Examples include hip dysplasia, slipped upper femoral epiphysis (SUFE) or Legg-Calve-Perthes disease.

Non-operative treatment options include activity modification and weight loss, pharmacological agents for analgesia and physiotherapy. Most operative treatments include variations of arthroplasty (joint replacement).

Case 3
History taking: Hand – Carpal Tunnel Syndrome

Task:	Achieved	Not Achieved
Introduces him/herself		
Clarifies who they are speaking to and establishes age		
Checks occupation		
Positions themselves at appropriate distance from patient and maintains eye contact		
Uses open questions to begin the history		
Elicits history of pain, paresthesia and weakness		
Asks about distribution		
Asks about chronology of symptoms		
Enquires about alleviating and exacerbating factors		
Enquires specifically about impact on daily activities and function, including employment		
Asks about symptoms at night		
Asks about constitutional upset (e.g. anorexia, weight loss and fevers)		
Asks about past medical history including precipitators such as diabetes and hypothyroidism		
Asks about drug history and allergies		
Asks about relevant family history		
Asks about smoking, alcohol and recreational drug use		
Elicits patient's concerns		
Summarises clinical history		
Offers diagnosis and relevant differential diagnoses		
Suggests initial investigations including X-Ray of hands, blood tests for thyroid function, inflammatory markers and FBC, Renal and Liver profiles		
Examiner's Global Mark	/5	
Actor's Global Mark	/5	
Total Station Mark	/30	

Learning Points

When assessing a patient with potential carpal tunnel syndrome be aware of potential risk factors associated with the condition such as female gender, pregnancy, obesity, hypothyroidism, diabetes and rheumatoid arthritis.

When asking about pain always remember that apart from the classical distribution of pain and paraesthesia in the hand, patients may report some pain radiating into the forearm due to recurrent innervation.

Remember with all hand cases to ask about clumsiness and ask specific probing questions about the ability to perform activities requiring fine dexterity such as doing up short buttons or picking up coins.

Case 4

History taking: Back pain - Ankylosing Spondylitis

Task:	Achieved	Not Achieved
Introduces him/herself		
Clarifies who they are speaking to and establishes age		
Checks occupation		
Positions themselves at appropriate distance from patient and maintains eye contact		
Uses open questions to begin the history		
Elicits inflammatory pattern of lower back and buttock pain and stiffness		
Asks about chronology of symptoms		
Asks about alleviating and exacerbating factors relating to pain and stiffness		
Asks about impact on daily activities and function, including employment and recreation		
Asks about associated disease manifestations including psoriasis, inflammatory bowel disease, uveitis, Achilles tendonitis, interstitial lung disease symptoms and aortic valve disease		
Asks about peripheral arthritis, enthesitis and dactylitis		
Asks about red flag symptoms of back pain including unexplained weight loss, fevers, night sweats, neurological symptoms and bladder or bowel dysfunction		
Asks about past medical history including current drug therapy and allergies		
Asks about family history of inflammatory or autoimmune diseases		
Asks about smoking, alcohol and recreational drug use		
Elicits patient's concerns		
Summarises clinical history		
Offers diagnosis and relevant differential diagnoses		
Suggests initial investigations including MRI of spine and sacroiliac joints or Sacroiliac joint X-Ray, blood tests for inflammatory markers and FBC, Renal and Liver profiles +/- HLAB27 gene testing		
Advises a trial of an alternative anti-inflammatory medication, a physiotherapy referral and if sustained disease activity, consideration for escalating drug therapy to biologics		
Examiner's Global Mark	/5	
Actor's Global Mark	/5	
Total Station Mark	/30	

Learning Points

Ankylosing spondylitis is diagnosed according to modified New York criteria. Patients must satisfy at least one clinical and radiological criteria. Clinical criteria include low back pain and stiffness for > 3 months which improves with exercise but is not relieved with rest. Other clinical diagnostic criteria include a limitation of motion of the lumbar spine in both sagittal and frontal planes or a limitation of chest expansion relative to normal values corrected for age and sex. Radiological criteria include sacroiliitis on plain film imaging > grade 2 bilaterally or grade 3-4 unilaterally. MRI of spine and sacroiliac joints can detect early inflammatory lesions including bone oedema and erosive changes

Initial therapies for ankylosing spondylitis include non-steroidal anti-inflammatory drugs (NSAIDs) and land and water-based physiotherapy programmes. Anti-TNF drugs may be indicated if disease activity is not adequately controlled with non-steroidal anti-inflammatories.

HLA B27 gene testing is not required to make a diagnosis of ankylosing spondylitis.

Case 5
History taking: Back pain - malignancy

Task:	Achieved	Not Achieved
Introduces him/herself		
Clarifies who they are speaking to and establishes age		
Checks occupation		
Positions themselves at appropriate distance from patient and maintains eye contact		
Uses open questions to begin the history		
Elicits pattern of back and specifically nocturnal symptoms		
Asks about chronology of symptoms		
Asks about alleviating and exacerbating factors relating to pain		
Asks about impact on daily activities and function		
Asks about weight loss		
Asks about change in bowel habit		
Asks about bladder dysfunction		
Asks about other red flag symptoms of back pain including fevers, night sweats and peripheral motor/sensory deficits		
Asks about past medical history including current drug therapy and allergies		
Asks about smoking, alcohol and recreational drug use		
Elicits patient's concerns		
Summarises clinical history		
Offers diagnosis and relevant differential diagnoses		
Suggests initial management plan including full clinical examination including breast exam and neurological examination and digital rectal examination for anal tone		
Suggests investigations including MRI of thoraco-lumbar spine, chest X-Ray (or CT chest, abdomen, pelvis) and haematological investigations including FBC, Liver, Renal, Bone profiles and a Myeloma screen		
Examiner's Global Mark	/5	
Actor's Global Mark	/5	
Total Station Mark	/24	

Learning Points

Cauda equina syndrome is a medical emergency and requires immediate attention. Red flag symptoms including severe back pain, saddle anaesthesia, bladder or bowel dysfunction need to be assessed promptly with urgent clinical assessment and imaging (ideally MRI scan) of the lumbar-sacral spine. Cauda equina syndrome may be due to non-malignant processes including central disc prolapse, but in the clinical vignette described, the opinion of a clinical oncologist would be appropriate.

The management of cauda equina syndrome may include surgical decompression, high dose intravenous steroid therapy and/or radiotherapy if neoplasia is the likely cause

Red flag signs and symptoms of back pain include:

Saddle anaesthesia	Urinary retention or faecal incontinence
Reduced anal tone	Non-mechanical pain
Hip or knee weakness	Thoracic pain
Generalised neurological deficit	Fevers or rigors
Progressive spinal deformity	General malaise

Case 6
Examination: GALS Examination

Task:	Achieved	Not Achieved
Introduces self to the patient and gains consent for examination		
Washes hands or uses alcohol gel		
Explains the examination to the patient and offers a chaperone		
Exposes patient appropriately or described appropriate exposure		
Asks patient 3 appropriate screening questions eg 1) do you have any pain or stiffness in your muscles, joints or back? 2) do you struggle to dress yourself? 3) do you find climbing stairs difficult?		
Undertakes initial inspection of patient whilst standing in the anatomical position from all planes. Note should be made of muscular bulk, scoliosis, spinal curvatures, abnormal swellings or obvious joint deformity or asymmetry		
Gait: assess for smoothness, symmetry and ability to turn quickly		
Spine: assess lumbar spine flexion (placing two fingers on the lumbar spine) and asking the patient to bend forward with legs shoulder width apart and keeping knees straight		
Spine: assess lateral flexion of cervical spine		
Assess temporomandibular joint movement		
Arms: assess shoulder abduction and external rotation		
Arms: assess for swelling and deformity of wrist and hands		
Arms: assess finger grip strength		
Arms: assess fine precision pinch movements		
Arms: performs metacarpophalangeal joint squeeze		
Legs: whilst the patient is supine, examines knee flexion and internal rotation of the hip		
Legs: performs patella tap		
Legs: inspects the soles of the feet for callous formation		
Legs: performs metatarsophalangeal joint squeeze		
Summarises clinical findings concisely		
Actor's Global Mark	/5	
Examiner's Global Mark	/5	
Total Station Mark	/30	

Learning points

The GALS assessment is a screening test for mechanical or inflammatory musculoskeletal disease. If there are abnormalities noted, a comprehensive regional musculoskeletal examination should be performed. The absence of abnormalities on GALS assessment does not exclude significant pathology.

Knowing the correct content of the GALS assessment is key. To minimise inconvenience for the patient, after initial inspection, the gait, arms and spine can be performed whilst the patient is standing. Examination of the legs should be performed whilst the patient is supine.

The results of the GALS assessment should be documented in a table. Assuming all facets of the assessment are normal, they should be recorded as below:

	APPEARANCE	MOVEMENT
GAIT	✓	
ARMS	✓	✓
LEGS	✓	✓
SPINE	✓	✓

Case 7
Examination: Shoulder – Rotator Cuff Tea

Task:	Achieved	Not Achieved
Introduces self to the patient and gains consent for examination		
Washes hands or uses alcohol gel		
Explains the examination to the patient and offers a chaperone		
Exposes patient appropriately or described appropriate exposure		
Observes patient in a standing and exposed from waist up		
Palpates for temperature of the joint using back of hand		
Palpates for tenderness in joint line systematically		
Specifically palpates SCJ, ACJ, spine of scapula		
Takes the chance to test tenderness at LHB with resisted flexion of the elbow		
Asks patient to demonstrate global compound movements (hands behind head, hands behind back) – excludes frozen shoulder		
Performs passive movements of one shoulder standing behind the patient and feeling for crepitus. Should do Flex/ Ext/ Abd/ Add/ Int/ Ext rot		
Performs ACJ Scarf test		
Performs Neer's impingement test		
Assesses rotator cuff function focusing on abduction in the mid-range of motion with and without resistance		
Assesses rotator cuff function of TM/IS with resisted external rotation		
Assesses rotator cuff function of Subscapularis with resisted external rotation		
Assesses for or describes how to assess apprehension test for instability		
States that would perform neurovascular examination of the arm		
Summarises findings and further investigations		
Offers a diagnosis and other differential diagnoses		
Examiner's Global Mark	/5	
Actor's Global Mark	/5	
Total Station Mark	/30	

Learning Points

In older patients with restricted range of shoulder movements the two key differentials are degenerative cuff tear vs frozen shoulder. Frozen shoulder affects all planes of movement both active and passive and should be easily differentiated from RCT.

Remember that RCT pathology can be acute tears in young athletic injury or degenerative in older patients. Supraspinatus is the most important musculotendinous unit to assess and affects abduction in mid-range of arc (deltoid initiates abduction).

Management of RCT varies between patient depending upon pathology. Be aware that tenderness of LHB or ACJ are important to determine prior to surgery as it may warrant surgical excision/ release.

Case 8
Examination: Hip – Osteoarthritis

Task:	Achieved	Not Achieved
Introduces self to the patient and gains consent for examination		
Washes hands or uses alcohol gel		
Explains the examination to the patient and offers a chaperone		
Exposes patient appropriately or described appropriate exposure		
Inspects around bedside for aids or adaptations		
Observes patient in a standing position from 3 sides		
Asks patient to walk and observes gait		
Performs and explains Trendelenburg sign		
Asks patient to lie of the bed and completes observations		
Measures and explains true and apparent leg length discrepancy		
Palpates for temperature over hip and groin crease		
Palpated for tenderness systemically around join		
Assesses passive movements of the hip including internal and external rotation		
Performs active movements of the hip including flexion, internal, external rotation, ABduction and ADduction		
With patient in prone position checks passive hip extension		
Performs Thomas' test for fixed flexion deformity		
Performs FABER / Figure 4 test		
Performs Straight leg raise test / Lasegue's test		
Suggests neurovascular exam of lower limbs		
Offers a diagnosis and other differential diagnoses		
Examiner's Global Mark	/5	
Actor's Global Mark	/5	
Total Station Mark	/30	

Learning Points

The Trendelenburg sign is said to be positive if, when standing on one leg, the pelvis drops on the side opposite to the stance leg to reduce the load by decreasing the lever arm. By reducing the lever arm, this decreases the workload on the hip abductors. The muscle weakness is present on the side of the stance leg. A positive Trendelenburg sign could indicate abductor weakness from disuse secondary to osteoarthritis but is also present in neuromuscular weakness.

Ensure you know the landmarks for True and Apparent leg length measurements and make sure you know how to interpret the results.

FABER or Figure 4 tests and Straight leg raises tests are looking for differential diagnoses for the hip pain such as Ankylosing Spondylitis or Sciatic nerve impingement respectively.

Case 9
Examination: Knee – Meniscal tear

Task:	Achieved	Not Achieved
Introduces self to the patient and gains consent for examination		
Washes hands or uses alcohol gel		
Explains the examination to the patient and offers a chaperone		
Exposes patient appropriately		
Inspects around bedside for aids or adaptations		
Observes patient in a standing position from 3 sides - anterior, side, posterior		
Asks patient to walk and observes gait		
Palpates for temperature using back of hand		
Palpates the quadriceps tendon		
Palpates for tenderness in joint line systematically		
Palpates for masses in the popliteal fossa eg Baker's cyst		
Assesses for a joint effusion; 'tap' or 'milk'		
Performs active then passive movements of the knee - flexion & extension		
Checks for posterior sag (PCL)		
Examines ACL using anterior draw or Lachmann's		
Examines MCL and LCL		
Performs MacMurray's meniscal tests		
Assesses for patella apprehension		
Summarises findings and further investigations		
Offers a diagnosis and other differential diagnoses		
Examiner's Global Mark	/5	
Actor's Global Mark	/5	
Total Station Mark	/30	

Learning Points

Demographics and mechanism of injury are key deciding whether a patient is likely to have a sport knee injury such as meniscal tear or ACL injury compared to degenerative disease.

Remember that symptoms and signs can fluctuate so even though patients may experience 'locking' of the knee this may not occur during the examination.

McMurray's meniscal tests are the classical exacerbation test to assist in the diagnosis of a meniscal tear. Remember that internal rotation affects the lateral meniscus, and external rotation the medial meniscus.

Case 10
Examination : Spine – Sciatica

Task:	Achieved	Not Achieved
Introduces self to the patient and gains consent for examination		
Washes hands or uses alcohol gel		
Explains the examination to the patient and offers a chaperone		
Exposes patient appropriately or described appropriate exposure		
Observes patient from front and behind looking for symmetry of muscle bulk, scars, scoliosis, abnormal hair tufts or evidence spina bifida		
Observes from the side of the patient looking for normal curvature specifically commenting on kyphosis or lordosis		
Palpates along bony margin of spinous processes identifying any areas of tenderness		
Palpates paraspinal musculature for tenderness		
Asks patient to perform active cervical spine movements (flexion, extension, rotation and lateral flexion)		
Asks patient to perform active lumbar spine movements (flexion, extension, lateral flexion)		
Performs Modified Schober's Index correctly using finger tips above and below sacral dimples/ PSIS		
Assesses thoracic spine rotation with the patient is a seated position with arms across the chest		
Performs Straight Leg Raise test on ONE leg and comments on presence of radicular pain		
Follows up SLR test with either Bragard's or Lasegue's test		
Assess ankle motor function		
Assess sensation around foot and ankle		
Assesses knee and ankle reflexes using tendon hammer appropriately		
Thanks patient and ensures patient is comfortable		
Summarises findings and further investigations		
Offers a diagnosis and other differential diagnoses		
Examiner's Global Mark	/5	
Actor's Global Mark	/5	
Total Station Mark	/30	

Learning Points

Radicular symptoms are common and history and examination should exclude red flags for cauda equina syndrome

The sensitivity of the SLR test is aid to be increased by Lasegue's and Bragard's modifications

Lumbar disc degeneration and root impingement can present with variable lower limb weakness or sensory loss but bilateral symptoms are a red flag

Case 11
Examination: Foot & Ankle – Hallux Valgus

Task:	Achieved	Not Achieved
Introduces self to the patient and gains consent for examination		
Washes hands or uses alcohol gel		
Explains the examination to the patient and offers a chaperone		
Exposes patient appropriately or described appropriate exposure		
Undertakes initial observation of both feet while weight bearing from front, side and behind		
Observes medial arch and position of calcaneus in standing and tip toe position		
Asks patient to walk and observes gait		
The candidate describes signs of posture, muscle wasting, scars, nodules and nail changes		
Assess temperature between feet using back of own hand		
Palpates the foot and ankle systematically from forefoot, midfoot, hindfoot		
Palpates the ankle joint circumferentially including medial and lateral malleoli		
Palpates specifically the 1st MTPJ		
Asks patient to perform specific active movements of dorsiflexion, plantarflexion, inversion and eversion at the ankle		
Performs passive movements of IPJs, MTPJs		
Performs passive movement of midfoot, hindfoot		
Performs passive ankle movements		
Palpates dorsalis pedis and posterior tibial pulses		
Assesses distal neurology including sole of foot		
Summarises findings and further investigations		
Offers a diagnosis and other differential diagnoses		
Examiner's Global Mark	/5	
Actor's Global Mark	/5	
Total Station Mark	/30	

Learning Points

Hallux Valgus is a complex deformity of the first digit. The condition is associated with lesser toe deformity such as 'hammer toe' and callosities on the pressure points

Examination of the foot and ankle is daunting and infrequently practised in isolation. It is important to remember that there are multiple joints to assess for passive and active ranges of movement. The tibio-talar joint, subtalar joint and midtarsal joints should each be tested independently

Compared to other examination stations observation and gait during assessment of the foot and ankle provide a greater proportion of the information needed to form a differential diagnosis. Ensure that you can describe the appearance of common foot and ankle pathologies.

Case 12
Examination: Upper Limb Neurology

Task:	Achieved	Not Achieved
Introduces self to the patient and gains consent for examination		
Washes hands or uses alcohol gel		
Explains the examination to the patient and offers a chaperone		
Observes patient from front and behind looking for symmetry of muscle bulk, scars, scoliosis, abnormal hair tufts or evidence spina bifida		
Observes from the side of the patient looking for normal curvature specifically commenting on kyphosis or lordosis		
Ask the patient to sit down and examine tone in both arms		
Tests power in C5 (Shoulder abduction)		
Test power in C6 (Wrist extension)		
Tests power in C7 (Elbow flexion)		
Tests power in C8 (Grip)		
Tests power in T1 Finger abduction)		
Tests reflexes in Elbow flexion, Wrist extension and Hoffman's reflex		
Tests sensation to light touch in C5		
Tests sensation to light touch in C6		
Tests sensation to light touch in C7		
Tests sensation to light touch in C8		
Tests sensation to light touch in T1		
Offers to test pin prick sensation		
Summarises findings and further investigations		
Offers a diagnosis and other differential diagnoses		
Examiner's Global Mark	/5	
Actor's Global Mark	/5	
Total Station Mark	/30	

Learning Points

General inspection is essential for any physical examination but in particular for the upper limb neurological examination. Check for Scars, Wasting, Involuntary movements, Flickering or Fasciculations and Tremors (SWIFT). This may give you early clues to the overall diagnosis.

Having a solid core knowledge of the dermatome and myotome map for neurology examination is essential. A good example to follow has been produced by the American Spinal Injury Association

In the Orthopaedic OSCE stations you are most likely to encounter upper limb pathology with Lower Motor Neuron signs. Ensure you are confident about differentiating between Lower and Upper Motor Neuron signs. Lower Motor Neuron signs are typically reduced tone, weakness and hyporeflexia

Case 13

Skills and data interpretation: Trauma – Pelvis X-rays

Task:	Achieved	Not Achieved
States that they would confirm patient's name		
States that they would confirm patient's DOB/ hospital number		
States that they would confirm date of the radiograph		
Identifies AP of pelvis		
Identifies lateral of left hip		
Comments on rotation		
Comments on adequacy		
Comments on penetration		
Identifies fracture of left neck of femur		
Identifies that this is a displaced fracture		
Identifies that this is an intracapsular fracture		
Comments on bone and joint alignment		
Comments on joint space of the hip		
Comments on cortical outline of all bones to exclude other injury		
Comments on soft tissues		
Demonstrates understanding of need for urgent orthopaedic referral		
Suggests examination of joints above and below		
Suggests need for medical clearance for underlying cause of fall		
Demonstrates understanding of need for surgery		
Summarises findings to examiner		
Answers all questions logically and clearly	/5	
Examiner's Global Mark	/5	
Total Station Mark	/30	

Learning Points

Reviewing two different views of any injury is essential – subtle fractures may only be easily identified on one of the views.

Even if there is an obvious fracture or abnormality, ensure you systematically assess the rest of the radiograph to avoid missing other abnormalities.

Displaced intracapsular neck of femur fractures in the elderly are serious injuries with a high risk of non-union and avascular necrosis – they are usually managed with urgent surgery in the form of a hemiarthroplasty or a total hip replacement.

Case 14
Skills and data interpretation :: Metabolic bone profile

Task:	Achieved	Not Achieved
Introduces him/herself to the CNS		
Elicits the current situation		
Elicits the concerns of the CNS		
States that they would confirm patient's name		
States that they would confirm patient's DOB/ hospital number		
States that they would confirm date of the blood test results		
Identifies raised creatinine consistent with renal failure		
Checks and confirms normal Na+ and K+		
Identifies abnormally high PTH level		
Identifies high ALP		
Identifies high phosphate and normal Ca++ levels		
Gives the correct diagnosis – secondary hyperparathyroidism		
Identifies that this is due to the underlying renal failure		
Correctly identifies that calcium supplements would be useful		
Agrees that vitamin D supplementation should be given		
Identifies the correct form of vitamin D replacement – alfacalcidol		
Suggests the use of cinacalcet		
Advises that parathyroid surgery may be required if the patient fails to respond to the above measures		
Agrees a plan of action with the nurse specialist		
Summarises appropriately		
Examiner's Global Mark	/5	
Actor's Global Mark	/5	
Total Station Mark	/30	

Learning Points

In end stage renal failure replacement of correction of vitamin D with conventional preparations of cholecalciferol or ergocalciferol will not work as these preparations require hydroxylation in the kidney to become active. Alfacalcidol or calcitriol should be used instead.

If untreated patients can develop tertiary hyperparathyroidism in end stage renal failure and hypercalcaemia will develop.

Cinacalcet can lead to hypocalcaemia it is important to repeat the bone biochemistry readings after starting it and adjust the dose accordingly.

Case 15
Skills and data interpretation: Scrubbing and gowning

Task:	Achieved	Not Achieved
Opens gown pack using appropriate technique		
Opens gloves onto sterile field using appropriate technique		
Puts on surgical mask		
Turns on taps and checks flow and temperature		
Uses scrubbing brush to clean under nails		
Applies appropriate volume of scrub solution		
Scrubs palm to palm		
Scrubs palm to dorsum each side		
Scrubs backs of fingers to palms with interlocked fingers		
Scrubs bases of thumbs		
Scrubs fingertips to palms		
Scrubs both wrists		
Scrubs both forearms		
Turns off taps using elbows		
Appropriate drying technique		
Picks up gown appropriately and puts arms into sleeves without revealing hands		
Dons gloves using closed or open technique		
Scrubs for appropriate time		
Keeps fingers above elbows at all points		
Avoids touching anything non-sterile throughout		
Answers all questions logically and clearly	/5	
Examiner's Global Mark	/5	
Total Station Mark	/30	

Learning Points

The first scrub of an operating list should be at least five minutes long. Further scrubs between cases can be shorter – around three minutes.

If at any point during the scrubbing process the hands or forearms come into contact with anything non-sterile then the entire process must be restarted from the beginning

Double gloving is commonplace in orthopaedic operating theatres – the risk of a glove perforation is high and two layers reduces the risks of contamination to both patient and surgeon.

Case 16
Skills and data interpretation : Cervical spine immobilisation

Task:	Achieved	Not Achieved
Introduces self		
Clarifies patient's name		
Checks name and expertise of assistance		
Puts of gloves/apron		
Asks patient to lie on bed		
Holds patient's head in neutral position		
Requests assistance from assistant to hold head		
Measures size of collar using fingers from lower chin to trapezius		
Adjusts cervical collar to appropriate size		
Slides collar under neck		
Closes collar applying appropriate tension		
Asks if patient is comfortable		
Applies blocks to sides of patient's head		
Applies tape/Velcro strap to immobilise head with blocks		
Ensures assistant applying in line immobilisation until blocks and tape applied		
Advises patient that collar will need to remain until injury has been excluded		
Organises Xray in timely manner to minimise time in collar		
Confident manner with patient		
Remains calm		
Appropriate communication with assistant		
Examiner's Global Mark	/5	
Actor's Global Mark	/5	
Total Station Mark	/30	

Learning Points

Even if a patient has walked away from an accident they could still have significant neck injuries and require cervical spine immobilisation until an injury can be excluded. The NICE guidelines can guide on which patients require plain film imaging and immobilisation.

Safe application of a cervical spine immobilisation collar requires teamwork with one team member applying manual in line immobilisation whilst another sizes and applies the collar.

The first line investigation of a patient with a painful neck following significant trauma would be a CT scan as this is less likely to miss subtle injuries and is readily available in most hospitals now. The NICE Head and neck injury guidelines exist to advise clinicians on the criteria for higher imaging.

Case 17
Emergency cases: Ward – Compartment Syndrome

Task:	Achieved	Not Achieved
Describes ABC approach to patient assessment		
Establishes the background of tibial nailing for a closed fracture earlier today		
Elicits the chronicity and progression of pain		
Elicits the severity of pain		
Assesses the previous use of analgesia and recognises high levels of opioid have failed to control pain		
Asks about neurovascular symptoms including tingling, pins and needles or numbness		
Recognises the potential for compartment syndrome and states the terminology		
States an initial plan of high elevation, release of plaster cast and analgesia		
States signs to observe on examination eg; patient in extremis, severe swelling of the limb, pale limb in advanced compartment syndrome		
Offers examination of the affected limb including neurovascular examination		
Demonstrates palpation of the limb to elicit tense compartments (cues given by the examiner)		
Demonstrates assessment of pain on passive stretch of the anterior compartment of the leg		
Demonstrates assessment of pain on passive stretch of the deep and superficial posterior compartment of the leg		
Demonstrates assessment of neurovascular status of the limb		
Recognises need for urgent surgical decompression recommends patient kept nil by mouth		
States would contact senior team, anaesthetist and book patient onto emergency theatre list		
Candidate defines compartment syndrome when asked		
Candidate states the signs of compartment syndrome as tense compartment with pain, exacerbation on passive stretch, paraesthesia, pallor, pulselessness, paralysis		
Able to state the underlying problem in compartment syndrome		
Able to outline the BOAST protocol for management of compartment syndrome		
Examiner's Global Mark	/5	
Actor's Global Mark	/5	
Total Station Mark	/30	

Learning Points

The British Orthopaedic Association have produced guidelines for diagnosis and management of compartment syndrome under their BOAST series. The following are selected key guidelines that are important to consider in the OSCE scenario and clinical practice;

Assessment for compartment syndrome should be routine after significant injury or surgery to a limb.

Key clinical findings are pain out of proportion to the injury and pain on pain passive movement of the muscles within the affected compartment.

Compartment syndrome is an emergency and operation should be performed within 1 hour of the decision to operate.

Further information can be found at:
https://www.boa.ac.uk/wp-content/uploads/2014/12/BOAST-10.pdf

Case 18
Mark scheme– Open Fracture Management

Task:	Achieved	Not Achieved
Introduces self to the patient and gains consent for examination		
Washes hands or uses alcohol gel		
Recognises the mechanism of injury warrants major trauma centre management		
Describes ATLS approach to primary survey		
States that airway should be assessed and inline c-spine immobilisation maintained		
States that thoracic trauma should assessed		
States that circulation including major source of bleeding should be assess eg, abdomen, pelvis and long bones		
Describes safe resuscitation of the patient including oxygen, analgesia, fluids +/- transfusion		
States that bloods including group and save and cross match should be taken along with radiographs of the chest and pelvis		
Able to describe the radiograph of a tibial fracture		
Able to describe appearance of an open wound		
Describes appropriate examination of the affected limb for neurovascular status		
Correctly identifies this as an open tibial fracture and recognises the importance in management of these injuries		
Describes the need of temporary wound coverage with saline and gauze followed by splinting		
Recognises need for administration of antibiotics and tetanus		
Recognises need for urgent surgical debridement		
Summarises situation to the examiner		
Candidate is able to describe the Gustilo Anderson Classification for open fractures		
Able to outline the BOAST protocol for management of open fractures		
States the indications for immediate out of hours surgery as neurovascular injury or gross contamination eg; farm waste		
Actor's Global Mark	/5	
Examiner's Global Mark	/5	
Total Station Mark	/30	

Learning Points

The British Orthopaedic Association have produced guidelines for diagnosis and management of open fractures under their BOAST series. The following are selected key guidelines that are important to consider in the OSCE scenario and clinical practice;

Administration of antibiotics. Any vascular impairment should be treated within 3-4 hours
Definitive management should be performed in a trauma centre with the input of multiple disciplines including plastic surgery

Gustilo Grade	Definition
I	Open fracture, clean wound, wound <1 cm in length
II	Open fracture, wound > 1 cm but < 10 cm in length without extensive soft-tissue damage, flaps, avulsions
III	Open fracture with extensive soft-tissue laceration, damage, or loss or an open segmental fracture. Any open fractures caused by farm injuries are Type II
IIIA	Type III fracture with adequate periosteal coverage of the fracture bone despite the extensive soft-tissue laceration or damage
IIIB	Type III fracture with extensive soft-tissue loss and periosteal stripping and bone damage
IIIC	Type III fracture associated with an arterial injury requiring repair

Further information can be found at: http://www.boa.ac.uk/publications/boast–4-the-management-of-sever-open-lower-limb-fractures/

Case 19

Emergency cases: ED – Neurovascular Injury

Task:	Achieved	Not Achieved
Describes ABC approach to patient assessment		
Establishes the background injury		
Elicits the timing of injury		
Elicits the severity of pain		
Asks about neurovascular symptoms including tingling, pins and needles, numbness, weakness		
Recognises the potential for neurovascular injury		
States signs to observe on examination eg; position of wound, pallor of limb, lack of movement		
Offers examination of the affected limb including neurovascular examination		
Demonstrates palpation of the limb to elicit temperature difference or tense compartments		
Demonstrates assessment distal pulses eg; radial and ulnar artery		
Demonstrates assessment of capillary refill time		
Demonstrates assessment of neurological function		
Recognises need for urgent surgical intervention		
States would contact senior team, anaesthetist and book patient onto emergency theatre list		
Candidate states the signs vascular injury when asked		
Able to describe signs of radial nerve injury		
Able to describe signs of median nerve injury		
Able to describe signs of ulnar nerve injury		
Describes 'ischaemia' time and urgency of repair within 4 hours		
Summarises the situation to the examiner		
Examiner's Global Mark	/5	
Actor's Global Mark	/5	
Total Station Mark	/30	

Learning Points

Anatomical knowledge of the area of injury can guide examination and management. Gauging the direction of injury and the weapon can also help.

Detailed neurovascular examination with clear documentation is important and referral onto specialty services will require this.

Ischaemia time of four hours is the approximate cut off where tissue begins to become non-viable. Thus, it is important to know the time of injury as it may guide surgical intervention.

Case 20
Emergency cases: Ward – Neck of Femur fracture

Task:	Achieved	Not Achieved
Describes ABC approach to patient assessment		
Establishes the injury and background with patient or nursing staff		
Attempts to elicit duration of time on the floor with patient or nursing staff		
Attempts to ask about non-mechanical fall symptoms such as chest pain, shortness of breath with patient or nursing staff		
Attempts to ask about past medical history and risk factors with patient or nursing staff		
Attempts to ask about pre-injury functional level		
Recognises dementia with AMTS level of 6		
Offers examination to assess for head injury and states that they would assess GCS score		
Demonstrates assessing chest examination		
Demonstrates assessing cardiac examination		
Demonstrates assessing abdominal examination		
Demonstrates assessment of pressure areas		
States that they would look for signs of fracture neck of femur including shortening and internal rotation of limb		
Demonstrates neurovascular examination of affected limb		
Requests further investigations including bloods, ECG, Pelvis and hip xrays		
Confirms fracture neck of femur on radiographs and recognises need for operative intervention on the next available trauma list		
States that they would offer analgesia, IV fluids and thromboprophylaxis and ensure patient isnil by mouth from midnight		
States would contact senior member of the team or Medical Registrar for review depending upon local policy		
Recognises the significance of a potential 'long-lie' on the floor and suggests catheterisation, urine output monitoring and U&E check		
Summarises the situation to the examiner		
Examiner's Global Mark	/5	
Actor's Global Mark	/5	
Total Station Mark	/30	

Learning Points

Patients with a fractured neck of femur present a significant workload to orthopaedic departments and the NHS. They suffer from significant comorbidities and have long inpatient stays. A more joined up approach with orthogeriatric multidisciplinary teams is now becoming the norm.

They must be carefully assessed for other medical issues that may have precipitated the fall. It is important to know the 10 point scoring system of the AMTS. Patients in this age group may have a background of dementia but always consider that a reduced AMTS could indicate a delirium and consider excluding additional problems such as head injury, urine infection or chest infection.

Management of these patients includes optimisation for early surgery, operative intervention and multidisciplinary rehabilitation.

Case 21
Emergency cases: ATLS scenario

Task:	Achieved	Not Achieved
Introduces self		
Checks patient's name and DOB		
Washes hands/uses alcohol gel		
Puts on gown and gloves		
Assesses airway		
Looks for obvious chest injuries		
Assesses trachea position		
Palpates chest wall bilaterally		
Percusses chest wall bilaterally		
Auscultates chest bilaterally		
Checks respiratory rate and saturations		
Assesses radial pulse		
Checks pulse and blood pressure		
Examines abdomen		
Assesses pelvis		
Examines long bones		
Assesses for external haemorrhage		
Assesses GCS		
Does not remove cervical collar and blocks		
Avoids focusing on painful feet/ sticks to ABCDE		
Examiner's Global Mark	/5	
Actor's Global Mark	/5	
Total Station Mark	/30	

Learning Points

When performing a primary survey, you must not become distracted by other injuries (such as the likely calcaneal fractures in this scenario). These are assessed in the secondary survey, once the primary survey, and any appropriate interventions, have been undertaken

Always consider the possibility of vertebral fractures in patients with calcaneal fractures. Given the common mechanism of a fall from height up to 10% of patients with a calcaneal fracture will have a concomitant vertebral fracture.

The cervical spine immobilisation collar should not be removed during the primary survey unless required to undertake an intervention for the airway.

Case 22
Communication: Consent for theatre

Task:	Achieved	Not Achieved
Introduces him/herself		
Clarifies who they are speaking to, establishes age and occupation of the patient		
Positions themselves at appropriate distance from patient and maintains eye contact		
Explains the purpose of the consultation and what they expect to achieve		
Establishes what the patient knows so far and elicits concerns		
Clearly states the procedure and confirms with the patient the correct side and site of surgery		
Offers to mark/checks marking of surgery site		
Lists (and explains if needed) - Infection risk		
Lists (and explains if needed) - Bleeding risk		
Lists (and explains if needed) – Risk or damage to local important structures i.e. nerves, blood vessels etc.		
Lists (and explains if needed) – VTE risk		
Lists (and explains if needed) – Malunion/non-union risk		
Lists (and explains if needed) – Repeat operation risk and/removal of metalwork		
Is able to explain the options for non-surgical treatment along with the risks of not treating an unstable ankle fracture		
Uses consent form and obtains appropriate signature		
Appears professional during consultation		
Gives clear and understandable information without excessive use of jargon or acronyms		
Allows the patient to talk and ask questions without talking over them		
Ensures all patient's concerns are dealt with		
Summarises the consultation to the examiner		
Examiner's Global Mark	/5	
Actor's Global Mark	/5	
Total Station Mark	/30	

Learning Points

Knowing the basics risks of a general orthopaedic trauma procedure are the crux of this station. Being able to explain them in simple terms to the patient rather than just listing them is what is required and what will happen in the real world.

A knowledge of the consent process including confirming the site and nature of the operation and being able to offer advice about alternative treatment makes the candidate safe.

Being able to obtain consent whilst stating often concerning risks (infection, repeat operation, damage to nerves) is aided by stratifying the list of risks into common (pain and swelling), less common (removal of metalwork) and rare (nerve damage).

Case 23

Communication: Counselling about thromboprophylaxis

Task:	Achieved	Not Achieved
Introduces him/herself		
Clarifies who they are speaking to, establishes age and occupation of the patient		
Positions themselves at appropriate distance from patient and maintains eye contact		
Explains the purpose of the consultation and what they expect to achieve		
Establishes what the patient knows so far and elicits concerns		
Explains that assessing someone's VTE risk is a balanced risk of developing a DVT versus bleeding risk of treatment		
Establishes risk of being immobilized and non-weight bearing in plaster cast		
Establishes risk of medication eg; Oral contraceptive pill		
Establishes no major bleeding risks		
Asks about personal history of VTE		
Asks about family history of VTE		
Makes appropriate judgment of the patients DVT risk and gives the appropriate advice		
Explains how low molecular weight heparin works in simple terms and describes a typical dose regimen		
Explains how compression stocks work		
Suggests other methods to lower risk (hydration, staying mobile, avoiding alcohol)		
Appears professional during consultation		
Gives clear and understandable information without excessive use of jargon or acronyms		
Allows the patient to talk and ask questions without talking over them		
Ensures all patient's concerns are dealt with		
Summarises the consultation to the examiner		
Examiner's Global Mark	/5	
Actor's Global Mark	/5	
Total Station Mark	/30	

Learning Points

Knowing the basics of a VTE risk assessment are key – you have to make your own judgment call for this particular patient balancing her risk factors against any bleeding risk.

A basic knowledge of the action and prescription of enoxaparin and compression stockings is also important as these details are important to the patient (when do I take it? How often? When can I stop?)

While this isn't a particularly confrontational consultation there is the need here to stand by your convictions and not change your advice when the patient doesn't necessarily like the medical advice you have given them (doesn't like needles, stocking make them too hot and would quite like to fly abroad!)

Case 24

Communication: Counselling about bisphosphonates

Task:	Achieved	Not Achieved
Introduces him/herself		
Clarifies who they are speaking to, establishes age and occupation of the patient		
Positions themselves at appropriate distance from patient and maintains eye contact		
Explains the purpose of the consultation and what they expect to achieve		
Establishes what the patient knows so far and elicits concerns		
Allows the patient time to talk without interruption		
Recommends that the patient start an oral bisphosphonate (alendronate would be first line)		
Explains that the medication is only taken once per week		
Advises that the medication is taken on an empty stomach at least 30 minutes before breakfast		
Advises the patient to drink plenty of water alongside when taking their bisphosphonate		
Advises that the patient should remain upright for 30 minutes after taking the medication		
Reassures the patient appropriately that the risk of osteonecrosis of the jaw is extremely low		
Addresses the patient's concerns about atypical femoral fractures appropriately		
Advises that the patient should take oral supplementation of calcium and vitamin D alongside the bisphosphonate		
Addresses patient's questions about denosumab appropriately		
Appears professional during consultation		
Gives clear and understandable information without excessive use of jargon or acronyms		
Allows the patient to talk and ask questions without talking over them		
Ensures all patient's concerns are dealt with		
Summarises the consultation to the examiner		
Examiner's Global Mark	/5	
Actor's Global Mark	/5	
Total Station Mark	/30	

Learning Points

Atypical femoral fractures have been seen in patients with prolonged bisphosphonate use but the risk is low. The risk of osteoporotic fragility fracture in a patient like this far outweighs the risk of atypical femoral fracture and treatment should therefore be given. The MHRA advice states "The risk of osteonecrosis of the jaw is substantially greater for patients receiving intravenous bisphosphonates in the treatment of cancer than for patients receiving oral bisphosphonates for osteoporosis or Paget's disease".

Current NICE guidelines on secondary prevention of osteoporotic fractures [TA161] do not require a DEXA scan to be performed before commencing a bisphosphonate in women over the age of 75 who have suffered a fragility fracture.

Denosumab is licensed for the treatment of osteoporosis in the UK but current NICE guidelines only recommend its use in patients who have a contra-indication or intolerance to oral bisphosphonates which are still the first line treatment for osteoporosis.

Case 25

Communication: Counselling - new diagnosis of rheumatoid arthritis

Task:	Achieved	Not Achieved
Introduces him/herself		
Clarifies who they are speaking to, establishes age and occupation of the patient		
Positions themselves at appropriate distance from patient and maintains eye contact		
Explains the purpose of the consultation and what they expect to achieve		
Establishes what the patient knows so far		
Explains the diagnosis of rheumatoid arthritis. Avoids the use of jargon – if technical terms are used they must also be explained in lay terms		
Reassures the patient that nothing they have done has caused them to develop arthritis		
Elicits concern that the patient will end up like her grandmother.		
Re-assures the patient that with modern treatment outcomes are much improved and she is very unlikely to be as severely affected by the disease as her grandmother		
Explains briefly how rheumatoid arthritis is treated (must mention either methotrexate or DMARDs)		
Discusses a multidisciplinary approach to the treatment of RA (involving pharmacist, physiotherapist, podiatrist etc.)		
Lists some of the side effects of methotrexate or other DMARDs (nausea, hair thinning, liver toxicity, increased risk of infections, need for blood test monitoring) – must mention at least two to score the mark		
Identifies that methotrexate is teratogenic and explains that a different treatment should be used instead		
Re-assures the patient appropriately about her risk of her children developing the condition		
Elicits concern that the patient will have to give up cycling and reassures the patient about the benefits of exercise in RA		
Appears professional during consultation		
Gives clear and understandable information without excessive use of jargon or acronyms		
Allows the patient to talk and ask questions without talking over them		
Ensures all patient's concerns are dealt with		
Summarises the consultation to the examiner		
Examiner's Global Mark	/5	
Actor's Global Mark	/5	
Total Station Mark	/30	

Learning Points

Rheumatoid arthritis commonly presents as a symmetrical polyarthritis affecting predominantly the small joints

Early treatment with disease modifying anti-rheumatic drugs is associated with better clinical outcomes and as such contemporary treatment algorithms advocate prompt referral to a specialist and early initiation of DMARDs.

Rheumatoid arthritis affects approximately 1% of the population. If you have a first degree relative with the condition your risk of developing RA is increased by approximately 3-5 times. However, this means you are still much more likely to never get the condition than you are to develop it.

Psychiatry

Case 1
Markscheme:OCD

Task:	Achieved	Not Achieved
Introduces self and clarifies who they are speaking to		
Gains consent		
Establishes nature of obsessions (onset, thoughts, images, ruminations, doubts)		
Establishes nature of compulsions (counting, washing, checking, rituals)		
Asks about physical symptoms (palpitations, breathlessness, sweating, dizziness) and biological symptoms (sleep, appetite)		
Elicits any triggers (friend who was in hospital)		
Asks about core depressive symptoms (low mood, anhedonia, fatigue)		
Asks about past psychiatric history		
Asks about past medical history		
Asks about social history (drug, alcohol, smoking, employment)		
Asks about personal history (childhood, relationships, school)		
Asks about family history, including specifically about mental health and suicide		
Asks about medication history including allergies		
Asks about forensic history		
Performs a risk assessment in a sensitive manner (self-harm and suicidal ideation)		
Reassures patient in non-judgmental way		
Summarises consultation concisely		
Provides suitable primary diagnosis and relevant differentials (e.g. OCD, adjustment disorder, panic disorder, obsessive personality disorder)		
Explains basic steps for management (reassurance, support, CBT, behaviour therapy, 'flooding technique,' SSRIs)		
Establishes rapport with patient		
Examiner's Global Mark	/5	
Actor / Helper's Global Mark	/5	
Total Station Mark	/30	

Learning points:

Obsessions are one's own thoughts and can be repetitive, intrusive and unpleasant. Compulsions are used to neutralize or prevent obsessions.

Depression is commonly seen alongside OCD and other anxiety disorders, it is important to ask screening questions about the three core symptoms of depression, including low mood, reduced energy and lack of interest, in every anxiety disorder.

Demonstrating empathy and reassurance is key with an anxious patient. Offering to bring the patient back in a week's time, perhaps with their sibling or carer, will signify this.

Case 2
Markscheme – "I only want to speak to the consultant'

Task:	Achieved	Not Achieved
Introduces self		
Clarifies who they are speaking to and gains consent		
Establishes rapport		
Listens attentively to patients concerns		
Invites the relative to sit down to avoid confrontation		
Apologises early for the consultant's absence and thanks the patient for speaking with them		
Explains their role within the ward and offers to be of help or gives patient option of coming back to speak to consultant at another time		
Makes empathetic statements "it must be very difficult to see a relative in hospital"		
Modifies speech and body language to de-escalate confrontation		
Appears to be non-defensive regarding the relatives complaint "I completely understand why that would upset you", "I'm very sorry your father had that experience"		
Explains the importance of the nursing handover process including passing on important information		
Offers to speak with the nurse about the incident		
Does not implicate nursing staff or collude with patient		
Explain that relatives views and opinions are considered very important to the team and any complaints are taken very seriously		
Explains there is a formal complaints procedure that the relative can follow if they wish, offers telephone number or leaflet for Patient Advice Liaison Service (PALS)		
Does not become flustered after threat of suing or talking to the press and explains taking legal action is within their rights.		
Explains that it is not possible to use images taken on their phone with people in without their consent		
Reassure relative that you will relay the information to the consultant as soon as possible		
Remains calm		
Non-judgemental approach		
Examiner's Global Mark	/5	
Actor / Helper's Global Mark	/5	
Total Station Mark	/30	

Learning points:

When dealing with an angry patient or relative always try and encourage them to sit down, having a conversation standing up can appear confrontational.

In communication terms anger has a purpose - to gain the listener's attention. In this case, it is wise for the doctor to give the patient their full attention.

To increase the sense of empathy lower the tone and volume a bit of your voice and look extra attentive with eye contact at the patient/relative. This makes you sound much more convincing! The NHS has a Zero Tolerance policy for physical aggression from patients or relatives, this should be reported immediately to security team immediately if you feel your safety is being compromised.

Case 3
Markscheme – "The Self-harmer"

Task:	Achieved	Not Achieved
Introduces self and explains purpose of discussion		
Clarifies to whom they are speaking and gains consent		
Asks about the presenting complaint of self-harm to determine if it was a suicide attempt		
Asks about previous self-harm and suicidal ideation		
Attempts to identify triggers for the episodes of crisis		
Enquires about relationships (childhood, family, partners) and their stability		
Asks about education (schooling) and employment		
Asks about impulsivity and unpredictability		
Asks about bouts of anger/outbursts of temper		
Asks about low mood/feelings of emptiness		
Excludes symptoms of psychosis (hallucinations/delusions)		
Asks about past medical and psychiatric history		
Asks about family history (mental health and suicide)		
Asks about illicit drug use / alcohol misuse		
Performs a risk assessment		
Maintains a calm and non-judgemental approach		
Gains the patient's trust (as evidenced by the patient revealing her full story)		
Avoids "down-playing" the current crisis which was not an actual suicide attempt		
Summarises consultation and offers a differential diagnosis		
Explains a basic management plan (e.g. referral to community mental health services, crisis plan, psychotherapy)		
Examiner's Global Mark	/5	
Actor / Helper's Global Mark	/5	
Total Station Mark	/30	

Learning points

The key to eliciting a meaningful history in a patient with EUPD is to establish a rapport and gain their trust.
Don't be tempted to "down-play" their suicide risk on the basis that they have made repeated threats. One in ten people will EUPD will die from suicide.

Psychotherapy (such as teaching tools to deal with difficult emotions) is one of the most effective forms of treatment but is not a short-term solution and a patient may require twice-weekly sessions for one to two years.

You may find it helpful to offer the patient a questionnaire. A diagnosis can usually be made if the patient answers "yes" to five or more of the following questions: 3
- Do you have a fear of being left alone?
- Do you have intense and unstable relationships?
- Do you ever feel you don't have a strong sense of your own self?
- Do you engage in impulsive activities in two areas that are potentially damaging, such as unsafe sex, drug   abuse or reckless spending?
- Have you made repeated suicide threats or attempts in your past and engaged in self-harming?
- Do you have severe mood swings, such as feeling intensely depressed, anxious or irritable, which last from a few hours to a few days?
- Do you have long-term feelings of emptiness and loneliness?
- Do you often find it difficult to control your anger?
- When you find yourself in stressful situations, do you feel like you're disconnected from the world or from your own body?

Case 4

Markscheme – postpartum

Task:	Achieved	Not Achieved
Introduces the conversation and confirms the patient's identity		
Elicits history from patient in a concise manner		
Asks about presenting complaint		
Asks about depressive symptoms – low mood, energy levels and sleep disturbances (early morning wakening)		
Asks about psychotic symptoms - delusions, auditory, visual and tactile hallucinations		
Asks about preconception period – young, first time mothers, support system, planned or unplanned pregnancy		
Asks about antenatal period – medical problems, social issues, support		
Asks about the birth – traumatic delivery, medical intervention, support		
Asks about postnatal period – support, bonding, mood, coping		
Asks specifically about self harm and suicidal ideation – thoughts of suicide, plans, final acts (writing a will, leaving a note, ensuring you wouldn't be found)		
Asks about risk of harm to child – emotional, physical, sexual abuse and neglect		
Asks about protective factors to prevent suicide – family support, carers, partners		
Asks about past medical history		
Asks about past psychiatric history		
Asks about family history		
Asks drug and alcohol history		
Assesses insight – ability to recognize there is a problem and accept treatment		
Presents the Mental State Examination fluently		
Structured management plan: conservative therapies – CBT, admission to mother-baby unit, paediatric team involvement, safeguarding, social services, community psychiatry nurses, midwife input. Medical management – anti-psychotics, anti-depressants, ECT for persistent symptoms		
Examiner's Global Mark	/5	
Actor / Helper's Global Mark	/5	
Total Station Mark	/30	

Learning Points

Differentiate between baby blues, postpartum depression and postpartum psychosis. Post partum depression can occur up to 1 year postpartum, symptoms of low mood, reduced energy and anhedonia. This requires treatment unlike baby blues, which lasts a few days to a week. Postpartum psychosis usually presents in the first 2 weeks postpartum with florid psychotic features. These are extremely high risk and vulnerable patients, and are often all admitted to Mother & Baby Units.

Determine the timeline of events from pre-conception through to the post partum period to find risk factors for post partum psychosis. These include unsupported first time mothers, antenatal medical problems, traumatic delivery, prematurity and difficulties during the post partum period.

Be as specific as you can with regards to suicidal risk, you need to assess if the patient is likely to harm themselves or their child. Ascertain if they have made a plan or committed any final acts such as writing a will.

Case 5
MSE STATION – Nasty neighbours

Task:	Achieved	Not Achieved
Introduces self		
Confirms patient identity and gains consent		
Asks about mood		
Asks about suicidal ideation and plans		
Asks about thought disorder (insertion, broadcasting and removal)		
Asks about delusional thought content (control, grandiose, reference, persecutory)		
Elicits persecutory delusion and confirms absolute certainty		
Elicits risk to self and others		
Asks about hallucinations (visual, tactile, olfactory, auditory, gustatory)		
Elicits characteristics/content of the hallucinations		
Differentiates if the voices are 2nd or 3rd person		
Assesses cognition (orientation, attention/concentration, recalling events)		
Asks about insight		
Summarises the MSE fluently		
Comments on positive findings (see examiner's instructions)		
Identifies correct delusions and hallucinations		
Gives appropriate diagnosis of paranoid schizophrenia		
Provides appropriate differential diagnosis		
Suggests appropriate management plan (e.g referral to liaison psychiatry team for assessment/admission or high intensity community support, medication)		
Develops rapport and shows empathy		
Examiner's Global Mark	/5	
Actor / Helper's Global Mark	/5	
Total Station Mark	/30	

Learning Points

It is vital to assess suicide risk on every patient you see with psychiatric symptoms, even if this isn't the focus of the station. If you're unsure of their risk always involve a senior.

The first rank symptoms of schizophrenia were devised by German psychiatrist Kurt Schneider are a collection of symptoms, commonly seen in, but not pathognomonic of patients with schizophrenia. Their presence can therefore aid with diagnosis.

They can be broadly categorised into four types which include:

Auditory Hallucinations: particularly third person, commentary or thought echo
Thought disorder: thought broadcasting, insertion or withdrawal
Delusions of control: Passivity phenomena including passivity of impulse, volitions or affect. Somatic passivity may also occur.
Delusional perception: A delusionary belief where a patient attributes meaning or a message to an everyday perception

Illusions are not true hallucinations. For example, this patient thinking there are cameras in/on ordinary objects is an illusion secondary to the delusion. If this was a 'true' visual hallucination, he would be able to see the cameras

Case 6

History taking- Anxious Anne

Task:	Achieved	Not Achieved
Introduces self		
Clarifies who they are speaking to and gains consent		
Asks about precipitating events/triggers		
Elicits at least 2 psychological symptoms (fatigue, sleep pattern, irritability, worry, concentration, guilt, feeling of doom)		
Elicits at least 2 somatic symptoms (sweating, palpitations, butterflies, restlessness, hyperventilation, palpitations)		
Impact on daily living and social function		
Asks about symptoms that differentiate anxiety disorders (obsessions, compulsions, repetitive thoughts, avoiding public places, previous trauma)		
Asks about symptoms of depression (low mood, anhedonia, fatigue, lack of concentration)		
Elicits details of premorbid personality – (e.g before these attacks did she have any problems leaving the house		
Past psychiatric history		
Past medical history and medication history		
Briefly asks about birth/development/school		
Elicits substance use (alcohol, smoking, drugs)		
Assess risk of suicide/self harm		
Summarises fluently		
Provides correct diagnosis (agoraphobia) and suitable differential (panic disorder, social phobia, generalised anxiety disorder)		
Appropriate initial management and follow up offered		
Builds rapport with patient		
Empathetic		
Reassures patient		
Examiner's Global Mark	/5	
Actor / Helper's Global Mark	/5	
Total Station Mark	/30	

Learning Points

Agoraphobia is a fear of crowds/open spaces and the patient usually feels safer at home. Agoraphobia is distinguished from general anxiety disorder by predominantly phobic symptoms rather than constant worry/anxiety.

75% of patients with agoraphobia are women between late teens and mid 30's.

First line treatment includes reassurance, providing diagnosis and education. If symptoms fail to improve then refer for psycho-educational groups or individual guided self help before considering step 3. However, if a patient has marked functional impairment then one can skip to step 3 (individual high intensity psychological intervention and/or medication).

Case 7
Medication counseling - Clozapine

Task:	Achieved	Not Achieved
Introduces self		
Clarifies who they are speaking to and gains consent		
Explains reason for consultation		
Explains rationale behind starting clozapine (e.g for schizophrenia when 2 other anti-psychotics have been ineffective)		
Briefly explains mechanism of action ("works by blocking overactive brain messengers and balancing hormone levels in the brain")		
Explains can take few weeks to have full effect		
Explains risk of low white cell count, agranulocytosis		
Explains it can interfere with the heart causing palpitations and cardiomyopathy/myocarditis		
Mentions 2 further side effects including: weight gain, constipation, dry mouth, flu-like symptoms, nausea, sleepiness, dizziness		
Explains need for regular blood tests (once weekly for 18 weeks, every 2 weeks for a year then once monthly thereafter) to monitor WCC		
Explains must avoid drinking alcohol and caffeine		
Stresses importance of compliance and must not stop suddenly and to inform medical staff if they have missed a dose		
Safety netting - Informs to seek immediate advice if any adverse side effects or takes too many tablets		
Advises to seek medical help immediately if they develop a sore throat (due to risk of agranulocytosis)		
Explains they start at a low dose and slowly up-titrate dose		
Offers patient leaflet/information		
Summarises consultation		
Builds rapport with patient		
Avoids medical jargon		
Clear and concise		
Examiner's Global Mark	/5	
Actor / Helper's Global Mark	/5	
Total Station Mark	/30	

Learning Points

Clozapine is an atypical antipsychotic only given if 2 other anti-psychotics have been trialled and have either been ineffective or if the patient develops a tolerance.

Agranulocytosis is a potentially life-threatening side effect and will develop in 1-2% of patients, in a dose independent manner. Full blood count must be performed weekly for the first eighteen weeks, fortnightly for a year, and then monthly thereafter. The Clozapine Patient Monitoring Service (CPMS) keeps a close track of all patients on clozapine and will only allow for its release by pharmacy if the full blood count is normal.

Despite the extensive side effect profile, clozapine is a very effective drug and one third of patients with chronic schizophrenia respond to treatment within 6 weeks and two thirds within a year.

Case 8
BIPOLAR AFFECTIVE DISORDER STATION OSCE – "Healing hands"

Task:	Achieved	Not Achieved
Introduces self		
Clarifies to whom they are speaking and gains consent for interview		
Elicits history in a concise manner: Onset of behavioural change Possible triggers e.g. lack of sleep or life events Impact on daily life (e.g. work, studies, finances, relationships) Change in sleeping/eating patterns		
Explores risk-taking behaviours/vulnerability (such as sex with strangers, excessive spending, sexual disinhibition)		
Elicits psychotic symptoms (delusions of grandeur/special powers, thought interference, religious preoccupations)		
Excludes suicidal ideation/thoughts of self-harm (Performs basic suicide risk assessment)		
Enquires about the patient's social situation (e.g. source of income for current spending pattern, living arrangements etc.)		
Enquires about forensic history/involvement with the Police		
Asks about personal history (childhood, relationships, education) and pre-morbid personality		
Asks about past medical history		
Asks about past psychiatric history		
Asks about regular medication and allergies		
Excludes illicit substance use and alcohol use		
Asks about family history, including mental health issues		
Explores insight into present mental state and behaviour		
Summarises and presents findings concisely		
Correctly identifies the diagnosis (bipolar affective disorder)		
Offers at least two other differential diagnoses including: schizophrenia, schizoaffective disorder, personality disorder, ADHD, stimulant substance abuse or endocrine disturbance		
Explains basic steps for management Drug therapy (Antipsychotics in acute episodes and mood stabilisers for prophylaxis e.g. lithium) Psychotherapy		
Employs a professional and calm approach		
Examiner's Global Mark	/5	
Actor / Helper's Global Mark	/5	
Total Station Mark	/30	

Learning Points

According to the ICD-10 criteria, a diagnosis of Bipolar Affective Disorder (BPAD) can be made when there have been at least two episodes of significant mood (depressive, manic or hypomanic) and behavioural disturbance. At least one of these episodes must be manic or hypomanic.

Manic episodes differ from the hypomanic type in that there are particularly severe (therefore having an impact on relationships, work, studies etc.) and involve psychotic symptoms.

It is important to remember that BPAD carries one of the highest lifetime risk for suicide attempts and suicide completion of all psychiatric illnesses. Lithium has been shown to reduce this risk.

Case 9
MEDICATION STATION OSCE – Lithium counselling

Task:	Achieved	Not Achieved
Introduces self, clarifies to whom they are speaking		
Explains the purpose of the discussion and gains consent to proceed		
Explains the benefits of lithium treatment (mood stabilisation)		
Explains that lithium is taken once a day, usually at night		
Discusses common side effects (such as weight gain, tremor, metallic taste, nausea, vomiting)		
Explains that most side effects can be treatable (e.g. propranolol for tremor, healthy diet and exercise for weight gain)		
Explains need for baseline tests (U&Es, TFTs, ECG)		
Explains need for long-term blood monitoring (TFTs, U&Es and lithium levels)		
Explains risks of teratogenicity (such as congenital cardiac abnormalities)		
Describes the signs of toxicity (worsening side effects as above plus ataxia, reduced consciousness, myoclonus, seizures)		
Explains risk of sudden cessation of the drug (may cause mania)		
Asks about current medication		
Checks for drug allergies		
Asks about alcohol use (when taken with lithium can cause drowsiness/cognitive impairment)		
Asks about past medical history		
Asks about family history (such as thyroid, renal or cardiac disease)		
Gives the patient an opportunity to ask questions		
Counsels the patient in a clear and concise manner		
Offers an information leaflet		
Examiner's Global Mark	/5	
Actor / Helper's Global Mark	/5	
Total Station Mark	/30	

Learning Points

Lithium can be extremely effective in stabilising mood in acute mania and in the prevention of recurrence. It has also been shown to reduce suicide risk both in bipolar and unipolar depression.

Remember the '4 T's' of Lithium side effects: Tremor, Thirst, thyroid dysfunction and teratogenicity.

If levels and side-effects are not closely monitored it can lead to renal and cardiac damage, and in severe cases can cause lasting cognitive and cerebellar dysfunction. Careful counselling including contraception advice is therefore essential.

Case 10
SUICIDE RISK STATION OSCE - Worried Colleague

Task:	Achieved	Not Achieved
Introduces themselves and establishes rapport		
Elicits history of presenting complaint from patient in a concise manner		
Asks about depressive symptoms		
Asks specifically about current suicidal ideation		
Asks about self harm		
Elicits the patient's isolation		
Asks about plans for suicidal act and the future		
Asks about a suicide note/financial planning		
Asks about precautions against being found		
Elicits suicide plans are premeditated rather than impulsive		
Asks about alcohol and substance abuse		
Asks about past psychiatric history		
Asks about past medical history		
Asks about medication		
Asks about anxiety symptoms		
Rules out psychosis		
Summarises consultation fluently		
Advises that the patient is high risk of suicide		
Gives examples of what determines the patient at being high risk (male, single, isolated, previous attempts, history of depression and anxiety, alcohol use, health care worker, plans for future attempts)		
Non judgmental approach		
Examiner's Global Mark	/5	
Actor / Helper's Global Mark	/5	
Total Station Mark	/30	

Learning Points

Knowing the suicide risk stratification is essential at determining level of risk and need for further management. A usual acronym is SADPERSONS (Juhnke, 1994 and Patterson et al. 1983)

> S - Male Sex
> A - Age <18 and >50
> D - Depression
> P - Prior history of attempts
> E - ethanol/drug use
> R - Rational thinking loss (psychosis/organic disorder)
> S - Social Support (lack of)
> O - Organised plan
> N - No spouse/significant other
> S - Sickness (medical/psychiatric co-morbidities).

Mental illness can affect anyone including members of staff around you. As a medical professional it might only be you that has noticed a member of staff that is of high risk. As soon as this is identified, senior support is essential at managing these cases appropriately and safely.

The ethical dilemma comes from breaking confidentiality in order to take the patient out of the working role to gain appropriate mental health support. Clearly in this case, some members of the nursing staff are not providing the patient with support and are provoking their low mood. Therefore, the patient should be asked who is a trusted member of the senior nursing team to be informed.

Health care professionals are at a high risk category of suicide and mental illness. There is often fear arising from disclosing mental illness on the implications it has on employment. However, according to the GMC, if a doctor is open about their illness and seeks means to have it well controlled it will not affect future employment.

Case 11
Bulimia Nervosa STATION OSCE – 'Antisocial and Irritable'

Task:	Achieved	Not Achieved
Introduces self		
Clarifies who they are speaking to and gains consent		
Elicits history of presenting complaint with a focus on psychiatric history		
Establishes the nature of the eating disorder including binge eating, vomiting and purging.		
Asks about physical symptoms (palpitations, SOB, sweating, dizziness) and biological symptoms (weight changes, appetite, libido)		
Asks about past medical history		
Asks about past psychiatric history		
Asks about personal history (childhood, relationships)		
Asks about family history with focus on mental health and suicide		
Asks about drug history and allergies		
Asks about comorbid drug / alcohol misuse		
Asks about forensic history		
Risk assessment: suicide and self-harm risk, considers hospitalization if malnourished.		
Explains a differential diagnosis to patient using lay terms: likely bulimia nervosa with aspects of anorexia nervosa and/or muscle dysmorphia		
Further investigations: BMI, FBC, iron studies, cortisol, TFT, U+E's including PO3+ and Mg2+, ECG		
Offers treatment such as family psychotherapy and CBT. SSRI's may be indicated if severe.		
Discusses how best to tell family		
Offers a second consultation as follow-up		
Clear and concise consultation		
Non judgmental approach		
Examiner's Global Mark	/5	
Actor / Helper's Global Mark	/5	
Total Station Mark	/30	

Learning Points

Use the SCOFF criteria for an easy way to remember the questions you should ask when considering an eating disorder:
SCOFF
Sick: have you ever made yourself sick? (remember to ask about other compensatory behaviours such as over exercise and laxative abuse)
Control: have you ever had a feeling of loss of control when you eat?
One stone: have you lost/gained weight?
Fat: Do you feel fat?
Food: does it dominate your life?

Muscle dysmorphia, (AKA bigorexia) is a recently acknowledged body dysmorphic anxiety disorder associated with a preoccupation of increasing muscle mass and a delusion that muscles are too small. Much like bulimia, this disorder is associated with a poor self-esteem. The disorder can interfere with ALD and patients may prioritize weight lifting and exercise over their family, social life and work commitments. This condition is seen as similar to anorexia in that there is body dysmorphia and obsession with body shape. This condition is associated with anxiety and depression and there is an increased suicide risk and risk of self-harm.

Sometimes it is best to see adolescence without their parents to enable them to express themselves fully and to prevent conflict from interfering with the consultation. Always remember to do what is best for the patient.

Case 12
EXAMINATION OSCE STATION- The rigid lady

Task:	Achieved	Not Achieved
Inspects surroundings/checks for danger		
Checks for patient response (patient is rousable)		
Introduces self		
Confirms patient name and DOB		
Gains consent		
Examines patient from end of bed		
Assesses airway		
Assesses breathing, offers to listen to the chest, asks for respiratory rate/oxygen sats		
Circulation – palpates pulse, asks for blood pressure/HR/Capillary refill time/listens to heart		
Asks for temperature		
Assesses mental state – AVPU or GCS		
Assesses tone and power of upper or lower limbs (examiner notes rigidity and tremor in both hands)		
Asks about/inspects for incontinence		
Palpates abdomen AND asks for glucose		
Summarises findings		
Gives correct diagnosis – neuroleptic malignant syndrome		
Gives appropriate differential diagnosis e.g. catatonia, malignant hyperthermia, serotonin syndrome or encephalitis/meningitis		
Lists appropriate initial investigations including any 4 of FBC, Blood cultures, CK, ABG, LFTs, U+E, clotting, ECG, CXR, consider LP/CT head		
Give appropriate initial management plan at least 2 of: Cooling, IV fluids, antipyretics, Senior review/ICU referral, consider benzodiazepines		
Explicitly asks for haloperidol to be stopped		
Examiner's Global Mark	/5	
Actor / Helper's Global Mark	/5	
Total Station Mark	/30	

Learning Points

Neuroleptic malignant syndrome is a rare but life threatening reaction to neuroleptic medication, and is thought to be secondary to blockade of dopaminergic neurons. IT is typically caused by either antidepressants, anti-psychotics or anti-Parkinsonian medications.

The four cardinal features are muscular rigidity (lead pipe), pyrexia >38C, autonomic instability and altered mental state. If the muscular rigidity is severe and sustained it can result in muscle breakdown (rhabdomyolysis) which is why creatinine kinase (CK) is an important investigation in their initial workup.

Management is mainly supportive, ideally, in an ITU setting to prevent respiratory failure. The most important step is to stop all neuroleptic agents and typically patients will recover in 1-2 weeks unless they have been given a long acting depot, where it can last up to 3 weeks.

Case 13

MILD-MODERATE DEPRESSION STATION OSCE - "Feeling blue"

Task:	Achieved	Not Achieved
Introduces self		
Clarifies who they are speaking to		
Establishes rapport		
Elicits history of symptoms (nature, onset, triggers, timing)		
Establishes timing (most of the day for >2 weeks)		
Establishes core symptoms of depression – (low mood, anhedonia, fatigue)		
Asks about *at least three* biological symptoms of depression (diurnal variation in mood, appetite and weight loss, disturbed sleep, early morning waking, reduced libido)		
Asks about *at least two* other symptoms of depression (guilt, hopelessness, poor concentration or indecisiveness, low Self-confidence, slowing of movement)		
Asks about symptoms of anxiety		
Asks about previous episodes of low or elated mood		
Asks about psychotic symptoms (delusions or hallucinations)		
Asks about self-harm or suicidal thoughts		
Asks about past psychiatric history		
Asks about past medical history		
Asks about medication history and allergies		
Asks about family history (depression, suicide)		
Asks about social history (alcohol, smoking, drugs, employment)		
Asks about personal history (childhood, school, relationships)		
Summarises consultation concisely		
Provides appropriate diagnosis (depression), including the severity (mild-moderate) based on duration and symptoms		
Examiner's Global Mark	/5	
Actor / Helper's Global Mark	/5	
Total Station Mark	/30	

Learning Points

Depression is an extremely common mental health disorder, affecting 350 million people worldwide and affecting one in five people at some point in their lives. It is likely to present in all healthcare environments.

A depressive episode can be categorized as mild, moderate or severe depending on the number of symptoms and symptom severity. Symptoms should be present for two weeks or more and every symptom should be present for most of every day. Symptoms can be divided into core, biological and other.

Case 14

PARANOID SCHIZOPHRENIA OSCE - "They are controlling us"

Task:	Achieved	Not Achieved
Introduces self		
Clarifies who they are speaking to and gains consent		
Establishes rapport		
Elicits history of symptoms (nature, onset, triggers, timing)		
Establishes timing of psychotic symptoms (>1month)		
Hallucinations: establishes presence of auditory hallucinations –running commentary and 3rd person auditory hallucinations		
Delusions: establishes presence of persecutory delusions		
Asks about thought insertion, withdrawal, echo and broadcast		
Asks about symptoms of low or high mood		
Asks about suicidal thoughts, risk to self and others		
Asks about past psychiatric history		
Asks about past medical history		
Asks about medication history and allergies		
Asks about family history		
Asks about social history (alcohol, smoking, drugs, employment)		
Asks about personal history (childhood, relationships, school)		
Asks about forensic history		
Summarises consultation concisely		
Provides appropriate diagnosis and suitable differential (delusional disorder, mood disorder with psychosis, organic causes such as epilepsy, drug induced psychosis)		
Non-judgmental approach		
Examiner's Global Mark	/5	
Actor / Helper's Global Mark	/5	
Total Station Mark	/30	

Learning Points

Paranoid schizophrenia is the most common type of schizophrenia in most parts of the world. Symptoms should be present for most of the time, during a period of 1 month or more.
ICD 10 diagnosis guidelines for schizophrenia include:

One or more of the followings symptoms	Two or more of the following symptoms
Thought echo, insertion, withdrawal, or broadcast Delusions of control or passivity; delusional perception Hallucinatory voices Persistent delusions of other kinds that are culturally inappropriate and completely impossible	Persistent hallucinations in any modality, with fleeting or half-formed delusions or by persistent over-valued ideas Thought disorder Catatonic behaviour Negative symptoms such as marked apathy, paucity of speech, and blunting or incongruity of emotional responses Significant and consistent change in overall quality of personal behaviour

In the patient with auditory hallucinations, remember to ask about 'command hallucinations' where they are being directly talked to or instructed. Always explore whether the patient would act on these. If they are being told to kill someone, and are unable to resist their hallucinations, this is very high risk!

Case 15
Mark scheme - "That thingamybob"

Task:	Achieved	Not Achieved
Introduces self to patient		
Clarifies who they are speaking to and obtains consent		
Establishes rapport		
Establishes history of symptoms (nature, onset, timing, slow or step-wise, examples, exacerbating factors)		
Rules out physical causes (head injury, hypothyroidism, B12 deficiency, Parkinsonism, space occupying lesion)		
Asks about behavioural change (agitation, aggression, disinhibition, calling out)		
Asks about cognitive change (aphasia, apraxia, agnosia, planning and organising)		
Asks about depressive symptoms – (low mood, anhedonia, fatigue, sleep, energy levels, appetite, self-care)		
Asks about psychotic symptoms (delusions, hallucinations)		
Performs risk assessment, including dementia-related risk (wandering, leaving taps running / oven on, driving, neglect and asking specifically about suicidal ideation).		
Asks about past psychiatric history		
Asks about medical history, medication and allergies, compliance		
Asks about alcohol and drugs		
Asks about psychotic symptoms (hallucinations, delusions – particularly delusions of worthlessness, neglect etc.)		
Asks about family history		
Asks about social history (home support, type of accommodation, personal [self-care, dressing] and domestic [finances, cooking, cleaning] activities of daily living)		
Is sensitive towards patients concerns throughout, counsels patient appropriately		
Summarises consultation fluently, including risk		
Provides at least 3 possible differential diagnoses (E.g. Alzheimer's dementia, vascular dementia, Lewy Body Dementia, depression, hypothyroidism, B12 deficiency)		
Lists a plan: MMSE or Addenbrookes Cognitive Assessment (ACE), dementia bloods screen (FBC, U&Es, LFTs, TFTs, B12 and Folate), CT head, collateral history, memory clinic, functional assessment		
Examiner's Global Mark	/5	
Actor / Helper's Global Mark	/5	
Total Station Mark	/30	

Learning Points

If you have ruled out delirium and suspect dementia, then perform a dementia screen. The purpose of this is to rule out reversible causes. This should include: FBC, U&Es, Calcium, Glucose, LFTs, TFTs, Serum Vitamin B12 & Folate.

It is important to have an understanding of the stages of dementia, and the typical features of memory impairment as the disease progresses. Mild dementia is characterised by symptoms such as word-finding difficulties and misplacing objects. In moderate dementia patients can often become disorientated and go wandering from their homes and may become agitated or aggressive. Severe dementia is characterised by problems such as swallowing difficulties, incontinence and speech loss [1]. With these symptoms in mind, it is important to evaluate the level of risk by asking about common incidents such as wandering, leaving the oven on or taps running, and any acts of aggression.

A common comorbidity of dementia is depression, and low mood or anhedonia can be a presenting symptom, often before memory problems are noticed. It is important to screen for symptoms of depression, as patients are likely to benefit from some form of anti-depressant treatment.

Case 16
Delirium station - The Good Wife

Task:	Achieved	Not Achieved
Introduces the conversation		
Confirms relatives identify and gains consent		
Elicits history of symptoms in a concise manner (acute or chronic, timing, nature, onset, triggers e.g. change in medication)		
Elicits symptoms of delirium: agitation, disorientation to person		
Slowly progressive or step-wise		
Asks about delusions and hallucinations		
Asks about mood (low mood, anhedonia, fatigue)		
Asks about circadian rhythm disturbance		
Asks about recent falls or head injury		
Asks about recent infective symptoms: fever, cough, shortness of breath, urinary symptoms, frequency, urgency		
Asks about past medical history		
Asks about medication history and allergies		
Asks about baseline cognition		
Finds out about pre-morbid function (dressing, cooking, cleaning, mobility, finances)		
Asks about social history (alcohol, drugs, previous employment)		
Q: Defines confusion as a delirum/acute confusion		
Q: Acute causes (any three): Infective: UTI, LRTI, sepsis, encephalitis Metabolic/endocrine: electrolyte disturbance, constipation, urinary retention, AKI/uraemia, hypothermia, hypoxia, hypoglycaemia. Drug induced: Opiates (co-codamol), steroids Intracranial: Head injury, Chronic or acute subdural bleed, SAH, raised ICP.		
Q: Chronic causes: Dementias (Vascular/Alzheimer's/Lewy Body/Fronto-temporal Metabolic: Vitamin deficiency (Wernicke's Encephalopathy), hypothyroidism Psychiatric: Depression		
Q: Management. Conservative, medical and social domains (e.g. well lit area, investigating and treating the underlying cause, CT head, MDT approach including physiotherapy, social services and occupational therapy involvement)		
Non judgmental approach		
Examiner's Global Mark	/5	
Actor / Helper's Global Mark	/5	
Total Station Mark	/30	

Learning Points

Delirium is defined as an acute, fluctuating change in mental status, disorganised thinking and altered levels of consciousness. It carries with it a high morbidity and mortality.

There are three main subtypes:
Hyperactive: associated with high levels of arousal, agitation, hallucinations and delusions
Hypoactive: associated with reduced energy, motor retardation and incoherent speech. Often overlooked as patients are quiet and do not draw attention to their behaviour.
Mixed delirium
(Bestpractice BMJ: Delirium (2015)

This case touches upon capacity and best interests. According to Good Medical Practice (GMC), in cases where patients do not have capacity around treatment choices, the clinician must consider the patient care their first concern. They must support and encourage the patient to be as involved as possible around treatment choices. They should consider if the capacity status is temporary or permanent. What treatment would provide overall benefit to the patient. Where there is a legally binding advanced statement/decision, the view of family members and close friends' should be considered.

If there is disagreement between family/friends and the healthcare team, it can normally be resolved by a case conference/family meeting and involving senior members of the team. If despite these measures, the conflict remains, legal advice should be sought in making sure the best interests of the patient are met.

Case 17
LEWY BODY DEMENTIA STATION OSCE - confused elderly patient

Task:	Achieved	Not Achieved
Introduces self		
Confirms patient identity and gains consent		
Elicits history from patient in a concise manner		
Asks about presenting complaint with an open question		
Asks about memory – short term memory, long term memory, names, faces		
Asks about onset and progression of symptoms e.g is it stepwise, gradual or sudden		
Asks about risky behaviour – wandering out, leaving the hob on, locking up		
Asks about triggers – illness, stroke, trauma, medications, seizures, bereavement, social stressors		
Asks about symptoms of low mood		
Asks about daily activities – washing, dressing, cooking, shopping, driving		
Asks about Parkinsonism symptoms – tremor, slow movements, difficulty writing/initiating movement		
Asks about hallucinations – Auditory or visual		
Asks about past medical history – diabetes, blood pressure, strokes, epilepsy, clotting disorders		
Asks about medication history and allergies		
Asks drug and alcohol history		
Conducts the AMTS exam fluently and correct score (4/10)		
Non judgmental approach		
QUESTION 1: Offers primary diagnosis of Lewy Body dementia and at least one other differential including Fronto-temporal Dementia, Alzheimer's disease, vascular dementia		
QUESTION 2: Investigations to rule out organic cause, confusion or dementia screen – urine dip, U+Es, TFTs, vitamin deficiencies, LFTs, CRP, Consider CT Head, MMSE		
QUESTION 3: Bio-psychosocial management. Conservative therapies – memory clinics, occupational therapist at home, education for family, Social services if care needs are not met, Referral to Parkinson's clinic if motor features are found. Medical management – Rivastigmine may help. Social support		
Examiner's Global Mark	/5	
Actor / Helper's Global Mark	/5	
Total Station Mark	/30	

Learning Points

Assess the 5 A's of Dementia – agnosia, aphasia, apraxia, amnesia and abnormal behaviour.

Be aware of how to differentiate between different types of dementia. The most common is Alzheimer's, but ensure you ask questions to rule out Vascular dementia (hypertension, diabetes, strokes, TIA, clotting disorders), Lewy Body Dementia (visual hallucinations, fluctuating symptoms, disrupted sleep-wake cycle, associated with Parkinsonian features) and rarer forms of dementia such as Fronto-temporal Dementia (disinhibition, personality and behaviour changes)

Depression in the elderly can sometimes mimic dementia, cognitive decline can be seen with low mood. When the mood disorder is treated, cognition returns to normal.

Core features essential for diagnosis of probable LBD (Two needed for Diagnosis)
Fluctuating cognition with significant variation in alertness and attention
Recurrent florid complex hallucinations, often well formed and detailed (Visual 60%, auditory 20%)
Motor symptoms of Parkinsonism (Bradykinesia, tremor and rigidity)

Case 18

HISTORY TAKING OSCE STATION- overdose

Task:	Achieved	Not Achieved
Introduces self		
Clarifies patient identity and gains consent		
Asks open question (elicits presenting complaint)		
Elicits events precipitating overdose – preparation, planning, suicide note, triggers		
Circumstance of overdose – alone/intoxicated and when the tablets were taken (simultaneously/ staggered)		
Asks about additional alcohol or drugs used		
Elicits type of medication and number of tablets taken		
Asks about events after the overdose – regret, hid evidence, told someone		
Asks about ongoing suicidal ideation, plans, protective factors, suicide note		
Assesses mood and elicits depressive symptoms– low mood, anhedonia, fatigue		
Asks about psychiatric history		
Asks about past medical history		
Asks about medications and allergies		
Social history –family, school, relationships, social activities, home life, smoking		
Summarises consultation appropriately		
States risk of self harm/suicide as low risk		
Suggests appropriate management plan including baseline bloods (including liver function, clotting profile) and taking paracetamol levels 4 hours post ingestion.		
States if levels are above the treatment line they will need to start an N-Acetylcysteine infusion.		
Mentions referring to the Child and Adolescent Mental Health Service for assessment.		
Non-judgemental approach		
Examiner's Global Mark	/5	
Actor / Helper's Global Mark	/5	
Total Station Mark	/30	

Learning points

Paracetamol overdose is one of the most common psychiatric presentations to the emergency department. The important factors to ask regarding the overdose are what medication, how many tablets, what dose, staggered or simultaneous overdose, and was there a delay in presentation?

Paracetamol undergoes breakdown in the liver to a toxic metabolite called N-acetyl-p-benzoquinoneimine (NAPQI) which depletes the liver's supply of glutathione stores. NAPQI can then cause hepatic necrosis once glutathione stores reach zero. Liver failure is therefore the biggest medical concern in patient presenting with paracetamol overdose and care needs to be taken when monitoring their paracetamol levels. N-acetylcysteine (NAC) is the antidote given to anyone above the treatment line on the paracetamol treatment graph or that presents with a significant overdose: over 12 grams (24 x 500mg tablets) or >75mg/kg. NAC can produce hypersensitivity reactions so is best given by slow intravenous infusion.

Alcoholics and those who are chronically malnourished (e.g. anorexia nervosa, cachexia) are at higher risk of liver damage due to reduced glutathione stores.

Case 19

Psych OSCE – Deliberate Self-Harm History

Task:	Achieved	Not Achieved
Introduces self to patient		
Clarifies who they are speaking to and obtains consent		
Establishes rapport		
Elicits history of symptoms (nature, onset, timing, exacerbating factors)		
Establishes trigger for DSH (row with mother)		
Establishes severity / intent: did not intend to end her life		
Asks about core symptoms of depression (low mood, anhedonia, fatigue)		
Asks about psychotic symptoms		
Asks about past psychiatric history		
Asks about past medical history, medication and allergies		
Enquires about drug and alcohol use		
Asks about social history (alcohol, smoking, childhood)		
Asks about personal history (childhood, relationships, school, brief birth and developmental history)		
Asks about family history (mental illness, suicide)		
Risk assessment: asks about current suicidal ideation, likelihood to self-harm		
Risk assessment: asks about other risk factors; e.g. risk to others or from others.		
Question: What do you consider the risk to be? Factors to consider (nature of attempt – i.e. impulsive, no current suicidal ideation, social support (parents/ boyfriend), alcohol use – increased risk, age places her in higher risk category.)		
Question: What options would you consider in your management plan? Offering an informal admission, or discharging with follow-up from the community team or crisis team involvement, telephone or home visit. Discharge would be considered if family or friends would be able to stay with her and keep an eye on her. Advising to see GP for follow up in next few days.		
Question: Who else would you speak to? Parents, patient's mental health team if available, care coordinator, or liaison team if out of hours.		
Non-judgmental approach		
Examiner's Global Mark	/5	
Actor / Helper's Global Mark	/5	
Total Station Mark	/30	

Learning Points

"Self-harm" covers a broad range of behaviours. Cutting is the commonest form seen in adolescents in the community, whilst in inpatient units self-poisoning (e.g. paracetamol overdose) is commoner. *Remember that self-harm can be with or without suicidal intent.*

10% of adolescents report having self-harmed, but only about 1 in 8 of these will present to services. It is therefore particularly important for healthcare professionals to talk to young people about the issues of self-harm and suicide.

Some key risk factors for suicide in adolescents are:

Male gender (although females are more likely to self-harm - particularly between the ages of 12 and 15, when the female-to-male ratio is approximately 5:1)
Family history of suicide
Lower socioeconomic status
Parental separation, divorce or death
A co-existing mental disorder – particularly depression, anxiety and ADHD
Alcohol and drug misuse
Case 20

BULLYING STATION OSCE - Cyberbullying

Task:	Achieved	Not Achieved
Introduces self		
Clarifies patient identify and obtains consent		
Elicits history of symptoms a concise and logical manner		
Establishes nature of the bullying (onset, triggers, timing, duration, exacerbating factors)		
Establishes severity of bullying		
Establishes core symptoms of depression (low mood, anhedonia, fatigue)		
Asks about *at least three* biological symptoms of depression (diurnal variations in mood, appetite and weight loss, disturbed sleep including early morning waking, reduced libido)		
Asks about *at least two* other symptoms of depression (guilt, hopelessness, poor concentration or indecisiveness, low self-confidence, agitation or slowing of movement)		
Asks about symptoms of anxiety		
Asks about previous episodes of low mood		
Asks about any previous episodes of mania		
Asks about psychotic symptoms		
Asks about self harm or suicidal thoughts		
Asks about past psychiatric history		
Asks about past medical history, medications and allergies		
Asks about family history		
Asks about social history (alcohol, smoking, drugs, occupation)		
Asks about personal history (childhood, relationships, school, brief birth and developmental history)		
Provides appropriate diagnosis, including severity (depression, mild-moderate)		
Gives clear explanation as to why mild-moderate depression (duration, symptoms)		
Examiner's Global Mark	/5	
Actor / Helper's Global Mark	/5	
Total Station Mark	/30	

Learning Points

Bullying is defined as repeated behaviour that is intended to hurt someone either physically or emotionally. There are many different types of bulling including:

> Verbal- e.g.- name calling, teasing and threats
> Physical bullying- e.g.- hair pulling, hitting, pushing
> Social bullying- e.g.- social excluding people, spreading rumours
> Cyberbullying- any bullying that involves the use of digital technology such as phone harassment, abusive messages, writing rude comments on social media, imitating others online

Supporting young people with low mood who are the victims of bullying can be thought of at the individual, class, and school level:

Individual level- the bullying should be reported and serious discussions should be help with bullies and the victim. Role-play and group therapy have been shown to be helpful.
Class level –The class rules should include a clear message that bullying won't be tolerated and a curriculum that promotes kindness and conflict resolution
School- bullying awareness week, regular education sessions for staff, increased supervision in playground and cafeterias, ongoing meetings between parents and staff, a central group of psychologists, counsellors, school nurses who are responsible for the antibullying programme
If there is no response and they are suffering with moderate to severe depression a multidisciplinary review is required before offering a trial of fluoxetine. Any children or young person started on fluoxetine should be reviewed closely for suicidal behaviour, self-harm or hostility

Surgery

Case 1
Markscheme - Acute Abdomen (Aortic Aneurysm)

Task	Achieved	Not Achieved
Wash hands & Introduces self		
Clarifies who they are speaking to		
Elicits presenting complaint		
Offers reassurance and calms patient		
History of presenting complaint		
Explores differentials – asks about pain (SOCRATES)		
Explores associated symptoms		
Asks about whether the symptoms fluctuate		
Explores differentials – asks about red flags of malignancy		
Asks about past medical & surgical history		
Asks about Drug History, allergies		
Ask about Family History & Social History		
Summarises history concisely		
Explains further immediate management (Approach using an ABCDE technique)		
Leaking AAA top of differentials, name three more		
Mentions this is an emergency & resuscitation		
Mention the need for close monitoring, Access, Blood markers, G&S clotting and order units of RBC		
Escalate to your senior		
Notify Emergency theatres and anaesthetist on call		
If patient is clinically stable, discuss forms of imaging such as CT angiogram		
Examiner's Global Mark	/5	
Actor/Helper Global Mark	/5	
Total	/30	

Learning Points:

Learn by heart the differential diagnoses of the acute abdomen presentation. SOCRATES is a mnemonic acronym for pain assessment, Site/Onset/Character/ Radiation/ Associations/ Time course/ Exacerbating/relieving factors/ Severity of pain score. Remember this tool for every history taking

Make sure your History taking includes important negatives to help you work towards your top diagnosis.

Always immediately manage acutely unwell patients using the
A B C D E approach.

Case 2
Markscheme - Right Iliac Fossa Pain in a Female

Task	Achieved	Not Achieved
Wash hands & Introduces self		
Clarifies who they are speaking to		
Elicits presenting complaint		
Offers reassurance and calms patient		
History of presenting complaint		
Explores differentials – asks about pain (SOCRATES)		
Asks about exacerbating/relieving factors		
Asks about urinary symptoms		
Asks about sexual history		
Asks about menstrual history		
Asks about past medical & surgical history		
Asks about Drug History, allergies		
Ask about Family History & Social History		
Explore Ideas, Concerns, Expectations		
Summarises history concisely		
Presents a reasonable differential diagnosis (3 of ectopic pregnancy, appendicitis, ovarian pathology, urinary tract infection)		
Next management steps to include examination of the patient's abdomen		
Specifically mentions the need for urine dip test and pregnancy test		
Specifically mentions the importance of inflammatory marker blood tests		
Discuss imaging, organising ultrasound abdomen/pelvis		
Examiner's Global Mark	/5	
Actor/Helper Global Mark	/5	
Total	/30	

Learning Points:

Appendicitis is the most common surgical emergency but in women of childbearing age ectopic pregnancy must always be considered. A joint care approach with Gynaecology may be needed in the first instance as delay must never occur with disagreements around which team should be in charge.

For women with normal inflammatory markers and sudden onset right iliac fossa pains consider gynaecological causes.

The Alvarado score has a low sensitivity but remembering the points of the score helps to collect many of the clinically relevant pieces of information.

Case 3
Markscheme - Abdominal pain and vomiting

Task	Achieved	Not Achieved
Wash hands & Introduces self		
Clarifies who they are speaking to		
Elicits presenting complaint		
Offers reassurance and calms patient		
History of presenting complaint		
Explores differentials – asks about pain (SOCRATES)		
Explores associated symptoms		
Explores a full gastro-intestinal history from mouth to anus		
Explores differentials – asks about red flags of malignancy		
Asks about change in bowel habits, absolute constipation, oral intake		
Asks about past medical & surgical history		
Asks about Drug History, allergies		
Ask about Family History & Social History		
Summarises history concisely		
Explores patient's Ideas, Concerns and Expectations		
Addresses patient's belief re diagnosis and desire to leave		
Explains further immediate management (Approach using an ABCDE technique)		
Bowel obstruction top of differentials, name three more		
Mention the need for close monitoring, Access, Blood markers, G&S clotting and order units of RBC		
Recommend NGT, catheter 'drip & suck', IVI, CT abdomen/pelvis		
Examiner's Global Mark	/5	
Actor/Helper Global Mark	/5	
Total	/30	

Learning Points:

Bowel cancer especially caecum pathology is often associated with a new anaemia. Don't forget to ask about anaemia symptoms in your system's enquiry.

Be specific when providing a management plan in an OSCE. Don't just state the test you would order but add why you are doing it and what you are looking for to gain the full marks. Also include name, route and dose of drugs where possible.

Do not neglect the points you will receive for your communication skills. In such a station taking notice of the patient's desire to leave and exploring his Ideas, Concerns and Expectations (ICE) can gain you numerous marks and importantly project a better global impression to the actor and examiner. Ultimately practicing this now will make you a much better doctor too as the success of most consultations rest upon ICE.

Case 4
Markscheme - Change in bowel habit

Task	Achieved	Not Achieved
Wash hands & Introduces self		
Clarifies who they are speaking to		
Elicits presenting complaint		
Explores patient's pain (SOCRATES)		
Explores associated symptoms		
Elicits timeline of symptoms		
Asks about red flags - Elicits weight loss symptoms		
Asks about red flags – PR bleeding and mucus, tenesmus		
Asks about red flags – appetite		
Asks about red flags – abdominal pain		
Asks about past medical & surgical history		
Asks about Drug History, allergies		
Ask about Family History & Social History		
Asks about past medical & surgical history		
Identifies patient's concerns		
Summarises history concisely		
Explains further immediate management (abdominal and PR examination)		
Provides differential diagnoses (name three)		
Malignancy at top of differentials		
Mentions need for colonoscopy, tumour markers and CT CAP in view of weight loss and staging		
Examiner's Global Mark	/5	
Actor/Helper Global Mark	/5	
Total	/30	

Learning Points:

Colorectal cancer is the 3rd most common malignancy in the UK. Change in bowel habit in the over 50s is bowel cancer until proven otherwise.

Always ask about red flag symptoms. Red flags for colorectal cancer are change in bowel habit, PR bleeding, weight loss, abdominal pain, mucus passed PR and loss of appetite.

Differential diagnoses do exist including diverticulitis, inflammatory bowel disease, irritable bowel disease and local pathologies such as haemorrhoid disease however if red flags exist key investigations for bowel cancer such as colonoscopy with biopsies will be undertaken.

Case 5
Markscheme - Upper GI Bleed

Task	Achieved	Not Achieved
Wash hands & Introduces self		
Clarifies who they are speaking to		
Elicits presenting complaint		
Offers reassurance and calms patient		
History of presenting complaint		
Explores haematemesis – volume, appearance,		
Explores associated symptoms		
Explores differentials – asks about pain		
Explores differentials – asks prior vomiting		
Explores differentials – asks about red flags of malignancy		
Elicits chronic alcohol history		
Elicits reasons for alcoholism		
Asks about past medical & surgical history		
Asks about Drug History, allergies		
Ask about Family History & Social History		
Summarises history concisely		
Explains further immediate management (Approach using an ABCDE technique)		
Variceal Bleeding top of differentials, name three more		
Mentions this is an emergency & resuscitation		
Urgent endoscopy within 4 hours and mention scoring system for UGI Bleeds		
Examiner's Global Mark	/5	
Actor/Helper Global Mark	/5	
Total	/30	

Learning Points:

Oesophageal Variceal bleeding carries a very high mortality rate and requires intravenous terlipressin and urgent endoscopic intervention within 4 hours.

If a patient with haematemesis presented shocked then they will need to be resuscitated and stabilised before endoscopy can occur, remember bleeding severity can be assessed by extent of blood loss and degree of shock. This requires large bore access and fluid resuscitation. Where blood loss is the obvious cause the resuscitation fluid should be blood with O negative blood used if type specific or fully cross matched isnt readily available.

Recommendations emphasise early risk stratification, using the Blatchford score at first assessment and the full Rockall score after endoscopy.

Case 6
Markscheme - Obstructive Jaundice

Task	Achieved	Not Achieved
Wash hands & Introduces self		
Clarifies who they are speaking to		
Elicits presenting complaint		
Offers reassurance and calms patient		
History of presenting complaint		
Explores differentials – asks about pain (SOCRATES)		
Explores associated symptoms		
Pain radiating to the shoulder tip or scapula		
Explores differentials – asks about pain		
Symptoms of obstructive jaundice		
Asks about past medical & surgical history		
Asks about Drug History, allergies		
Ask about Family History & Social History		
Explores patient's Ideas, Concerns and Expectations		
Summarises history concisely		
Explains further immediate management (Approach using an ABCDE technique)		
3 of Acute Cholecystitis, Cholangitis Pancreatitis, Choledocholithiasis, top of differentials, name three more		
Suggests managing the patient immediately using the ABCDE approach		
Specifically mentions 2 of: erect CXR, serum amylase, inflammatory markers or abdominal USS, MRCP (Intraductal stones), ERCP,		
Recommends giving analgesia and antibiotics		
Examiner's Global Mark	/5	
Actor/Helper Global Mark	/5	
Total	/30	

Learning Points:

Acute cholecystitis patients can be very unwell with sepsis & jaundice – management of sepsis starts with an A to E assessment and resuscitation following the sepsis 6 care bundle. The main difference from biliary colic and cholecystitis is the inflammatory component (local peritonism, fever, raised white cell count. If the stone moves to the CBD, jaundice may occur.

Use targeted investigations to make a diagnosis following a thorough examination. Ultrasound is the key technique in distinguishing medical from surgical jaundice, and should be performed on all cases of acutely unwell jaundice.

Recommend diagnostic flow chart for patients for intraductal Common bile duct stone is firstly perform MRCP, then ERCP and early laparoscopic cholecystectomy.

Case 7

Markscheme - Leg pain

Task	Achieved	Not Achieved
Wash hands & Introduces self		
Clarifies who they are speaking to		
Elicits presenting complaint		
Offers pain relief promptly		
Explores patient's pain (SOCRATES)		
Explores appearance of the leg		
Elicits leg feels cold		
Elicits previous symptoms of peripheral vascular disease		
History of claudication		
Asks about peripheral risk factors: TIA/IHD/High cholesterol		
Asks about past medical & surgical history		
Asks about Drug History, allergies		
Ask about Family History & Social History		
Smoking History		
Exercise Tolerance		
Summarises history concisely		
Provides differential diagnoses (name three)		
Explains further immediate management ABCDE, full neurovascular examination		
Recognises Acute Limb Ischaemia		
Mentions likely emboli due to acute onset and plan for urgent emergency surgery (limb salvage)		
Examiner's Global Mark	/5	
Actor/Helper Global Mark	/5	
Total	/30	

Learning Points:

Acute limb ischaemia is a surgical emergency characterised by the '6 P's' Pain!!!! paralysis, paraesthesia, pulseless, pale and perishingly cold. These findings can be picked up in any clinical setting (primary or secondary care) so there should be no excuse for not considering this diagnosis early and directing the patient to the appropriate vascular opinion.

The majority of cases are caused by a thrombus of an atheroma or by an embolus in those prone to clot formation. Acute scenarios are commonly due to an embolus and atrial fibrillation.

Critical ischaemia can be defined by the presence of ischaemic pain at rest, or tissue loss in the form of gangrene or ulcers. It is consistent with an ABPI of < 0.4. Candidates should reacquaint themselves with the method to perform an ABPI.

Case 8
Markscheme - Haematuria

Task	Achieved	Not Achieved
Wash hands & Introduces self		
Clarifies who they are speaking to		
Elicits presenting complaint		
Offers reassurance and calms patient		
History of presenting complaint		
Explores Heamaturia		
Explores associated symptoms		
Explores differentials – asks about pain (SOCRATES)		
Asks about storage symptoms- urgency, nocturia, frequency		
Asks about voiding symptoms- hesitancy, poor stream, terminal dribbling, incomplete voiding, dysuria		
Explores differentials – asks about red flags of malignancy		
Asks about previous occupational history		
Asks about past medical & surgical history		
Asks about Drug History, allergies		
Ask about Family History & Social History		
Summarises history concisely		
Explains further immediate management (Approach using an ABCDE technique)		
Offers to examine abdomen and perform Rectal Examination		
Bladder cancer top of differentials, name three more		
Frank haematuria, insertion of 3 way catheter and actively suction of clots with syringe		
Examiner's Global Mark	/5	
Actor/Helper Global Mark	/5	
Total	/30	

Learning Points:

When assessing a patient with haematuria remember that the most severe cause is cancer of the urinary tract but the most common cause in men is BPH.

Remember that painless haematuria can occur anywhere in the urinary tract not just in the bladder.

Assessment of this patient will include imaging of the upper tracts (ideally with a CT IVU), a flexible cystoscopy and in men a DRE and PSA (take PSA before performing DRE).

Case 9
Markscheme - Testicular pain

Task	Achieved	Not Achieved
Wash hands & Introduces self		
Clarifies who they are speaking to		
Elicits presenting complaint		
Offers reassurance and calms patient		
History of presenting complaint		
Explores patient's pain (SOCRATES)		
Explores associated symptoms- fever, rigors, urinary symptoms		
Asks about constitutional symptoms (lymphadenopathy, night sweats, weight loss)		
Asks about previous trauma		
Sexual health History		
Foreign travel History		
Asks about past medical & surgical history		
Asks about Drug History, allergies		
Ask about Family History & Social History		
Summarises history concisely		
Suggest performing abdominal, testicular and rectal examination		
Explains further immediate management		
Testicular cancer top of differentials, name three more		
Suggest urine dip, USS testes		
Name the tumour markers for testicular cancer		
Examiner's Global Mark	/5	
Actor/Helper Global Mark	/5	
Total	/30	

Learning Points:

Testicular cancer is usually a disease of the young have a high index of suspicion in patients with longstanding testicular pain particularly if they have a history of undescended testes. Testicular cancer can occur at any age but is most common between the ages of 15 and 40 years with testicular tumours the most common malignancy in men aged between 20 and 35 years.

A swollen high rising testis should give you a suspicion of testicular torsion. In this case urgent exploration is needed without delay for imaging.

An ultrasound scan of the testis is first line imaging to image any testicular lump however remember that an ultrasound can not rule out a testicular torsion.

Case 10
Markscheme - Breast Lump

Task:	Achieved	Not Achieved
Wash hands & Introduces self		
Clarifies who they are speaking to		
Elicits presenting complaint		
Offers reassurance and calms patient		
History of presenting complaint		
Ask about red flags- Lump, sudden increase in size, skin changes		
Ask about red flags- Nipple inversion/discharge/skin changes/ulceration		
Ask about pain (SOCRATES)		
Associated weight loss and back pain		
Gynecological History		
Asks about past medical & surgical history		
Asks about Drug History, allergies		
Ask about Family History & Social History		
Summarises history concisely		
Show empathy		
Address Ideas, concerns and expectations		
Breast cancer top of differentials, name three more		
Discuss 2 week referral to breast surgical one-stop clinic		
Triple assessment (examination, mammogram and core biopsy)		
Discuss Surgical and medical management for breast cancer		
Examiner's Global Mark	/5	
Actor / Helper's Global Mark	/5	
Total Station Mark	/30	

Learning Points:

Every patient with a breast lump should be referred to the one-stop breast clinic for triple assessment (examination, imaging, core biopsy)and review by a specialist.

Remember to ask about relevant gynaecological history such as age of menarche, menopause, parity, breastfeeding, contraceptive and hormone replacement therapy.

Have a systematic approach to history taking, covering the red flags for breast disease:
Breast lump
Nipple eczema or retraction
Skin distortion
Persisting, intense unilateral pain

Case 11
Markscheme - Post op confusion

Task:	Achieved	Not Achieved
Candidate introduces self		
Candidate confirms patient identity (this may be with a name band)		
Candidate establishes/explains role		
Candidate attempts to ask a symptom screen		
Candidate asks patient age		
Candidate asks patients the current time		
Candidate asks patient the current year		
Candidate asks patient the name of the building they are in		
Candidate asks the patient if they recognize two people/objects		
Candidate asks patient date of birth		
Candidate asks patient date recall question (what date was world war two etc)		
Candidate asks patient name of current monarch		
Candidate asks patient to count back from 20-1.		
Candidate attempts to ask patient to register and recall address (eg 42 west street)		
Candidate summarises discussion		
Candidate closes appropriately		
Candidate approaches discussion in structured manner		
Candidate listens actively		
Candidate allows appropriate silences and pauses		
Candidate demonstrates empathy and sensitivity		
Examiner's Global Mark	/5	
Actor / Helper's Global Mark	/5	
Total Station Mark	/30	

Learning Points:

Delirium is a clinical syndrome which is difficult to define exactly but involves abnormalities of thought, perception and levels of awareness. It typically is of acute onset and intermittent and can exhibit hypo and hyperactive episodes.

Post operatively remember to consider if there is an iatrogenic cause for the acute change - has the patient been prescribed anything that has made them confused. Blood sugars and infection screens can be initiated early to identify a cause.

The AMTS is absolutely key here. Once you have established the patient is confused and there is not much history to be gained, assessment of mental state should be the priority.

Case 12
Markscheme - Flexible Sigmoidoscopy

Task:	Achieved	Not Achieved
Candidate introduces him/herself and confirms patient identity		
Candidate explains their role to the patient		
Candidate confirms patient's current understanding, their worries and expectations of the consultation		
Candidate approaches explaining/addressing concerns in a clear structured manner		
Candidate explains that bowel preparation (enema/laxatives) is required		
Candidate explains that the procedure visualizes the rectum and the last portion of the large bowel (appropriate description of the endoscope used)		
Candidate explains general aspects of the procedure (a small camera with a similar width to a little finger with a light source is introduced to the back passage. Images from the camera are seen and assessed by the endoscopist as the procedure is carried out)		
Candidate explains the use of painkillers and/or sedatives to enable procedure and it should not be painful		
Candidate explain that if sedation is used the patient will not be able to drive themselves home and will require a friend/family member to supervise them after the procedure.		
Candidate explains that after the procedure they will be taken to the recovery area		
Candidate explains the benefits of the procedure – visualization of the bowel and acquisition of tissue samples for diagnostic purposes		
Candidate explains that there are risks, specifically bowel perforation, infection and bleeding but that these are rare		
Candidate explains that if polyps are removed there may be further fresh blood from the back passage over 12-24 hours after the procedure.		
Candidate explains that if samples are taken they will be processed in approximately 2 weeks.		
Candidate explains alternatives to flexible sigmoidoscopy, barium enema, ct colonography and briefly their benefits (non invasive) and limitations (no tissue diagnosis).		
Candidate summarises appropriately and prompts further questioning		
Candidate offers reading material		
Candidate demonstrates explanation in clear structured manner		
Candidate listens appropriately		
Candidate demonstrates empathy and sensitivity		
Examiner's Global Mark	/5	
Actor / Helper's Global Mark	/5	
Total Station Mark	/30	

Learning Points:

Explaining procedures and interventions is a common task for the foundation year doctor and so rightly many OSCEs are based around this. Having a structure is important - check understanding thus far, explain indications, contraindications, the location and duration of the procedure, the mechanics of the procedure itself and of course the potential side effects.

If formal written consent is required as per GMC guidelines this should only be done by someone that can actually carry out the procedure themselves. For procedures and interventions that only require verbal consent it is still good practice to explain all the sections above to ensure fully understanding.

Remember that in some situations patients may decline to give consent to a procedure. You may offer them more time, further reading materials and resources and senior to explain further however if they have capacity they are of course allowed to decline to give consent.

Case 13
Markscheme - Upset relative

Task:	Achieved	Not Achieved
Candidate introduces self		
Candidate confirmation of patient details		
Candidate explains their role & expresses sorrow for the situation		
Candidate establishes mother's current understanding of the situation		
Give reason for why she was not contacted		
Candidate explores their current concerns related to their clinical problem		
Candidate Breaks bad news that operation is an emergency signposting/appropriate warning shot		
Candidate allows the mother time to digest the news —severity of the situation		
Explain risks of procedure, avoid medical jargon		
Explore social background, ex-husband and father's drinking issue		
Child safety, child safeguarding procedure in a sensitive way		
Have to involve pediatric team and share information mother has given		
Not to collude with parent		
Discuss post-operative management of patient with splenectomy		
Candidate summarises discussion		
Candidate closes appropriately		
Candidate approaches discussion in a structured, clear manner		
Candidate listens actively and allows appropriate silences and pauses		
Maintains eye contacts, open body language, reassurance		
Candidate demonstrates empathy and sensitivity		
Examiner's Global Mark	/5	
Actor / Helper's Global Mark	/5	
Total Station Mark	/30	

Learning Points:

Good history taking is essential here to include a detailed social history around the child but also the parent and extended family circle too.

Always have a high suspicion for abuse and non-accidental injury and listen carefully to pick up on hidden cues and red flags such as a changing or inconsistent history, injuries that don't fit the mechanism stated, delayed presentations and children with disabilities to name a few.

Post-operative splenectomy management includes prophylactic antibiotics to mitigate against the risks of overwhelming post-splenectomy infection.

Case 14
Markscheme - Referral to ICU

Task	Achieved	Not Achieved
Introduction		
Clarifies who they are speaking to		
Remains polite and respectful throughout		
Purpose of referral		
Stress concern of patient safety		
Current Situation		
Background Information (blood test)		
Interprets ABG		
Explain patient has severe pancreatitis		
Mentions Glasgow Score for severity stratification		
Summarise your Assessment		
Does not make up results or investigations		
Stresses need for ITU review		
1. Invasive monitoring (Central Venous Pressure Line)		
2. Invasive monitoring (Arterial Line)		
3. Respiratory support		
Ask for Recommendation from ITU SpR		
1. 15 L oxygen		
2. Fluids, catheter hourly Urine output monitor		
Secure ITU review of patient		
Examiner's Global Mark	/5	
Actor/Helper Global Mark	/5	
Total	/30	

Learning Points:

Remember to clarify who you are speaking to and state the purpose of your call straight away. Sometimes 'headlining' with an opening statement like 'I have a patient I am worried about with probable pancreatitis' focuses the minds of both parties.

Always keep in mind that you are there representing your patient and act in their best interest to ensure they get the best quality care. Many specialist teams will be under pressure at work but you must be you patient's advocate and explain why you need that team's help.

Know the different reasons for referral to ITU. These include ventilatory support and haemofiltration and adopt a SBAR (Situation, Background, Assessment and Recommendation) approach

Case 15
Markscheme - Chest drain insertion

Task:	Achieved	Not Achieved
Introduces self, clarifies the name and age of the patient		
Gets verbal consent		
Prepares equipment: needle, syringe, local anaesthetic, sterile wound pack, skin prep, sterile gloves, scalpel, Roberts or similar instrument, 28-32F chest drain and under water collecting bottle.		
Asks about the patient's allergies		
Puts patient into a suitable position eg. 45° on a bed with their right hand behind their head		
Discusses the need for patient monitoring during the procedure – with or without sedation.		
Cleans hands and puts on gloves		
Keeps the sterile field		
Anatomically defines the safe triangle		
Cleans the skin prior to local anaesthetic		
Safely injects local anaesthetic (e.g. 1% lignocaine) first to the skin, then the intercostal muscles and down to the pleura		
Tests skin to check local anaesthetic has worked		
Makes an incision above an appropriate rib		
Bluntly dissects down to and through the pleura		
Finger sweep inside chest		
Introduces the drain a suitable distance atraumatically using Roberts		
Attaches drain to collecting system		
Checks that the drain is "swinging"		
Fixes (eg sutures) drain in place appropriately		
Gets a CXR to check position of the drain		
Examiner's Global Mark	/5	
Actor / Helper's Global Mark	/5	
Total Station Mark	/30	

Learning points:

It is important to appreciate the difference between a simple pneumothorax, which needs draining within hours and a tension pneumothorax with is an emergency and needs draining within minutes.

Careful consideration of the anatomical landmarks will reduce the risk of iatrogenic injury to surrounding structure. Beware of the neurovascular bundle below each rib.

This is not a routine procedure that a foundation doctor would be expected to perform. it is however essential to know the indications for thoracocentesis and chest drain insertion and also good practice to know the equipment and methodology as you may well assist your senior in these procedures.

Case 16
Markscheme - Abdominal radiograph interpretation

Task:	Achieved	Not Achieved
Introduces self & washes hands		
Clarifies whom they are speaking to.		
Comment on date of radiograph		
Correct Patient details (DOB & Hospital No)		
Projection of image – Anterior –Posterior		
Comments on adequacy of the image		
Comments on the rotation		
Comments on the penetration		
Comment on bowel gas pattern		
Bowel 3cm, 6 cm, 9 cm – normal anatomical width of small bowel, large bowel and caecum.		
Comment on Small bowel identified (i.e. Valvulae conniventes described if present)		
Comment on Large bowel identified (i.e.haustra described if present)		
Comment on pathology such as volvulus		
Comment on faecal loading		
Other organs: Soft tissue shadows – liver, spleen, kidneys, gall bladder, psoas shadow.		
Bone: The lower ribs, lumbar vertebrae, sacrum, coccyx, pelvic bones		
Comment on any calcification and artifact		
Summarize findings		
Provide differential diagnosis and further investigations		
Comment on your management plan for this patient		
Examiner's Global Mark	/5	
Actor / Helper's Global Mark	/5	
Total Station Mark	/30	

Learning Points

Example one demonstrates large bowel obstruction. The most common aetiology of large bowel obstructions are colorectal cancer and diverticular strictures. Dilatation of the caecum >9cm is considered abnormal.

Example two demonstrates sigmoid volvulus. The sigmoid colon is more prone to twisting than other segments of the large bowel because it is 'mobile' on its own mesentery. Treatment is decompression of the volvulus with rigid/flexible sigmoidoscopy.

Example three demonstrates small bowel obstruction. Plain radiograph will demonstrate centrally located multiple dilated loops of gas filled bowel. The valvulae conniventes are visible. This confirms small bowel involvement.

Case 17
Markscheme - CXR interpretation

Task	Achieved	Not Achieved
Introduces self and washes hands		
Clarifies whom they are speaking to		
Comment on date of radiograph		
Correct Patient Details (D.O.B. & Hospital No:)		
Projection of image – Anterior-Posterior		
Airway – Tracheal Deviation		
Breathing – Lung Fields, Pneumothorax, Lobar Collapse		
Hilar Lymphadenopathy		
Circulation – Heart Size, Heart Position		
Great vessels, Mediastinal Width <8cm on PA		
Diaphragm – Position and Shape, Costo-phrenic angles		
Air below diaphragm		
Bones, Artefacts		
Soft Tissues- Looking for masses, subcutaneous, calcification of aorta		
Summarize Findings		
Provides differential diagnosis and further investigations		
Comment on a management plan for the radiograph		
Examiner's Global Mark	/ 5	
Actor /Helper's Global Mark	/ 5	
Total Station Mark	/ 30	

Learning Points

Patient details are the most simple and important point. Always start with checking the film bears the patient's name, date of birth and hospital number and is the image taken today. With the advent of digital image banks it is very easy to open the wrong image.

Example one is an example of pneumoperitoneum, most likely due to a visceral perforation that is a surgical emergency. Example two shows rib fractures and a surgical drain placed likely due to trauma. Such a patient should be managed in an ATLS trauma call manner. Example three shows left pneumothorax, signs of early tension and example four shows aortic injury.

Being able to identify CXR findings is essential as a junior doctor but knowing the initial management of each of these diagnoses is even more important. Learning the BTS guidelines for management for pneumothorax treatment for example is a core piece of knowledge for doctors.

Case 18
Markscheme - Suturing under local anaesthetic

Task:	Achieved	Not Achieved
Introduces self		
Clarifies the name and age of the patient		
Asks about how the injury occurred		
Asks about the patient's allergies		
Comments on the neurovascular status of the hand		
Gain consent for procedure		
Prepare the sterile field		
Cleans hands with alcohol gel		
Puts on gloves		
Cleans the area around the wound		
Administers a suitable amount (e.g. 5mls) of local anaesthetic (e.g. 1% lignocaine) around the wound site		
Specifically shows he/she is aspirating before injecting the local anaesthetic		
Tests skin to check local anaesthetic has worked		
Uses non-touch technique when manipulating the needle		
Choose correct suture type		
Applies at least two sutures across laceration with at least 3 throws		
"Wet and dry" clean after administering suture		
Applies a dressing to the site		
Asks the patient about their tetanus status & gives injection if not covered		
Consider antibiotic cover and explains that they will need to have the suture removed in 7-10 days		
Examiner's Global Mark	/5	
Actor / Helper's Global Mark	/5	
Total	/30	

Learning points

It is important to check the neurovascular status of any laceration that you see as well as potential damage to any surrounding structures. Always check the tetanus status for any patient who comes to you with a laceration.

Take time to create a good sterile field for these procedures and take especial care not to contaminate this by touching anything that is not sterile.

Known maximum dosage calculation for Lidocaine 3ml/kg and with adrenaline 6ml/kg. When choosing a suture for wound, consider properties such as non-absorbable and monofilament and the most appropriate suture size for the area of the boy effected.

Case 19
Markscheme - Examination of the acute abdomen

Task:	Achieved	Not Achieved
Washes their hands, introduces themselves and obtains consent for the examination		
Examines patient from the end of the bed		
Checks hands and nails		
Pulse		
Examines the face / sclera for jaundice		
Examines the conjunctiva for pallor		
Examines the mucus membranes for hydration		
Exposes the abdomen and positions the patient flat then inspects for distension, scars and abnormal movements		
Palpates abdomen methodically in 9 sections		
Palpates abdomen for masses		
Palpates abdomen for Liver, Spleen and ballots the Kidneys		
Percusses abdomen		
Auscultates abdomen (bruits and bowel sounds)		
Examines hernial orifices		
Suggests DRE and examination of the external genitalia to complete the examination		
Thank patient and wash hands		
Summarize findings		
Asks for the patient's observations		
Requests sensible initial investigations to include Blood tests for FBC, CRP, LFTS, U&Es, Amylase and AXR / erect CXR or an ABG		
Differential Diagnosis – perforated peptic ulcer, pancreatitis, small bowel obstruction, mesenteric ischaemia, cholecystitis, gastritis, medical causes e.g. MI or LRTI		
Examiner's Global Mark	/5	
Actors Global Mark	/5	
Total Station Mark	/30	

Learning points:

Remember to adequately expose the patient. Examining around a patient gown can lead to missing pathology but the "Nipple to knee" approach is not appropriate for all patients – be guided by your findings.

Ensure you have a well-practiced slick method of examination. Start the examination of the abdomen by looking for peripheral stigmata of gastrointestinal disease.

Recognize that due to pain, your examination may need to be adapted so that you do not hurt the patient. Never forget that the genitalia should be examined as pain can radiate upwards and patients may feel shy in openly saying there is a problem.

Case 20
Markscheme - Hernial orifices

Task:	Achieved	Not Achieved
Introduces self, washes hands and checks patient identity		
Puts patient at ease by asking patient how they are feeling or another type of generic question		
States aim of the consultation: to perform an inguinal hernia examination		
Explains to patient why this examination is necessary		
Offers the presence of a same sex chaperone		
Describes level of undress required: trousers and underwear pulled down to knees		
Inspection of both inguinal regions, evaluating for size, induration and temperature check		
Observe cough impulse standing and lying		
Palpation of both inguinal regions		
Examination of the scrotum		
Feel for cough impulse on both sides		
Encourages the patient to tell you to stop if they experience any pain or discomfort		
Find deep inguinal ring		
Firmly press on lump and starting inferiorly lift the hernia up.		
Once reduced maintain pressure and assess cough impulse again		
Percussion of hernia		
Auscultation of hernia		
To complete examination- full abdominal and DRE required		
Summarize finding and investigations		
Able to differentiate between strangulated and incarcerated hernia		
Examiner's Global Mark	/5	
Actor / Helper's Global Mark	/5	
Total Station Mark	/30	

Learning points:

The difference between irreducible /incarceration/strangulation:
Irreducible – hernia that cannot be reduced to its original anatomical location.
Incarcerated – the contents of the hernia sac are stuck within the hernia sac
Strangulated –ischemia of the tissues contained within the hernia sac.

The mid-inguinal point is the halfway point between the anterior superior iliac spine and the pubic symphysis.

The anatomy borders for inguinal canal and femoral canal:
The inguinal canal is located above the medial half of the inguinal ligament. The inguinal ligament runs from the anterior superior iliac spine to the pubic tubercle. The inguinal canal has a deep inguinal ring located at the lateral aspect, and an external inguinal ring at the medial aspect.

The femoral canal is composed of:
Medial border – lacunar ligament
Lateral border – femoral vein
Anterior border – inguinal ligament
Posterior border – pectineal ligament, super pubic ramus and the pectineal muscle

The opening to the femoral canal is located at its superior border. This is known as the femoral ring.

Case 21
Markscheme - Breast examination

Task:	Achieved	Not Achieved
Wash Hands, Introduction and Consent		
Requests a chaperone		
Expose & Position Patient		
Inspection:		
Asymmetry, Scars, Skin Changes, Nipple changes		
At Rest		
Patient tensing Pectoralis Muscles		
Patient's Hands behind Head axillae and inframmary folds		
Ask patient if she is in any pain before palpating the breasts.		
Palpation:		
Position- ipsilateral arm behind their head and tilt towards the contralateral side to flatten breast against chest wall		
Palpates breasts in a systematic manner		
Palpate the four quadrants, nipple areolar complex and the inframammary fold		
Feeling a Lump:		
Site, Size, Surface, Skin Changes		
Tenderness, Temperature		
Mobility and underlying attachment		
Fluctuant, compressible, pulsatile, Consistency		
Palpate B/L axillary tail of Spence and supraclavicular nodes		
Cover the patient, thank them and wash your hands		
Summary of Findings		
Initial investigations		
Management Plan		
Examiner's Global Mark	/5	
Actor / Helper's Global Mark	/5	
Total Station Mark	/30	

Learning Points

On inspection remember to look for any past signs of breast cancer such as mastectomy, scars, hair loss, radiation burns and lymphedema. As well as inspecting the back for latissimus dorsi flap reconstruction scars and the abdomen for TRAM flap reconstruction scars

Triple assessment for Breast Lump would be History & Examination (P1-5), Imaging – Mammography/USS (M1-5, U1-5) and Histology – Core Biopsy (B1-5)

Differential diagnosis for a breast lump: cancer, firboadenoma, cyst, abscess, fibrocystic change, lipoma, fat necrosis (20yrs – fibroadenoma, 40s – cyst, 70s – cancer).

Case 22
Markscheme - Thyroid examination

Task:	Achieved	Not Achieved
Introduces self, washes hands and checks patient identity		
Explains examination, gains consent		
Asks patient to sit on a chair with neck and shoulders exposed		
Inspects hands, nails and skin		
Tests for fine tremor with a sheet of paper		
Looks for exophthalmos, lid lag and assesses eye movements		
Comments on clothing		
Inspects for signs of muscle wasting		
Looks for neck lump and scars		
Feels for radial pulse		
Feels for skin temperature		
Inspects for pre-tibial myxodema		
Palpates the thyroid and cervical nodes using a two handed technique and standing behind the patient asking them to tilt chin upwards.		
Asks patient to swallow water and observes/feels with one hand for movement of any neck lumps		
Asks patient to stick out tongue and observes/feels with one hand for movement of any neck lumps		
Auscultates for thyroid bruits		
Tests ankle reflexes		
Systematic presentation of findings		
Correctly identifies euthyroid state		
Identifies that: Both goitre and cyst move on swallowing but only cyst rises on tongue protrusion Cyst is soft whereas a goitre is hard +/- nodular		
Examiner's Global Mark	/5	
Actor / Helper's Global Mark	/5	
Total Station Mark	/30	

Learning Points

Practice presenting your examination findings in a systematic manner. Start by highlighting any obvious abnormality or state that this is a normal examination. Follow by summarising relevant positive findings and 2 to 3 significant negative findings. If it is a normal examination then state significant negatives and use opportunity to mention things you looked for but aren't necessarily obvious to the examiner. Conclude by offering a potential differential diagnosis or test that would help confirm diagnosis.

Know how to examine and describe a lump. There are many helpful mnemonics available. Most importantly always comment on site, size, shape, consistency and mobility. Top tip- soft is like your lips, firm is like the tip of your tongue and hard is like your nasal bridge.

When examining the cervical lymph nodes palpate using the pads of all four fingertips whilst standing behind the patient. Examine both sides at the same time. Walk your fingers along the pre-auricular, anterior cervical, posterior cervical, tonsilar, submandibular, submental and supraclavicular nodes.

Case 23
Markscheme - Genital examination

Task	Achieved	Not Achieved
Introduces self, washes hands and checks patient identity		
Consent patients for examination		
Asks whether patient would like a chaperone		
Adequately exposes patient		
Performs general inspection of the patient notifying whether they are comfortable at rest or show signs of distress/compromise		
Observation of the groin		
Scrotal swellings		
Skin changes e.g. erythema,		
Surgical scars		
Discharge		
Palpation of testes		
Lump- size, shape, consistency (hard, firm, soft), Tenderness, Transillumination, painful/painless		
Palpates both sides		
Auscultates for bowel sounds		
Examines patient lying down		
Examines patient standing up		
Palpates associated structures- epididymis, ductus deferens.		
Examines glans penis		
Assesses phimosis,		
Lesions on penis		
Examines inguinal canal-		
Attempts to reduce lump if present		
Cough impulse to differentiate between direct and indirect hernia		
Palpates for enlarged inguinal and para-aortic lymph nodes.		
Examiner's Global Mark	/5	
Actor / Helper's Global Mark	/5	
Total Station Mark	/30	

Learning Points

Typically a varicocoele (dilatation of the pampiniform plexus veins) is described as feeling like "a bag of worms".

The gonadal vein on the right side drains directly in the IVC, however the vein on the left side drains into the left renal vein. Dilatation of the plexus on the left side may be indicative of a renal malignancy obstructing the left renal vein and causing back pressure .

Other differentials for testicular lumps include hydrocele (which would transilluminate), and an indirect inguinal hernia (cough impulse, bowel sounds).

Case 24
Markscheme - ATLS

Task:	Achieved	Not Achieved
Airway: Notes airway in patent		
C-spine: Elicits pain in patient's neck		
Immobilises patient's neck with blocks		
Breathing: Asks for RR and Saturations		
Chest wall movement/Percussion/Auscultation		
Trachea position		
Asks for CXR		
Suggests 15L oxygen non-rebreathe mask		
Circulations: Asks for HR and BP		
Capillary refill + pallor		
Heart sounds		
ECG		
Suggests large bore IV lines x2 and fluid bolus		
Recommends suitable blood test		
Disability: Pupils + GCS		
Blood sugar + temperature		
Mentions need for CT head + Chest/Abdomen/Pelvis		
Mentions need for full secondary survey for completion		
Mentions need to go back to A and continually reassess		
Suggests chest drain insertion for the pneumothorax		
Examiner's Global Mark	/5	
Actor / Helper's Global Mark	/5	
Total Station Mark	/30	

Learning points:

Remember in ATLS that assessment of the c-spine ALWAYS come in parallel with the airway.

It is important to be methodical and if you encounter an abnormality during your assessment to attempt an intervention before moving on. Even if there appears to be an obvious abnormality eg a deformed limb, stick to the A to E approach to avoid missing other more life threatening injuries

It is vital in these scenarios that you constantly go back and assess the patient again from the beginning to check for deterioration or success of intervention.

Case 25
Markscheme - ABG interpretation

Task	Achieved	Not Achieved
Introduces self, washes hands and checks patient identity		
Consents patient for examination		
Asks whether patient would like a chaperone present		
Adequately exposes the patient's lower limbs		
Performs a general observation of the patient noting whether they are comfortable at rest		
Observation of the lower limb:		
Scars from previous surgery		
Skin changes in colour / tissue loss. Venous eczema		
Presence of ulcers ensures to look all around the feet including heel		
Palpates temperature of both legs beginning distally		
Assesses capillary refill		
Performance of Buerger's tests if capillary refill is >2secs		
Performs palpation of pulses:		
Aorta		
Femoral		
Popliteal		
PT		
DT		
Checks for radiofemoral delay		
Auscultates for abdominal aortic bruits		
Correctly performs Doppler examination of the DP and PT pulse		
Correctly calculates the ABPI on both legs		
Examiner's Global Mark	/5	
Actor / Helper's Global Mark	/5	
Total Station Mark	/30	

Learning Points

Presence of any varicose veins – often seen best with the patient standing up! Remember you should feel pulses on both sides and comment on their strength, comparing one side relative to the other.

Pulse Location:

Femoral - Mid inguinal point, halfway between the ASIS and the pubic symphysis

Popliteal - Deep in the popliteal fossa

Dorsalis Pedis - Between the head of the 1st and 2nd metatarsal

Posterior Tibial - Behind the medial malleolus

At the end, you should mention that you would perform a full cardiovascular system, examination the venous system in their legs and arrange an arterial duplex or angiogram.

Emergency medicine

Case 1
Moulage - ATLS

Task	Achieved	Not Achieved
Appropriate introduction and task allocation to team members		
Calls early for trauma team		
Ensures all members of the team wear appropriate PPE		
Ensures C-spine immobilisation throughout assessment		
Appropriate assessment of patient's airway		
Assessment of breathing - RR, oxygen saturations, work of breathing, auscultation, percussion		
Administers oxygen via appropriate device		
Assessment of circulation - BP, HR, capillary refill time		
States would like to gain IV/IO access and send appropriate samples to laboratory		
States would like to commence IV/IO fluids		
Assessment of neurological status		
Adequately exposes patient to look for other injuries or bruising		
Makes diagnosis of tension pneumothorax		
States would like to perform immediate needle decompression		
States correct anatomical landmarks for procedure (2nd ICS MCL)		
Reassesses patient after intervention has been made		
States definitive management is a chest drain		
Correctly identifies landmarks for insertion of chest drain		
Considers need for imaging (CXR)		
Demonstrates systematic A-E assessment		
Examiner's Global Mark	/5	
Actor / Helper's Global Mark	/5	
Total Station Mark	/30	

Learning points

Tension pneumothorax is a clinical diagnosis, which needs immediate management with needle decompression. This is performed by inserting a large-bore cannula in the 2nd intercostal space, in the mid-clavicular line on the affected side. This relieves the tension and converts the injury to a simple pneumothorax, which will subsequently need definitive treatment with insertion of a chest drain.

In a trauma scenario, it is important to have a systematic process to assessing patients. The A (and C-spine) BCDE technique is easy to remember and ensures that you do not miss any injuries. Remember to treat life-threatening injuries as you go along and reassess the patient after you have made an intervention. If there is a B problem then make an intervention before you move on.

In order to assess breathing and ventilation, adequately expose the patient's chest and use all information available to you, including inspection for any open injuries, bruising of the chest wall, work of breathing and movement of the chest. Oxygen saturations and respiratory rate provide valuable information as does thorough auscultation and percussion of the chest.

Case 2
Moulage - ALS PEA Arrest

Task	Achieved	Not Achieved
Checks it is safe to approach		
Establishes patient unresponsive, not breathing and pulseless (look,listen and feel for 10s)		
Calls for help/activates emergency buzzer		
Commences CPR (at correct position and depth)		
Attached defibrillator pads when help arrives/delegated		
Correctly assesses rhythm as PEA		
Asks for pulse check (3 point check)		
Continues chest compressions immediately - 100-120/min		
Switches to 30:2 now help has arrived w BVM		
Establishes intravenous access		
Gives 1mg of Adrenaline IV (1:10000)as soon as possible		
Secure the airway – iGel or intubation		
Switches from 30:2 to continuous CPR once airway secured		
Rhythm and pulse check after 2 minutes		
Continues CPR		
Ensures high quality of chest compressions (1/3rd of chest depth)		
Gives 1mg Adrenaline IV every 3-5 minutes		
Mentions reversible causes of cardiac arrest (4H's, 4T's)		
Identifies return of pulse		
Commences post resuscitation care		
Examiner's Global Mark	/5	
Actor / Helper's Global Mark	/5	
Total Station Mark	/30	

Learning Points

Be well versed with the ALS algorithm for shockable (VT/VF) and non-shockable (PEA/asystole) rhythms.

Have a good grasp of the reversible causes of cardiac arrest and their management:

Hypoxia
Hypovolaemia
Hyperkalaemia, hypokalaemia, hypoglycaemia, hypocalcaemia, acidaemia and other metabolic disorders
Hypothermia

Thrombosis (coronary or pulmonary)
Tension pneumothorax
Tamponade – cardiac
Toxins

If a diagnosis of asystole is made, check the ECG carefully for the presence of P waves. The patient may respond to cardiac pacing when there is ventricular standstill with continuing P waves. There is no value in attempting to pace true asystole.

Case 3
Moulage - ALS VF Arrest

Task	Achieved	Not Achieved
Introduces self to nurse on scene		
Confirms cardiac arrest		
Puts on defibrillating pads and pauses for rhythm check		
Identifies VF on monitor		
Identifies VF as a shockable rhythm		
Communicates the need for a shock to be delivered		
Requests chest compressions to be restarted immediately after rhythm has been identified		
Reassures compression nurse that she will not be shocked		
Selects a setting of at least 150J and charges the defibrillator		
Requests that everyone stand clear		
Requests that oxygen is kept clear		
Briefly checks that everyone is clear of the patient and safely delivers shock		
Requests for chest compressions to be started immediately after delivery of shock		
Knows that CPR should be continued for another 2 minutes after shock		
Inserts IV access or suggests alternative access		
Correctly identifies normal sinus rhythm and checks for pulse		
Communicates well with members of the team		
Knows that adrenaline should be administered after the third shock and every 3-5 minutes thereafter		
Knows that amiodarone 300mg should be administered after the third shock		
Correctly lists 4H's and 4T's		
Examiner's Global Mark	/5	
Actor / Helper's Global Mark	/5	
Total Station Mark	/30	

Learning points

As the clinician running the arrest the temptation is to get drawn in. Stand back, observe and delegate to the rest of the team. A team will function far better with an allocated leader to coordinate the multiple interventions that are ongoing. In addition to the leader, roles are needed for managing the airway, the defibrillator, performing chest compressions, delivering drugs and scribing.

Communication is imperative in this situation. It is very useful to use closed-loop communication. This means that you give an instruction to one person specifically and ask them to give you feedback when they have carried it out. This ensures that you are well informed about what your team members are doing.

Ask a competent assistant to manage the airway as much are they are able to. Early use of the supra-glottic airway allows for continuous compression and ventilation to take place. Once the airway is secure check for good bilateral air entry.

For the full ALS algorithm see www.resus.org.uk

Case 4
Moulage - Anaphylaxis

Task	Achieved	Not Achieved
Introduces self		
Call for help/bleep anaesthetists/senior review		
Assess patency of airway (speaking/GCS/additional sounds)		
OXYGEN 100% given immediately		
Asks for respiratory rate & pulse oximetry		
Chest auscultation for wheeze		
Salbutamol and ipratropium bromide nebs given		
Can consider an ABG and/or portable CXR		
GIVE ADRENALINE 500mcg of 1:1000 IM adrenaline (can be given earlier than this point)		
Lie flat and raise legs		
Checks BP, HR & CRT		
IV crystalloid fluid challenge through 2 wide bore cannulae		
Bloods to be sent off e.g. Mast cell tryptase		
Chlorphenamine 10mg IV		
Hydrocortisone 200mg IV		
GCS examination and glucose		
Expose patient looking for rashes		
Reassess patient after each intervention		
recognise need for airway manoeuvres or airway adjuncts (Correctly size and insert airway adjunct)		
Ask for anaesthetic review required urgently and considers 2nd dose of Adrenaline after 5 minutes		
Examiner's Global Mark	/5	
Actor / Helper's Global Mark	/5	
Total Station Mark	/30	

Learning Points

Practice, practice, practice! The A-E approach should become second nature to you so that every patient you approach (real or simulated), should be managed in the acute setting in the same way. It will ensure safe practice and good methods of managing and resuscitating unwell patients.

In moulage scenarios, expect the patient to go off! If they do, remember to remain calm and re-assess again. Anaphylaxis is a good example of where interventions need reassessment but that scenarios can deteriorate even despite treatments. Going back to A in the A-E approach will ensure that nothing is missed.

Adrenaline in this scenario should be given as soon as anaphylaxis is recognized regardless of which stage of the A-E assessment you are on. Imtramuscular adrenaline is the first line route and if a patient has their own adrenaline auto injector with them (eg Epipen, Jext) it is fine to use this in the first instance.

Case 5
Moulage - Acute Asthma

Task	Achieved	Not Achieved
Introduction and consent		
Takes appropriate history of presenting complaint		
Asks about medication and admission history		
Past medical history including atopy and smoking history		
Uses ABCDE approach		
Calls for help/ Provides O2		
Assess airway and trachea		
Assess breathing and ask for peak flow (ABG can be provided)		
Interprets peak flow chart		
Start nebuliser and steroid therapy		
Assess circulation and ask for IV cannula		
Assess disability (GCS and pupils) and exposure		
Reassess after initial treatment		
Knowledge of classifying severity of asthma attack		
Knowledge of admission criteria for asthma attack		
Knowledge of discharge criteria following asthma attack		
Aware of treatment ladder for asthma attack		
Criteria for chest xray/use of antibiotics/ ICU referral		
Early escalation for senior help		
An idea of appropriate follow up for asthma patients		
Examiner's Global Mark	/5	
Actor / Helper's Global Mark	/5	
Total Station Mark	/30	

Learning Points

The peak expiratory flow rate is useful to determine severity of asthma. It is expressed as a percentage of the patients' previous best. If this is unavailable, then one can refer to the predicted PEFR chart for the patient's age and height. After treatment is administered the PEFR can be rechecked to see if there has been any improvement.

Pulse oximetry determines the need for an arterial blood gas. Use supplemental oxygen to aim saturations between 94-98%. If the saturations drop below 92% an arterial sample should be obtained for analysis.

Blood gas analysis is useful as it can help diagnose the presence of life threatening asthma. This is when the PO_2 is below 8kPa (very low) or the CO_2 is normal (between 4.6 -6.0 kPa)

Case 6
Moulage - DKA

Task	Achieved	Not Achieved
Introduces themselves to the patient, establishes need for consult and seeks consent		
Introduces themselves to nurse and establishes experience		
Washes hands		
Requests monitoring		
Takes a focused history from patient		
Establishes airway is patient and not compromised		
Listens to the chest. Notes Raised respiratory rate		
Notes they are tachycardic		
Notes their GCS and that they are drowsy. Blood glucose is available.		
Abdominal examination. Checks for injuries and rashes.		
Requests an ECG - notes concerns regarding potassium		
Requests urinary/serum ketones to confirm diagnosis		
Obtains IV access		
Recognises DKA as likely diagnosis		
Initiates fluid therapy at appropriate rate		
Prescribes fluid therapy correctly		
Initiates/ notes the need for insulin infusion		
Communicates well with nursing colleague throughout		
Sets monitoring requirement for nurse and initial therapy goals		
Can identify 2 potential complication of DKA		
Examiner's Global Mark	/5	
Actor / Helper's Global Mark	/5	
Total Station Mark	/30	

Learning points

DKA is a potentially life threatening complication of diabetes and as doctors we need to be aware that it is easy to 'forget the glucose'. On an A-E approach D is for disability and should also be for *don't forget the glucose*.

Insulin is essential in the management of DKA, however, dehydration is often more immediately life threatening and thus takes priority. Patients can require remarkably large quantities of fluid to restore their circulating volume. This can risk causing sudden shifts between fluid compartments and can lead to the potentially fatal complication of cerebral oedema.

Electrolyte disturbance is another important complication to be aware of, as is hypoglycaemia! Therapy therefore requires a careful approach and regular reassessment. Local DKA protocols vary with regards to fluid resuscitation, insulin infusions and potassium control and it is always worth checking them.

Reference
Joint British Diabetes Societies Inpatient Care Group. The Management of Diabetic Ketoacidosis in Adults. March 2010

Case 7
Moulage - Status Epilepticus

Task	Achieved	Not Achieved
Appropriate introduction and task allocation to team members		
Calls early for senior help		
Ensures all members of the team wear appropriate PPE		
Appropriate assessment of patient's airway		
Makes attempt to suction patient's mouth and upper airway		
States would use airway adjunct (ie. nasopharyngeal airway) to maintain airway		
Commences high flow oxygen - 15L via non-rebreathe mask		
Assessment of breathing - RR, oxygen saturations, auscultation, percussion		
Assessment of circulation - BP, HR, capillary refill time		
States would like to gain IV/IO access and send appropriate samples to laboratory		
Explicitly states would like to check BM		
States would like to commence IV/IO dextrose (50ml of 50% solution)		
Assessment of neurological status		
Adequately exposes patient		
Makes diagnosis of status epilepticus		
States would administer IV/IO lorazepam or Diazepam		
States no response to benzodiazepines so commences loading with phenytoin		
Inform anaesthetist/ICU and prepares for intubation		
Appropriate handover to ICU colleague when they arrive		
Demonstrates systematic A-E assessment		
Examiner's Global Mark	/5	
Actor / Helper's Global Mark	/5	
Total Station Mark	/30	

Learning points

Status epilepticus is a medical emergency and is defined as continuous seizure activity lasting more than 30 minutes, or repeated tonic–clonic convulsions occurring over a 30 minutes period without recovery of consciousness between each convulsion. Any seizure however that lasts more than 5 minutes needs to be treated as status epilepticus as termination of the seizure can became increasingly difficult.

The first line of treatment for a seizure is benzodiazepines. Common preparations include rectal diazepam, buccal midazolam or intravenous lorazepam. If the first dose does not terminate the seizure within 5 minutes, administer a second dose.

On-going assessment of the patient whilst having a seizure includes a neurological examination to look for a focal intra-cranial lesion and to consider hypoglycaemia as both can cause seizures or as a result of prolonged seizure activity.

Case 8
Moulage - Hyperkalaemia

Task	Achieved	Not Achieved
Introduces themselves, consents and washes hands		
A – looks for signs of obstruction, attaches oxygen		
B - counts respiratory rate		
Attaches arterial saturations probe		
Inspects chest expansion & checks position of trachea		
Percusses chest & Auscultates thorax		
C – Colour, temperature, capillary refill time		
Comments on heart rate and blood pressure		
Looks for signs of haemorrhage		
Inserts IV access and takes blood including VBG		
Requests ECG		
Correctly identifies changes associated with high K^+		
Confirms with VBG		
Attach continuous cardiac monitoring		
Gives: 10mls of 10% Calcium chloride or calcium gluconate		
Insulin Dextrose – 10 units actrapid in 100mls 20% dextrose		
Suggests 0.9% Sodium chloride infusion		
Considers salbutamol nebulizer if delay in insulin dextrose		
D and E - Checks GCS and Blood glucose		
Mentions the possibility of dialysis or haemofiltration if hyperkalaemia refractory to insulin dextrose.		
Examiner's Global Mark	/5	
Actor / Helper's Global Mark	/5	
Total Station Mark	/30	

Learning Points

Classic causes of hyperkalemia include; Insulin insufficiency as insulin drives potassium intracellularly or the inability to excrete potassium through the kidneys.

In cardiac arrest, continue with resuscitation until potassium normalized. Once ROSC achieved, continue insulin and dextrose until the repeat blood gases demonstrate an improvement.

Consider dialysis or haemofiltration for hyperkalaemia that is resistant to routine medical therapy,

Case 9
History taking - shortness of breath DVT/PE

Task	Achieved	Not Achieved
Introduces self, washes hands and checks identity		
Elicits history from patient in a concise manner		
Asks questions to explore the possibility of other cases of shortness of breath: cough, fevers, exacerbating and relieving factors, associated chest pain.		
Asks about past medical history (previous history of clots or varicose veins)		
Asks family history (previous history of clots or sudden death or inherited factor disorders)		
Asks about drug history (anticoagulants or COCP)		
Asks about social history (smoking and recent travel)		
Asks about specific VTE risk factors: recent immobility, operations		
Asks about pregnancy or LMP		
Elicits concern about heart problems after her father's heart attack		
Reacts to patient's concerns in an empathic and non-judgemental manner		
Is able to summarise findings		
Generates a reasonable differential diagnosis including respiratory and cardiac complaints		
Discusses the need for basic blood tests and knows to consider a d-dimer in this context		
Can discuss the use of a d-dimer in risk assessment for VTE		
Discusses the need for imaging. Chest x-ray at least and knows to consider CTPA or V/Q		
Is able to give at least one scoring system for assessing PE risk.		
Identifies that this patient is likely high risk for a PE.		
Is aware of the need for anticoagulation with LMWH followed by warfarin		
Is aware of thrombolysis as a management option in a life threatening PE.		
Examiner's Global Mark	/5	
Actor / Helper's Global Mark	/5	
Total Station Mark	/30	

Learning points

Scoring systems for a PE include the popular Well's score, the Geneva score and the Pulmonary Embolism Severity Index or PESI score.

A d-dimer is useful to exclude a PE in the low risk patient. If a patient is low risk and has a negative d-dimer they are unlikely to have a PE. If they are low risk with a raised d-dimer they may have a PE but the test may be raised for a variety of other reasons. If they are high risk they should have further investigations for a PE by way of a CTPA (or V/Q in certain cases) even if their d-dimer is normal making it an unnecessary test.

Other causes of a raised d-dimer include: Aortic dissection, malignancy, sepsis, acute coronary syndromes, upper GI bleeds, disseminated intravascular coagulation (DIC), stroke and AF.

Case 10
History taking - Febrile neutropenia

Task	Achieved	Not Achieved
Introduces themselves, seeks consent for consultation and washes hands		
Offers analgesia		
Establishes the patient's main issue (presenting complaint)		
Explores the nature of the headache site, onset, character, radiation, severity		
Establishes the onset, timeframe, associated symptoms, aggravating & relieving factors		
Specifically asks about head injury		
Specifically asks about focal neurology		
Specifically asks about visual symptoms		
Ascertains if there are symptoms of meningitis		
Check for other red flags		
Takes a past medical history		
Takes a drug history		
Takes a family and social history		
Explores the patient's ideas, concerns and expectations		
Establishes a safe and clear management plan		
Checks understanding & invites questions		
Closes the consultation appropriately		
Identifies three reasonable differential diagnoses		
Summarises and signposts during the consultation		
Appropriate language throughout. Avoids medical terminology		
Examiner's Global Mark	/5	
Actor / Helper's Global Mark	/5	
Total Station Mark	/30	

Learning points

Headaches are a common presenting complaint in the emergency department and these can be very rewarding consultations because most headache diagnoses can be made with a thorough history.

Headaches have a broad spectrum of underlying causes from the common and benign to the rare and life threatening and therefore need to be treated with a generous dose of suspicion. Some patients will need urgent investigation and treatment whereas others will require nothing more than reassurance, and a solid follow up plan that includes a clear safety net in case things deteriorate.

You cannot plan for every possible clinical scenario that may arise, but you can have a framework that guides your consultation. This should include appropriate introduction, informal consent, open questions followed by focused questioning, summarising and signposting to ensure accuracy and provide structure to the consultation as well as specifically addressing ideas, concerns and expectations. Give the patient time to talk and be sympathetic and considerate, you will find most consultations flow a lot easier if the patient's agenda is established near the start.

Case 11
History taking - Head injury (minor)

Task	Achieved	Not Achieved
Introduces self and clarifies patient's identity		
Offers analgesia / checks patient is comfortable		
Uses open questions to begin consultation		
Inquires about mechanism of injury		
Inquires about drops in GCS		
Mentions signs of basal skull fracture		
Mentions open or depressed skull fracture		
Asks about post traumatic seizure		
Loss of consciousness		
Focal neurological deficit		
Vomiting episodes		
Amnesia (30 minutes Retrograde or Antegrade)		
Asks about past medical history, medication history and social history		
Mentions need to perform full neurological examination of patient		
Enquires about patient's ideas, concerns and expectations		
Gives explanation of likely diagnosis to patient i.e. Concussion/minor head injury		
Advises no need for further imaging		
Reassures patient and alludes to NICE head injury guidelines		
Mentions provision of written head injury advice on discharge		
Closes the consultation appropriately with appropriate safety net advice		
Examiner's Global Mark	/5	
Actor / Helper's Global Mark	/5	
Total Station Mark	/30	

Learning points

Knowing the NICE head injury guidelines is essential and should guide your clinical practice when faced with head injury patients. Utilising evidence based guidelines allows the clinician to use validated decision making to reassure both the patient and the clinical team.

Try to elicit patient's ideas, concerns and expectations regarding their presentation to the department. Ensuring these are addressed will improve overall patient satisfaction. Communication here is the key to a happy patient.

Always provide both verbal and written head injury advice upon discharge from the department, appropriate safety-net advice is important.

Case 12
History taking - Paracetamol OD

Task	Achieved	Not Achieved
Introduces self and washes hand		
Is able to encourage the patient to give the history of the overdose attempt.		
Specifically asks about type and time of overdose and the number of pills taken to establish the need for medical treatment.		
Asks about the circumstances of the overdose.		
Asks about the history of the depressive episode. Duration and associated symptoms of depression.		
Asks about previous episodes and suicide attempts		
Asks about alcohol and other substance abuse		
Specifically asks about the intention of the attempt		
Asks about protective factors		
Establishes how the patient is feeling now		
Establishes the patient's willingness to comply with treatment		
Reacts to the patient in a professional, empathic and non judgmental manner		
Is able to summarise findings		
Correctly identifies the high-risk nature of the suicide attempt and knows that this patient should not be permitted to leave the hospital.		
Is aware of the treatment nomogram for a paracetamol overdose and knows that it is based on the time since the overdose and the paracetamol level.		
Knows that over a certain mg/kg dose treatment should not be delayed if the paracetamol level is not available quickly.		
Outlines the baseline investigations including LFTs, paracetamol level, coagulation profile, blood gas for lactate and pH.		
Suggests N-Acetylcysteine as the treatment for the overdose		
Suggests trust guidelines and toxbase as resources to help establish whether treatment is required.		
Knows that a psychiatric referral is required for this patient.		
Examiner's global mark	/5	
Actor's global mark	/5	
Total station mark	/30	

Learning points

A paracetamol level is only useful if the patient is presenting 4 hours or more since ingesting the paracetamol. Their mg/kg dose of paracetamol should be calculated. Once the paracetamol level is known it should be plotted on the paracetamol overdose nomogram.

Any evidence of liver damage in the form of newly deranged ALT/AST and clotting also requires treatment.

Have an idea how you are planning on asking the questions. These questions are quite clearly of a sensitive nature which may cause you to tumble over your words. For example; If you want to know if someone is suicidal, try an open question such as, 'how do you feel now?' and then 'do you still feel like you want to end your life?' as supposed to something very blunt like 'do you want to die?'.

Case 13
History taking - Rectal bleeding

Task	Achieved	Not Achieved
introduces self and washes hands		
Clarifies who they are speaking to and gains consent		
Starts with an open question and then moves to closed questions.		
Clarifies that this Is not haematuria or vaginal bleeding		
Frequency and amount		
Asks if Blood is mixed in with the stool, around the stool, on the pan, or on the tissue paper		
Establishes character: fresh blood, melaena, clots, muscus, smell		
Asks about exacerbating or alleviating factors (relieved by defecation, dietary or foreign body history)		
Ask about associated symptom (dragging sensation, tenesmus, itching and pain)		
Elicits if important red flag symptoms are present (haemetemesis, weight loss, loss of appetite and change in bowel habit)		
Asks about bleeding from elsewhere		
Does a general systemic review for any other symptoms not previously mentioned.		
Asks about previous medical history		
Asks about any surgical history		
Asks about any family history of cancer and GI disorders (e.g. angiodysplasia or IBD)		
Gets an accurate drug and allergy history (specifically NSAIDS or anticoagulants)		
Asks about job, smoking and alcohol.		
Elicits the patient's ideas, concerns and expectations.		
Manages the patient in a caring yet professional manner when upset or worried.		
Forms a good relationship with the patient along the course of the history.		
Examiner's Global Mark	/5	
Actor / Helper's Global Mark	/5	
Total Station Mark	/30	

Learning points:

GI bleeding can originate anywhere from the mouth to the anus and can be overt or occult. How this presents depends on the location and rate of bleeding.

Red flags of PR bleed include: Weight loss, altered blood PR, change in bowel habit, abdominal pain, mucus passed PR and anorexia.

If the patient is initially haemodynamically unstable the first action must be to do an A to E assessment with appropriate interventions along the way - two large bore cannula, bloods, venous blood gas and Group and Save. Always call for help.

Case 14
History taking - Syncope

Task	Achieved	Not achieved
Washes hands, Introduces self to patient and confirms identity		
Begins with open ended questions		
Asks about aura/indications		
Asks about what patient was doing preceding the collapse		
Asks about preceding chest pain, dizziness, headache		
Asks if there was any head trauma		
Asks if the collapse was witnessed and what was the account		
Asks questions about a possible seizure, loss of bladder or bowel control, tongue biting		
Asks about conscious level after collapse, was there a period of unresponsiveness (Post-Ictal)		
Asks about past medical history and history of syncope		
Ask after symptoms of meningitis		
Ask about symptoms of malignancy		
Asks drug history including allergies and recreational drugs		
Asks family history- epilepsy, heart valve or heart rhythm problems		
Asks about occupation		
Summarises findings		
Differential diagnosis: vasovagal syncope, arrhythmia, epilepsy		
Investigations: ecg, blood gas,		
Asks for blood sugar level		
Management plan can go home if all tests normal		
Examiners Global Mark	/5	
Patient's Global Mark	/5	
Total station Mark	/30	

Learning points

Collapse is a very common presentation with a mixture of benign and sinister causes. Have a list of the sinister causes and how to rule them out. E.g. cardiac arrhythmia, check an ECG for conduction abnormalities.

Categorise collapse into main aetiologies e.g. cardiac valve problems, conduction problems, Neuro: epilepsy, Cardiovascular: vasovagal, micturition syncope, Endocrine: hypoglycaemia. Coareful histroy taking is required and enquiry about the events before, during and after the episode will go a long way in narrowing down your differential diagnoses.

Collapse in the elderly patients should have infection ruled out, anticoagulation status checked and skeletal injuries considered and excluded, especially the potential for pelvic and neck of femur fractures.

Case 15
Examination - Respiratory Exam

Task	Achieved	Not achieved
Introduces themselves and washes hands		
Consents patient and confirms identity		
Asks if the patient has pain & offers analgesia if appropriate		
Positions at 45º and exposes appropriately		
General inspection. Respiratory rate.		
Hands - tobacco staining, tremor, flap, stigmata of disease. Pulse.		
Face - eyes and mouth. Cyanosis, ptosis, conjunctival pallor		
Neck - JVP, tracheal position and lymphadenopathy		
Palpation - chest expansion		
Percussion - clavicles, anterior and posterior		
Auscultation - anterior and posterior		
Checks for either vocal resonance or tactile vocal fremitus		
Pedal and sacral oedema		
Performs examination in a considerate way, maintaining communication and safeguarding patient decency throughout.		
Performed in a systematic and sensible order. Compares the left and right sides.		
Presents their finding in a systematic and clear way		
Identifies the need for vital signs and can name three bedside tests		
Identifies pneumonia as a likely diagnosis		
Formulates an appropriate management plan		
Able to name two clinical findings consistent with pneumonia. Aware of CRB-65/CURB-65 assessment.		
Examiner's Global Mark	/5	
Actor / Helper's Global Mark	/5	
Total Station Mark	/30	

Learning points

A rehearsed and methodical examination of the respiratory system is a basic clinical skill and you should aim to be comfortable performing this examination. A systematic approach looks professional, helps you to remember all areas to be covered and ensures you aren't moving the patient around unnecessarily.

CURB 65 is a clinical prediction rule. Each criteria is valued with a point. Points are linked to a 30-day mortality and are used for deciding how to treat the patient. They are marked as follows:
Confusion of new onset (defined as an AMTS of 8 or less),
Blood Urea nitrogen greater than 7mmol/l (19 mg/dL)
Respiratory rate of 30 breaths per minute or greater
Blood pressure less than 90 mmHg systolic or diastolic blood pressure below 60mmHg
Age 65 or older

Although ideal, it is not essential to detect all of the clinical signs present in an OSCE examination. It is more important to show that you can perform the examination thoroughly, maintain a professional and polite approach and to show that you are aware of the necessary next steps to ensure that the patient is managed safely.

References
Lim et al. BTS guidelines for the management of community acquired pneumonia in adults:update 2009. A quick reference guide. Thorax 2009.

Case 16
Examination - Cardiovascular Exam

Task	Achieved	Not achieved
Introduces self and washes hands		
Consents Patient and Checks identity		
Checks patient is comfortable and obtains verbal consent		
Exposes patient adequately and positions patient lying at 45 degree angle		
Performs general inspection from the end of the bed		
Inspects hands - peripheral cyanosis, temperature, nicotine staining, clubbing, signs of infective endocarditis		
Palpates radial pulse (rate, volume, character – slow rising)		
Mentions checking blood pressure		
Assesses Jugular Venous Pressure (JVP) +/- hepatojugular reflux		
Inspects face – corneal arcus, central cyanosis, conjunctival pallor, malar flush		
Palpate carotid artery (volume, character)		
Inspects the precordium – no visible scars		
Palpates for heaves, thrills and apex beat		
Auscultates in correct regions - apex, pulmonary, aortic, tricuspid, mitral		
Performs manoeuvre to accentuate murmur - sits patient forwards and listens with diaphragm in expiration		
Auscultates for radiation of murmur into carotid		
Auscultates lung bases, checks for sacral and ankle oedema		
Thanks patient, offers help in redressing/covering		
Demonstrates systematic approach		
Correctly summarises findings – ejection systolic murmur loudest in aortic region, radiates to carotids		
Examiner's Global Mark	/5	
Actor / Helper's Global Mark	/5	
Total Station Mark	/30	

Learning points

When approaching examination stations in the OSCE, always take the time to introduce yourself to the patient and ask them if they are in pain. Being kind and courteous throughout will ensure you pick up the allocated global marks.

Clinical features specific to aortic stenosis include: a slow rising pulse, narrow pulse pressure, an ejection systolic murmur heard loudest in the aortic region with radiation into the carotids. There may or may not be signs of heart failure.

The correct regions for auscultation are as follows:
Apex – 5th intercostal space, anterior-mid axillary line
Pulmonary – left sternal edge, 2nd-4th intercostal space
Aortic – right sternal edge, 2nd-4th intercostal space
Tricuspid – left sternal edge, 4th-6th intercostal space
Mitral – mid-clavicular line, 4th-6th intercostal space

Case 17
Moulage - Acute coronary syndrome

Task	Achieved	Not Achieved
Introduces self, washes hands and checks patient identity		
Explicitly comments on patient airway patency		
Starts 15L oxygen via non-rebreathe mask		
Comments on respiratory effort		
Asks for oxygen saturations and RR		
Percusses and auscultates the chest		
Requests ABG and CXR		
Asks for HR, BP, Temp, urinary catheter, ECG and cardiac monitoring, blood tests including troponin		
Assess radial pulse, CRT, auscultates for heart sounds		
Starts ACS protocol- Morphine, Oxygen, Nitrates, Aspirin, Clopidogrel, mentions doses and routes. -		
Comments on rational for holding IVF and starting IV furosemide.		
Comments on referral to cardiology/cath lab		
Explicitly mentions GCS or AVPU		
Examines pupils		
Asks for BM		
Explicitly mentions examining the rest of the body		
States pull crash button and place 2222 arrest call		
Correctly identifies diagnosis of ACS		
Flash pulmonary oedema		
Demonstrates systematic ABCDE approach		
Examiner's Global Mark	/5	
Actor / Helper's Global Mark	/5	
Total Station Mark	/30	

Learning Points

Being familiar with utilising an A to E approach in the assessment and management of the sick patient. Remember to treat each finding before moving on to the next step.

Be familiar with the treatment of ACS - MONAC

Morphine sulphate 10mg PO or 5mg IV
Oxygen- high flow via non-rebreath mask
Nitrates- 1 puff S/L GTN spray (400mcg)
Aspirin- 300mg PO
Clopidogrel- 300mg PO

Communicating your assessment, impression and plan of the patient is key to getting your patient treated promptly. In the exam scenario you must get into the habit of describing your findings out loud and asking for observations and treatments in order to get your marks, a bit like a driving test. In the clinical setting, this same approach will ensure you and your team are all on the same page, ensuring treatments are started in a timely manner.

Case 18
History taking - Renal stones

Task:	Achieved	Not Achieved
Introduces self, washes hands and checks patient identity		
Opens consultation with use of open questions		
Explores pain history in a systematic manner		
Asks about haematuria		
Explores urinary symptoms		
Asks specifically about previous renal stones		
Explores past medical and surgical history		
Takes a thorough drug history including over the counter and illicit drugs		
Asks about smoking and alcohol history		
Asks about family of renal stones		
Explores a brief system's enquiry		
Explores patient's Ideas, Concerns and Expectations		
Recognizes need for analgesia and reassures patient		
Correctly identifies diagnosis of renal colic		
Asks for a urine dip and justifies to check for microscopic haematuria		
Asks for an FBC and CRP and justifies to check for signs of infection		
Asks for U&Es and justifies to check for acute kidney injury		
Asks for CT KUB and justifies to check for renal stones and urinary obstruction		
States would give Per Rectum diclofenac as first line analgesia		
States next step would require urology inpatient or outpatient review depending on CT scan result and renal function		
Examiner's Global Mark	/5	
Actor / Helper's Global Mark	/5	
Total Station Mark	/30	

Learning Points

Have a systematic approach to taking a pain history, such as SOCRATES. This will show the examiner that you can take an organized history. It is also vital clinically to get all the information from the patient. Every aspect of pain is a clue to the diagnosis.

Be specific when providing a management plan in an OSCE. Don't just state the test you would order but add what you are looking for.

When presenting a history to a senior or colleague having a systematic approach can help you remain concise and still report all the relevant information. SBAR is a commonly used acronym for this

The Situation is the Presenting problem and suspected likely diagnosis (or main medical problem)

The Background contains 2 or 3 main facts from the history highlighting the suspected diagnosis and 1 or 2 important negatives that exclude other important differentials. Go on to explain Assessment findings.

Recommendation can be when you outline your management plan or conclude by saying that you would now do a focused examination of the patient.

Case 19
Examination - Lower limb neurology

Task:	Achieved	Not Achieved
Introduces self and washes hands		
Check identity and gains consent		
Explains examination and what it will entail		
Begins by inspection, commenting on wasting, fasciculation's etc		
Assess gait		
Tone bilaterally tested		
Power of the hip		
Power of knee		
Power of ankle		
Power of toes		
Check for clonus		
Sensation: Dermatomal distribution - perform light touch and Mention Pin prick, hot/cold and vibration		
Suggest checking perianal sensation		
Mentions need for PR		
Reflexes - Knees and Ankles		
Coordination (Sliding ankle from knee to foot)		
Checks Babinski plantar reflex		
Checks Proprioception		
Mentions vibration sense		
Methodical approach comparing like for like on left and right side		
Examiner's Global Mark	/5	
Actor / Helper's Global Mark	/5	
Total Station Mark	/30	

Learning Points

Use the acronym SWIFT for remembering what to look for on inspection
Scars
Wasting of muscles
Involuntary movements – *dystonia / chorea / myoclonus*
Fasciculations – *lower motor neurone lesions*
Tremor – *Parkinson's*

It is important to revise and learn the myotomes and dermatomes.

In all patients presenting with back pain the clinician should always consider the possibility of cauda equina. This is an emergency and requires urgent MRI scan of the spine with neurosurgical input.

Case 20
Examination - Cerebellar Exam

Task	Achieved	Not Achieved
Introduces self and washes hands		
Gains consent and confirms patient identity		
Inspection around bed, patient appearance and posture		
Assesses gait- Stance and balance		
Assesses tandem walking		
Performs Rombergs test		
Assesses for dysarthria		
Checks for nystagmus		
Checks for dysmetric eye movements and poor pursuit		
Assesses / explains one would asses for pronator drift		
Checks for normal arm rebound		
Assess for dysdiadokinesia		
Assesses for past pointing (finger- nose coordination)		
Assesses tone and reflexes in upper limb		
Assesses tone and reflexes in lower limb		
Assesses heel shin coordination		
Thanks patient and summarises positive findings		
Explains would perform cranial nerve and peripheral nerve examination to complete neurological exam		
Suggests head thrust test as further examination for labyrinthine disorders		
Asks for further imaging, such as CT/MRI and referral to Stroke centre		
Examiner's Global Mark	/5	
Actor / Helper's Global Mark	/5	
Total Station Mark	/30	

Learning points

If caught early, strokes can be treated much more effectively. The presentations of posterior circulation stroke and labyrinthine disorders have some similarities. In cerebellar disease, there can be mild hyporeflexia. In unilateral cerebellar disease, there is deviation to the side of the lesion due to hypotonia.

In assessment of pronator drift, a slow upward movement of the arm indicates an ipsilateral lesion in the cerebellum. Tandem walking will exaggerate any unsteadiness - It is good at assessing function of the cerebellar vermis – the first to go with alcoholic degeneration. Romberg's test is a test of sensory, not cerebellar ataxia. Slurred staccato speech is typical of cerebellar dysfunction.

The head thrust test is useful for detecting unilateral vestibulopathy. The patient's head is turned left and right while the patient keeps a fixed gaze on a certain spot. When the head is turned towards the affected side, the vestibular ocular reflex fails and the eyes perform a corrective saccade to refocus on the target. This indicates a positive test for vestibular disease on that side. This is a good test to differentiate between vestibular and brainstem dysfunction.

Case 21
Examination - Knee Exam

Task	Achieved	Not-Achieved
Washes hands, introduces self.		
Checks identity and gains consent.		
Starts with inspection from the end of the bed: General appearances of patient - are they unwell?		
Quickly checks hands, mouth and eyes- for any signs of rheumatological disease.		
Inspects the knee from front and side comparing it to the right knee, for swelling, deformity, redness, bruising, symmetry, inflammation.		
Inspects the back of the knee & popliteal fossa		
Palpates the knee- along the joint line, at the back and over the patella, for tenderness.		
Palpates the knee temperature.		
Assess the knee for effusion- patella tap or brush test.		
Asks the patient to actively flex and extend the knee.		
Passively moves the joint.		
Tests the ACL, PCL, MCL and LCL.		
Completes McMurray's manoeuvre (or similar) to test for meniscal injury.		
Tests sensation of left leg in dermatomal regions, comparing to right leg.		
Tests motor power in lower limb myotomes.		
Checks all lower limb pulses.		
Specifies they would examine the joint above and joint below also.		
Assess the gait of the patient.		
Considers all causes of knee pain/swelling during the examination (i.e. septic arthritis, arthropathy)		
Covers the patient after the examination		
Examiner's Global Mark	/5	
Actor / Helper's Global Mark	/5	
Total Station Mark	/30	

Learning points

Maintaining the basic principles of Look, Feel, Move then Special tests will hold you in good stead in the OSCE but also in the clinical setting. You should also always remember to examine the joint above and joint below, especially in children and the elderly as it can be hard for them to localise where the pain is coming from.

The medial collateral ligament is found on the inside of the knee and any damage to it is called a sprain. There are different severities of sprain including:

First degree sprain: only a few ligament fibers are damaged and the knee will often heal in 3-4 weeks.
Second degree sprain: The ligament is still intact but there is more extensive damage to the ligament fibers.
Third degree sprain: Complete rupture of the ligament.

When there is third degree medial collateral ligament sprain, it is very important to also assess the anterior cruciate ligament and menisci also as there is a high likelihood that these are also damaged. Injury of all three is called the 'triad of O'Donoghue', which usually results from a lateral force to the knee while the foot is fixed on the ground.

Case 22
Examination - Shoulder Exam

Task	Achieved	Not Achieved
Introduces self, washes hands and checks identity		
Checks identity and gains consent		
Initiates consultation by asking if the patient has any pain and offers analgesia		
Inspects both shoulders for symmetry, swelling and bruising from the front, back and side		
Palpates both shoulders for temperature		
Palpates the sternoclavicular, acromioclavicular and glenohumeral joint lines for tenderness, swelling and crepitus		
Palpates the humerus, humeral head, acromion process, scapula and clavicle bilaterally for bony tenderness		
Palpates the muscle bulk of the deltoid, supra and infraspinatus and trapezius muscles		
Asks patient to perform screening movements (hands behind head and hands behind back)		
Assesses for painful arc		
Assesses active movement of flexion, extension, abduction, internal and external rotation for symmetry, pain and range of movement		
Assesses passive movements as above for range of motion, crepitus, subluxation and pain		
Assesses supraspinatus muscle by testing active abduction against resistance		
Assesses infraspinatus and teres minor muscles by testing active external rotation against resistance		
Assesses subscapularis muscle by testing active internal rotation against resistance		
Tests for acromio-clavicular joint pathology by placing the arm into forced adduction across the chest and palpating the ACJ		
States that they would also examine the C-spine and elbow for a complete evaluation		
States that they would also assess the neurovascular status of the limb		
Summarises examination succinctly		
Correctly identifies diagnosis of acromio-clavicular joint sprain/separation		
Examiner's Global Mark	/5	
Actor / Helper's Global Mark	/5	
Total Station Mark	/30	

Learning Points

Remembering the basics of most joint examinations will gain you plenty of marks in any joint examination OSCE: correctly expose the joints, always assess and compare both joints, remember to look, feel, move and perform special tests. Finish by stating you would examine the joints above and below as well as the neurovascular status of the limb.

It is not always possible for exam organisers to provide models with joint pathology, you may have to rely on the patient providing you with cues or you may be examining a normal joint. Do not hesitate to present your findings as those of a normal joint examination if that is the case.

You do not require an orthopaedic level depth of anatomy knowledge. However, you must know the correct anatomical names of the muscles, joint lines, bones and ligaments that you test in your examination.

Case 23
Procedures - Airway Manoeuvres and adjuncts

Task	Achieved	Not Achieved
Introduces themselves to the student and washes hands		
Establishes student's learning needs		
Establishes existing knowledge and experience		
Sets realistic and achievable learning objectives		
Briefly explains how to assess airway patency and adequate ventilation		
Uses suction to remove any liquid obstruction		
Demonstrates head tilt chin lift correctly		
Demonstrates jaw thrust correctly		
Demonstrates bag valve mask ventilation (one handed or two) correctly		
Explains rationale and demonstrates the use of nasopharyngeal airway		
Demonstrates how to size a nasopharyngeal airway		
Explains rationale and demonstrates the use of oropharyngeal airway		
Demonstrates how to size a oropharyngeal airway		
Explains rationale and demonstrates the use of a supraglottic device		
Explains correctly the process of escalation of airway management if an intervention is inadequate		
Aware of the need to escalate complex cases and the possible need for ET intubation by a senior colleague/ anaesthetist		
Checks the student's understanding		
Gives the student the opportunity to practice		
Encouraging and provides constructive feedback		
Asks if the student has any questions and answers them correctly		
Examiner's Global Mark	/5	
Actor / Helper's Global Mark	/5	
Total Station Mark	/30	

Learning points

Managing a patient's airway can be complex and frightening and a methodical escalating stepwise approach should be used. it is important to convey to an examiner that you understand that early involvement of senior colleagues/ an anaesthetist is always appropriate if there is potential for airway compromise.

A sound knowledge of airway manoeuvres, bag valve mask ventilation and basic airway adjuncts and devices is key. Know how they are selected, sized and notable contraindications. Be able to demonstrate how each is inserted.

Teaching is an integral part of a doctor's job. You need to be able to demonstrate the ability to establish learning objectives, communicate in a clear and appropriate manner and deliver teaching in a supportive and enthusiastic way. Always check the baseline knowledge to avoid over or under pitching your teaching and importantly set realistic and achievable objectives.

Case 24
Procedures - Urinary Catheter

Task	Achieved	Not Achieved
Introduces self and washes hands		
Check Identity and gains consent		
Takes history of presenting complaint and urological history		
Examines patient's abdomen		
Requests external genitalia and PR examination		
Asks for bladder scanner		
Explains the need for catheterisation to the patient and takes consent		
Washes hands and uses sterile technique (throughout)		
Prepares trolley with necessary equipment. Uses gloves and gown		
Exposes patient and drapes field around penis		
Retracts foreskin and cleans glans away from urethral meatus		
Changes gloves		
Applies anaesthetic gel and waits appropriate time		
Passes catheter fully and inflates balloon via syringe, asking about pain when inflating		
Pulls catheter until resistance is felt		
Attaches to reservoir bag		
Replaces foreskin over glans		
Thanks patient and recovers them		
Explains would document procedure and residual		
Asks for appropriate investigations (blood tests, Urine dip)		
Examiner's Global Mark	/5	
Actor / Helper's Global Mark	/5	
Total Station Mark	/30	

Learning points

When seeing patients with urinary retention, it is important to elicit the urinary symptoms as they will guide us in a differential diagnosis. Hesitancy, poor stream, and feeling of incomplete emptying is normally due to prostatic hyperplasia or prostate cancer. A PR exam is important to determine whether the prostate is Smooth or craggy. We can also check for anal tone during the PR as a cauda equina syndrome can present with urinary symptoms.

Replacing the foreskin is a must after urethral catheterisation as failure to do so may cause a paraphimosis. This is when the glans swells up and the foreskin cannot be replaced.

Check a urine dip and the renal profile (electrolytes, urea, and creatinine) after inserting a catheter. Patients can go into diuresis due to increased urea and salt retention, which needs to be lost. There is also as a reduced concentration gradient in the loop of Henle (due to low flow), which does not recover immediately after the obstruction is relieved. Sometimes patients in retention need IV fluids to aid subsequent losses.

Case 25

Investigations - ABG interpretation

Task	Achieved	Not Achieved
Introduces self and washes hands		
Establish student's current level of knowledge/understanding		
Sets specific objectives of this learning session		
Systematic approach to analysing ABG		
Brief overview of history/describes clinical context		
Confirms patient details from which ABG was taken		
Confirms time ABG was taken		
States oxygen rate delivered		
Determines PH status Acidotic/alkalosis		
Comments on level of hypoxia		
Explains respiratory component		
Explains metabolic component		
Explains base excess correctly		
Establishes primary disturbance (respiratory acidosis)		
Establishes compensation (metabolic)		
Gives overall diagnosis (Type 2 respiratory failure)		
Describes appropriate management plan		
Has some knowledge of other components displayed on typical ABG		
Summarises **learning points**		
Asks if student has any further questions		
Examiner's Global Mark	/5	
Actor / Helper's Global Mark	/5	
Total Station Mark	/30	

Learning points

Remember to compare the pO2 to rate of oxygen being delivered to determine level of hypoxia. As a rough rule of thumb the pO2 should be comparable to the percentage oxygen delivered minus 10 eg 15L via non re -breathe bag at a FiO2 percentage of 85% should manifest an approximate pO2 in the blood of 85-10 =75

Always do a Chest X-ray prior to starting NIV. One of the causes of COPD exacerbation can be a pneumothorax that will be made worse with NIV.

When teaching junior colleagues remember to establish their current level of knowledge/skill. State learning objectives prior to the session, summarise the points after and ask for any questions. Giving them resources such as websites or podcasts to go away and access is a good way to consolidate learning.

Obstetrics & Gynaecology

Case 1
Markscheme - Dysmenorrhea

Task	Achieved	Not Achieved
Introduces self, washes hands		
Confirms name, age & occupation of patient		
Establishes reason for consultation		
Asks about menstrual history and cycle		
Asks about change in periods over time		
Asks about pain ("SOCRATES" approach)		
Asks about associated heavy bleeding		
Asks about dyspareunia, post coital bleeding, intermenstrual bleeding and vaginal discharge		
Asks about non gynaecological symptoms (urinary/bowel symptoms)		
Asks about weight loss or systemic features		
Asks about smears, STIs and gynaecological procedures		
Elicits past medical history, drug and allergy history		
Elicits social and family history		
Asks about treatment offered so far and impact on symptoms		
Identifies patient's ideas, concerns and expectations in an empathetic manner		
Summarises history in clear and concise manner		
Suggests appropriate differentials (e.g. fibroids, adenomyosis, endometriosis)		
Suggests appropriate examination and investigation (FBC, USS)		
Suggests appropriate management options		
Completes station in a confident and professional manner		
Examiners Global Mark	/5	
Actors Global Mark	/5	
Total Station Mark	/30	

Learning points

Do not forget to ask about the impact on the patient's social and professional life. This will often guide patient's expectations of your management plan.

Primary dysmenorrhea is diagnosed *after* excluding any organic cause, and is most common at menarche

It is important to ask about the *progression* of symptoms, as your likely differentials would change depending on how the patient's symptoms have evolved over time.

Case 2
Markscheme - Menorrhagia

Task	Achieved	Not Achieved
Introduces self, washes hands		
Confirms name, age & occupation of patient		
Establishes reason for consultation		
Asks about menstrual history and cycle		
Asks about change in periods over time		
Asks about symptoms of anaemia		
Asks about symptoms/signs of clotting abnormalities		
Asks about dyspareunia, post coital bleeding and intermenstrual bleeding		
Asks obstetric history		
Asks about contraception, smears, STIs and gynaecological procedures		
Asks about weight loss or systemic features		
Elicits past medical history, drug and allergy history		
Elicits social and family history – asks about impact on social life		
Asks about treatment offered so far and impact on symptoms		
Identifies patient's ideas, concerns and expectations in an empathetic manner		
Summarises history in clear and concise manner		
Suggests appropriate differentials (e.g. fibroids)		
Suggests appropriate examination and investigation (Bloods, USS)		
Suggests appropriate management options – medical and surgical according to history		
Completes station in a confident and professional manner		
Examiners Global Mark	/5	
Actors Global Mark	/5	
Total Station Mark	/30	

Learning points

It is important to identify the impact that symptoms have on the patient's day-to-day life, as this is key to managing their expectation of your treatment plan.

Note that in the history, the patient was unsure of the long-term effects of hormone therapy. Giving the patient information and picking up on their concerns could make them more willing to accept hormonal treatment options, which can be very effective in the management of menorrhagia.

Establish whether the patient is trying to conceive or not or if they would like to in the future, as this would impact the appropriate management options. Many of the surgical treatment options can impact on fertility so careful counseling is important.

Case 3
Markscheme - Pain and Discharge

Task	Achieved	Not Achieved
Introduces self, washes hands		
Confirms name, age & occupation of patient		
Establishes reason for consultation		
Asks thorough history of pain ("SOCRATES" approach) and associated symptoms		
Asks about vaginal discharge		
Asks about urinary or bowel symptoms		
Asks about other systemic symptoms		
Takes full gynae history (IMB, PCB, dyspareunia)		
Elicits obstetric history/prior pregnancies/TOPs		
Gives warning shot re. sensitive questions and reiterates confidentiality		
Asks about sexual partners in last 6 months: gender, type of sex and contraceptive use		
Asks about high risk behaviour for HIV/Hepatitis		
Asks about previous and current STIs and completion of treatment		
Elicits past medical history, drug & allergy history		
Identifies patient's ideas, concerns and expectations in an empathetic manner		
Summarises history in clear and concise manner		
Suggests likely diagnosis of PID but *highlights* ectopic pregnancy to be excluded		
Suggests examination & investigations – *highlights* ectopic must be excluded first		
Suggests management options & appropriate antibiotics		
Completes station in a confident and professional manner		
Examiners Global Mark	/5	
Actors Global Mark	/5	
Total Station Mark	/30	

Learning points

Pelvic inflammatory disease (PID) is a general term for infection of the upper female genital tract, including the uterus, fallopian tubes, and ovaries. Risk factors for PID include multiple previous sexual partners, young age (<30), lack of barrier contraception, termination of pregnancy or miscarriage, and an IUCD inserted within the last 20 days.

Look over current guidelines for appropriate treatment of common STIs, as well as PID. This can occasionally be managed in the community but if severe, the patient should be admitted.

It is important to be sensitive and non-judgemental when discussing sexual history. Patients can often feel embarrassed and stigmatised as a result of this diagnosis. As their doctor, it is important to make them feel comfortable to open up so you can treat them quickly and appropriately.

Case 4
Markscheme - Fertility issues

Task	Achieved	Not Achieved
Introduces self, washes hands		
Confirms name, age & occupation of patient		
Establishes reason for consultation		
Asks about duration of difficulty conceiving		
Asks about previous conception or pregnancies		
Asks if male partner has been able to conceive with other women		
Asks about frequency of intercourse		
Asks about systemic symptoms and signs (galactorrhoea, hair growth, weight)		
Asks about smears and STIs		
Asks about stress and effect on relationship		
Asks specifically about menstrual cycle		
Elicits full gynaecological history		
Elicits past medical history, drug & allergy history		
Elicits social history and family history		
Identifies patient's ideas, concerns and expectations in an empathetic manner		
Summarises history in clear and concise manner		
Suggests differentials (endometriosis, fibroids, idiopathic subfertiliy)		
Suggests appropriate examination & investigations of both partners		
Suggests management options or follow up		
Completes station in a confident and professional manner		
Examiners Global Mark	/5	
Actors Global Mark	/5	
Total Station Mark	/30	

Learning points

History is pertinent here especially with respect to factors that directly impact fertility and those which do so indirectly, such as previous contraceptive choice, previous abdominal surgery and stress.

Always consider male subfertility. In this scenario, the partner has been able to successfully conceive twice. Despite this, it is still important to take a full history from the male partner to identify areas of concern. Drugs and alcohol can reduce male fertility, as well as infections, anatomical abnormalities and antisperm antibodies.

Positive evidence-based information can encourage an anxious couple. For example, 80% of couples will conceive within a year and 90% within two years, providing the woman is under 40 years old and they are having regular intercourse (*NICE, Aug 2016*). Fertility issues can be difficult to discuss and can often impact on a patient's self esteem and relationship. It is important to deal with this sensitively and explore the effects it is having on her personal life.

Case 5
Markscheme - Pruritis

Task	Achieved	Not Achieved
Introduces self, washes hands		
Confirms name, age & occupation of patient		
Establishes reason for consultation		
Asks about duration of symptoms		
Asks about specific locations of itching		
Asks about presence of rash with itching		
Asks about jaundice or change in colour of urine or stools		
Asks about other systemic symptoms		
Asks about environmental changes (e.g. detergent, clothing, dust)		
Asks about changes to medication including over the counter remedies		
Asks about effect on daily life		
Elicits current and previous obstetric history		
Elicits past medical history, drug & allergy history		
Elicits social history & family history		
Identifies patient's ideas, concerns and expectations in an empathetic manner		
Summarises history in clear and concise manner		
Suggests suitable differentials		
Suggests examination & investigations (bloods, USS abdomen)		
Suggests management options according to differentials e.g. ursodeoxycholic acid		
Completes station in a confident and professional manner		
Examiners Global Mark	/5	
Actors Global Mark	/5	
Total Station Mark	/30	

Learning points

Do not forget to ask about sites of pruritus – this is often a key indicator to the diagnosis. Obstetric cholestasis often affects the palms and soles, whereas Polymorphic Eruption of Pregnancy and Prurigo of Pregnancy often affect the abdomen and limbs.

Always consider pemphigoid gestationis, which is rare but can have serious complications such as IUGR and prematurity. It is characterised by a blistering vesicular rash and should be managed as a high risk pregnancy

Do not forget to consider other non-pregnancy related causes, including liver, renal or haematological disease.

Case 6
Antepartum haemorrhage

Task	Achieved	Not Achieved
Introduces self, washes hands		
Confirms name, age & occupation of patient		
Establishes reason for consultation		
Asks about bleeding: quantity, colour, duration of symptoms		
Asks about associated pain		
Asks about other associated PV discharge/fluid		
Asks about fetal movements		
Asks about precipitating abdominal or vaginal trauma, including sexual intercourse		
Asks about other systemic symptoms		
Asks about current pregnancy including complications and scans		
Elicits obstetric history and brief sexual history, including risk of STIs		
Elicits past medical history, drug & allergy history		
Elicits brief social history and enquires about home situation (e.g. domestic violence)		
Identifies patient's ideas, concerns and expectations in an empathetic manner		
Summarises history in clear and concise manner		
Suggests suitable differentials including placenta praevia or placental abruption		
Suggests abdominal and PV examination		
Suggests appropriate investigations to determine maternal and fetal wellbeing		
Suggests management plan – admit & observe, CTG, consider steroids, anti-D if Rhesus negative		
Completes station in a confident and professional manner		
Examiners Global Mark	/5	
Actors Global Mark	/5	
Total Station Mark	/30	

Learning points

Read the vignette carefully. This asks you to 'take a history' so do not forget to cover all aspects including past medical, drug and social history and not get carried away with just the antenatal history. As pregnancies progress, pre-existing medical issues can come to the forefront so it is important to be thorough in your history taking.

The main causes of antepartum haemorrhage should be revised. Placenta praevia is more common in this case because of the previous Caesarean section. This defines the insertion of the placenta, partially or fully, in the lower segment of the uterus but may remain asymptomatic during the pregnancy. Placental abruption, on the other hand, is premature separation of a normally placed placenta.

Make note of the risk of vaginal or abdominal trauma, which may not always be accidental. Domestic violence commonly presents for the first time in pregnancy, so do give the patient an opportunity to discuss this.

Case 7
Unwell postpartum

Task	Achieved	Not Achieved
Introduces self, washes hands		
Confirms name, age & occupation of patient		
Establishes reason for consultation		
Asks about fever – duration, if measured, response to antipyretics		
Asks about associated PV discharge/lochia		
Asks about urinary or bowel symptoms		
Asks about other systemic symptoms & pain		
Asks about breastfeeding or breast symptoms		
Asks about pregnancy, delivery and obstetric history		
Elicits past medical history, drug & allergy history		
Elicits brief social history		
Identifies patient's ideas, concerns and expectations in an empathetic manner		
Picks up on patient concerns regarding Paracetamol while breastfeeding		
Reassures patient it is safe to continue breastfeeding while being treated for mastitis		
Summarises history in clear and concise manner		
Recognises likely diagnosis of mastitis		
Suggests suitable differentials e.g. vaginal wound infection, endometritis		
Suggests appropriate examination (check uterus, IV sites, breast, legs) and investigations		
Suggests suitable management plan – *highlights* need to exclude sepsis		
Completes station in a confident and professional manner		
Examiners Global Mark	/5	
Actors Global Mark	/5	
Total Station Mark	/30	

Learning points

Pick up on cues given by the actor. The patient mentions that she is concerned about taking Paracetamol while breastfeeding – which is known to be safe in pregnancy. Use this as an opportunity to educate the patient. Additionally there are many antibiotics that are deemed safe whilst breastfeeding. A simple way to remember is that if you would give the antibiotic to the child directly it is safe to be exposed to via breastfeeding.

Consider all causes of surgical or hospital acquired infections – check IV sites, legs for a possible DVT, chest as well as breast, uterine and PV infections.

Maternal sepsis (in particular genital tract sepsis) remains one of the top five causes of maternal mortality in the last UK Confidential Enquiry into Maternal Deaths (CEMD) (*Nair & Knight, 2015*). Examine the patient thoroughly in order to exclude sepsis, but do not forget to 'safety net' appropriately.

Case 8
6 week post natal check

Task	Achieved	Not Achieved
Introduces self, washes hands		
Confirms name, age & occupation of patient		
Establishes reason for consultation		
Asks about delivery and any complications		
Asks about post delivery – wound healing/pain		
Asks about PV discharge, bleeding (including if menstrual cycle has resumed) or lochia		
Asks about urinary and bowel symptoms, including incontinence		
Asks about type of feeding and any issues		
Asks about breast soreness/infective symptoms		
Asks about sleeping pattern		
Asks about mood and emotional issues		
Asks about social support available to patient		
Asks about sexual activity and contraception		
Discusses contraceptive options if breastfeeding		
Takes brief medical, drug, allergy and social history		
Identifies patient's ideas, concerns and expectations in an empathetic manner		
Summarises history in clear and concise manner		
Suggests appropriate examination of abdomen and vaginal stitches		
Suggests suitable management or follow up		
Completes station in a confident and professional manner		
Examiners Global Mark	/5	
Actors Global Mark	/5	
Total Station Mark	/30	

Learning points

The 6-week postnatal check should cover physical, psychological and social health. It is an important time to screen for any signs of mental illness, which is relatively common in the postnatal period. It is also not restricted to depression, so consider other possibilities such as anxiety and PTSD.

Ask about bowel or urinary incontinence as a third of women experience urinary incontinence after childbirth but many feel too embarrassed to bring it up themselves. Regular pelvic floor exercises are a good way for patients to manage the symptoms as first-line option.

Always enquire about contraception and intercourse. The Lactational Amenorrhoea Method (LAM) can be effective, but only in the first 6 months, if totally amenorrhoeic, and if *fully* breastfeeding at least 4 hourly during the day and 6 hourly at night. If these three criteria are not met, additional contraception is required. After 6 weeks postpartum, fertility may return if breastfeeding reduces or stops.

Case 9
Cervical smear

Task	Achieved	Not Achieved
Introduces self, washes hands		
Confirms name, age & occupation of patient		
Establishes reason for consultation		
Establishes prior knowledge of cervical smear – why it is done and what it involves		
Explains that it is a screening test for cervical cancer and explains what 'screening' is		
Identifies who falls under the screening criteria		
Explains what the results of the test can be		
Explains what will need to be done if the tests are abnormal		
Explains what treatment can be done if there are abnormal cells		
Checks understanding of information given		
Offers/informs of presence of chaperone		
Explain what a speculum is and insertion		
Explain that a brush will be used inserted and turned three times		
Explains that sample will be sent to the lab and results directly by post		
Explain risks of procedure		
Explain benefits of procedure		
Identifies patients ideas, concerns & expectations in an empathetic manner		
Reassures patient that they will stop if in too much discomfort or changes her mind		
Checks understanding (asks patient to summarise) and obtains verbal consent		
Completes station in a confident and professional manner		
Examiners Global Mark	/5	
Actors Global Mark	/5	
Total Station Mark	/30	

Learning points

Understand how to clearly explaining what a screening programme is without the use of jargon. Patient information websites offer simple explanations that are worth reading over.

Cervical smears are offered to women aged 25-64 at 3 yearly intervals until age 49 and then 5 yearly intervals till age 64. Certain patient groups require more frequent smears or colposcopy – i.e. HIV patients and renal transplant patients.

It is now well known that human papillomavirus (HPV) causes the vast majority of cases of cervical cancer. In the UK and many developed countries, the HPV vaccine has been introduced for girls aged 12-13 but it will be many years before an impact on incidence of cervical cancer may be truly seen.

Case 10
Postmenopausal bleeding

Task	Achieved	Not Achieved
Introduces self, washes hands		
Confirms name, age & occupation of patient		
Establishes reason for consultation		
Takes brief history of recent symptoms and events leading up to consultation		
Establishes prior knowledge of what the procedure is and why it is done		
Explains causes of postmenopausal bleeding		
Explains the procedure usually a day case		
Can be done under general anaesthetic if preferred and a suitable candidate for this		
Explains preparation before surgery		
Explains what to expect during procedure and timescale		
Explains what to expect after the procedure – cramping, bleeding		
Advises to arrange transport home or to be with someone if under anaesthetic		
Discusses recovery time		
Explains procedure risks: bleeding, infection, injury to anatomy, anaesthetic risks		
Advise no sexual intercourse for 7 days or until bleeding stops to reduce risk of infection		
Explains will contact with results within a week		
Identifies patients ideas, concerns & expectations in an empathetic manner		
Summarises key points, checks understanding & avoids jargon		
Arranges follow up and offers take home info		
Completes station in a confident and professional manner		
Examiners Global Mark	/5	
Actors Global Mark	/5	
Total Station Mark	/30	

Learning points

Separate explaining procedure stations into before, during and after the procedure to deliver more manageable 'chunks' of information. The 'chunk-and-check' approach to information delivery is effective in ensuring understanding and paced well in real life, but also in the OSCE exam to ensure you are covering all your bases (and gathering marks!).

As is the case in this scenario, a balanced explanation should be given to the patient outlining both the benefits of the procedure but also the potential risks and complications. It may seem more stressful and difficult to describe potential complications, however informed consent cannot be given sufficient explanation of these facts.

Hysteroscopy can be performed both in the Gynaecology outpatient department and in theatres. It can be both diagnostic and therapeutic, as most polyps and some fibroids can be removed.

Case 11
Stages of labour

Task	Achieved	Not Achieved
Introduces self, washes hands		
Confirms name and stage of training		
Establishes students current knowledge base		
Identifies that there are 3 stages of labour		
Explains stage 1 is split: latent & active phase		
Explains latent phase is indicated by regular contractions and cervical changes		
Explains active phase is from 4cm dilation onwards to full dilation (10cm) and effacement		
Explains 2nd stage is from full dilation to delivery		
Explains the passage of the fetus through the canal		
Discusses engagement		
Discusses descent and flexion		
Discusses internal rotation		
Discusses extension and delivery		
Discusses Restitution and external rotation		
Explains 3rd stage is delivery of the placenta		
Uses model to clearly demonstrate stages of birth		
Summarises key points, checks understanding & avoids jargon		
Asks if any further questions		
Identifies causes of prolonged first stage: Power, Passage, Passenger		
Completes station in a confident and professional manner		
Examiners Global Mark	/5	
Actors Global Mark	/5	
Total Station Mark	/30	

Learning points

It is important to inspect the station before starting and look for any aids or props that might be available to you in order to explain the process clearly – use them! It is far easier in stations like this to demonstrate with a model than to simply talk out loud and expect the listener to be able to picture it all in their head.

This station involves time management – there are clearly definitive phases you need to cover and signposting is a useful way to inform the actor and examiner that you have taken note of the vignette.

A pictorial record of labour (partogram) can be used once labour is established to track the initial progress of the labour. Clinicians should keep in mind that birth is a 'normal' process and should not be unnecessarily medicalised. Clinical intervention should not be offered or advised where labour is progressing normally.

Case 12
Vaginal examination and swabs

Task	Achieved	Not Achieved
Introduces self, washes hands		
Confirms name, age & occupation		
Establishes purpose of consultation and seeks permission		
Requests chaperone, asks if patient prefers door locked		
Expose and Reposition patient		
Prepares equipment: cytobrush, lubricating gel, speculum (checks speculum and screw)		
Inspect vulva and mentions appearance or abnormalities seen		
Part labia and insert speculum using correct technique		
Inspect cervix for abnormalities		
Insert cytobrush into external os and rotate 360 degree 3 times		
Break off head of brush into specimen pot		
Unscrew and remove speculum, cover patient		
Label and date specimen pots		
Perform bimanual exam – two gloved & lubricated fingers close to posterior fornix		
Applies pressure to suprapubic area, comments on uterus, palpates adnexae		
Covers and thanks patient, clears workspace		
Safety netting, discusses results and follow up		
Summarises key points, checks understanding		
Asks if any further questions		
Completes station in a confident and professional manner		
Examiners Global Mark	/5	
Actors Global Mark	/5	
Total Station Mark	/30	

Learning points

In examination stations, remember to address the actor as the actual patient, as communication skills are still assessed. Most patients will appreciate you talking through what you are doing in real time both to prepare them for what is coming, but also to explain the reasons for why you are doing the various parts of the examination.

Always request a chaperone for any intimate examinations and ensure that their details are documented in the notes. Having another person present can ensure both the patient and doctor feel supported.

The bimanual examination is able to assess for abnormalities in the vaginal vault, to palpate the cervix for lumps or excitation, to assess the uterine position, size and tenderness and to examine the adnexae for swellings or tenderness.

Case 13
Examination of the gravid abdomen

Task	Achieved	Not Achieved
Introduces self, washes hands		
Confirms name, age & occupation		
Establishes purpose of consultation and seeks permission		
Exposes and repositions patient		
Asks if in any pain or discomfort		
Inspects abdomen for scars, striae & linea nigra		
Assesses fundal height – informs patient this may be uncomfortable		
Palpate contents or abdomen to locate head, back and limbs		
Comment on lie i.e.: transverse, longitudinal		
Comment on presentation (i.e. breech, cephalic)		
Determine position of head in pelvis (occiput in relation to anterior pelvis – i.e. LOA, ROA)		
Determine how many fifths palpable above pelvic brim		
Comments on liquor volume		
Offers to assess fetal heartbeat		
Covers & thanks the patient, clears workspace		
Comments on further assessments to complete exam (BP, peripheral oedema, urine dipstick)		
Summarises findings in clear and concise manner		
Identifies larger than expected fundal height		
Able to give causes of polyhydramnios		
Completes station in a confident and professional manner		
Examiners Global Mark	/5	
Actors Global Mark	/5	
Total Station Mark	/30	

Learning points

Assessing the fetal lie is something that comes with practice. By applying gentle but sustained pressure to either side of the uterus, one side should appear fuller indicating the fetal back is there, and the opposite side may allow you to palpate fetal limbs. The lie may be described as longitudinal, transverse or oblique.

Know the causes of polyhydramnios and oligohydramnios – fundal height from pubic symphysis to fundus in centimetres (+/-2cm) should correlate with the number of weeks gestation up till 20 weeks at least.

Examination of the fetal heart is often the most anticipated and stressful part of the examination for both patient and doctor. Use of a hand held Doppler or Pinard stethosope is essential and the fetal heart rate should be between 110-160bpm. Comparison with the mother's radial pulse can ensure you are happy it is indeed that of the fetus.

Case 14
Explaining smear results

Task	Achieved	Not Achieved
Introduces self, washes hands		
Confirms name, age & occupation of patient		
Establishes reason for consultation		
Discusses previous smear results or symptoms		
Establishes patient's current knowledge of cervical smear outcomes		
Explains CIN is cervical intraepithelial neoplasm and describes changes in the cervical squamous cells		
Sensitively explains 'mild dyskaryosis' and HPV positive		
Explains that changes in cells seen on smear could indicate CIN		
Reassures patient that CIN is NOT cancer		
Discusses that CIN I can progress to II or III		
Explains if CIN II or III are untreated, it can progress to cervical cancer		
Explains HPV is sexually transmitted		
Explains it is usually asymptomatic but certain types can increase risk of warts or cancer		
Explains plan to refer for routine colposcopy		
Explains colposcopy investigation, can take biopsy and treat if required		
Explains not hereditary, but vaccination given to 12-year-olds to prevent certain strains of HPV		
Identifies patient's ideas, concerns and expectations in an empathetic manner		
Summarises key points, checks understanding & avoids jargon		
Suggests follow up or take home information		
Completes station in a confident and professional manner		
Examiners Global Mark	/5	
Actors Global Mark	/5	
Total Station Mark	/30	

Learning points

Ensure the patient understands this is NOT a diagnosis of cancer, and be able to clearly explain the risks associated with untreated CIN. Approximately a third of women with CIN II or III will go on to develop cancer over the next 10 years. CIN I is less concerning as it commonly regresses, but can also progress to CIN II or III.

Learn about all possible outcomes of a cervical smear: negative, borderline, mild, moderate or severe dyskaryosis and relevant further investigation.

Understand how cervical cancer develops and pathophysiology including in relation to HPV. HPV inactivates important tumour suppressor genes and this, in conjuction with other mutations, can lead to cancer.

Case 15
Explaining OCP use

Task	Achieved	Not Achieved
Introduces self, washes hands		
Confirms name, age & occupation of patient		
Establishes reason for consultation		
Establishes patient's current knowledge of oral contraceptive methods		
Discusses 2 types of OCP – COCP or POP		
Explains the mechanism of the COCP		
Discusses advantages of COCP and efficacy (perfect and typical use)		
Discusses disadvantages of COCP – compliance, common side effects, risk of STIs		
Discusses differences and benefits of POP		
Takes focused history to elicit suitability for COCP, directly asking about contraindications		
Able to identify she is suitable for COCP		
Discusses initiating pill, also mentioning need for additional cover if starting after day 5 of cycle		
Discusses increased and reduced risks of different forms of cancer		
Discusses missed pill management		
Discuss need for caution with over the counter/prescription meds		
Informs patient long term fertility unaffected		
Identifies patient's ideas, concerns and expectations in an empathetic manner		
Summarises key points, checks understanding & avoids jargon		
Suggests follow up or take home information		
Completes station in a confident and professional manner		
Examiners Global Mark	/5	
Actors Global Mark	/5	
Total Station Mark	/30	

Learning points

Remember – the oral contraceptive pill slightly increases the risk of breast and cervical cancer but reduces the risk of ovarian, endometrial and bowel cancer.

Missed pill information is very easy to get confused about for patients. If the patient forgets to take a progestogen-only pill (POP), they must take it as soon as they remember. It is important to remind the patient that if they are more than three hours late in taking it (or more than 12 hours with a third generation POP) then the protection immediately fails. They must continue to take the POP each day, but will need to use extra contraception (such as condoms) for two more days before the POP becomes effective again.

VTE risk is notably higher in women on the COCP (2 per 10 000 women in general population, 5-12 per 10 000 in combined hormonal contraception users (*FSRH, 2014*)). It is true however that for most women the overall benefits outweigh the overall risks. Each woman should be risk assessed and then stratified for suitability.

Case 16

Sexual history & HIV counselling

Task	Achieved	Not Achieved
Introduces self, washes hands		
Confirms name, age & occupation of patient		
Establishes reason for consultation and identifies why they want to be tested		
Gives warning shot re sensitive questions and reiterates confidentiality		
Asks about sexual partners in last 6 months: gender, type of sex and contraceptive use		
Asks about high risk behaviour for HIV/Hepatitis e.g. IVDU, travel, background of partner		
Asks about previous and current STIs and completion of treatment		
Checks current level of understanding about HIV and knowledge of transmission risk		
Explains what HIV is		
Explains the test procedure		
Explains test limitation (3 month window period)		
Identifies implications of having a positive or negative test result		
Explains how long until results come back and how they will be communicated		
Checks how patient would cope with positive result, asks about support network		
Asks patient if still happy to have the test		
Identifies patient's ideas, concerns and expectations in an empathetic manner		
Summarises key points, checks understanding & avoids jargon		
Suggests follow up or take home information		
Completes station in a confident and professional manner		
Examiners Global Mark	/5	
Actors Global Mark	/5	
Total Station Mark	/30	

Learning points

Pre-exposure prophylaxis (PrEP) has been shown to be very effective in reducing the transmission of disease in high-risk individuals. This can either be taken daily if consistently at risk, or 'on-demand' before and after sex. Currently, this is not available on the NHS but can be purchased privately. It does not protect against other STIs or the risk of pregnancy.

Patients will need to be retested If exposure was within the last 3 months as there is a window period where a patient may test negative and the virus may not be detectable.

Ask about any recent non-specific symptoms that could represent a seroconversion illness. This usually occurs 1 to 4 weeks following exposure and is noted to be a 'flu-like' illness with non-specific symptoms. This includes lethargy, fever, rash, lymphadenopathy, and muscle/joint pains.

Case 17
Explaining HIV Management

Task	Achieved	Not Achieved
Introduces self, washes hands		
Confirms name, age & occupation of patient		
Establishes reason for consultation		
Establish what the patient remembers from the last meeting		
Ask how patient has been coping and what support they have		
Allows patient to lead discussion with questions		
Reassures patient that many patients have a normal lifespan with follow up and treatment		
Discusses the difference between HIV and AIDS		
Reassures patient that they can continue to have sexual intercourse with barrier protection		
Reassures patient that he can still have children and discusses options for doing so safely		
Discusses transmission methods and how to reduce risks		
Reassures about confidentiality, no need to inform workplace if irrelevant to job description		
Explores concerns about informing workplace		
Reiterates confidentiality in clinical session, within the parameters set by GMC		
Discusses general treatment options		
Explains monitoring viral load and CD4 count		
Identifies patient's ideas, concerns and expectations in an empathetic manner		
Summarises key points, checks understanding & avoids jargon		
Suggests follow up or take home information		
Completes station in a confident and professional manner		
Examiners Global Mark	/5	
Actors Global Mark	/5	
Total Station Mark	/30	

Learning points

You do not need to have extensive knowledge about specialist medications for the treatment of HIV, but an understanding of the mechanisms of action with 1-2 examples will help in this scenario and also in the written exam.

It is important to clarify what the patient can remember from their last meeting. When breaking bad news, patients rarely retain much information due to the shock of the diagnosis. Always check what needs to be covered again to make sure the patient is fully informed.

When counselling a patient, it is important to consider psychosocial issues in the OSCE and in real life. Explore their support network and concerns regarding the cultural and social stigma that still surrounds HIV. Confidentiality with friends, work colleagues and their other medical should be stressed. This diagnosis is not one that needs to be shared widely without the patient's consent.

Case 18
Explaining termination of pregnancy

Task	Achieved	Not Achieved
Introduces self, washes hands		
Confirms name, age & occupation of patient		
Establishes reason for consultation		
Asks open questions about patient's feelings towards the pregnancy		
Asks about factors impacting decision: personal, financial, social, family & professional		
Asks if partner is aware or if they have a support network		
Discusses alternative option to TOP: adoption		
Asks about LMP and estimates gestation		
Asks brief gynaecological and medical history		
Discusses/offers STI check		
Explains medical procedure & indications		
Explains surgical procedure & indications		
Discusses complications of pregnancy – Bleeding, infection, physical/mental trauma		
Explains that blood test required to check rhesus status as she may need Anti-D injection		
Discusses process of referring for termination		
Offers time to think about options or counselling services via family planning clinics		
Identifies patient's ideas, concerns and expectations in an empathetic manner		
Summarises key points, checks understanding & avoids jargon		
Suggests follow up or take home information		
Completes station in a confident and professional manner		
Examiners Global Mark	/5	
Actors Global Mark	/5	
Total Station Mark	/30	

Learning points

This is a difficult conversation and decision to make for the majority of patients. Encourage them to seek support from partner / friends / family and/or offer counselling to help make the decision.

The Human Fertilisation & Embryology Act 1990 (*HFEA, 1990*) states the current law allows termination of pregnancy to be granted if:

Pregnancy is <24 weeks and risk of injury to physical/mental health of woman or existing children in the family greater if it is continued than if it is terminated.
Termination is necessary to prevent grave permanent injury to physical/mental health of pregnant woman.
Pregnancy at any stage would involve risk to the life of the pregnant woman greater if it is continued than if it is terminated.
Substantial risk of severe mental/physical abnormalities in the unborn child causing serious handicap.

Remember to offer an STI check and follow-up to discuss contraceptive options. Often at the time of a surgical TOP, an IUD can be placed. Following a medical TOP, several methods including the OCP, depot or implant can be started on the day of prostaglandin administration. The IUD can be inserted following the next menstrual cycle.

Case 19
Explaining sickle cell inheritance

Task	Achieved	Not Achieved
Introduces self, washes hands		
Confirms name, age & occupation of patient		
Establishes reason for consultation		
Checks current knowledge of sickle cell disease		
Explains the difference between sickle cell disease and trait		
Establishes patient is a sickle cell carrier – asks about family history and symptoms		
Asks about her husband's sickle cell status		
Explains that it is an autosomal recessive condition and the pattern of inheritance		
Discusses disease/trait inheritance probability if partner is a carrier or not		
Suggests partner screening if status unknown		
Suggests importance of antenatal screening for other haemoglobinopathies		
Explains implications if the child develops sickle cell disease		
Explains implications if the child is a sickle cell carrier		
Explains diagnostic techniques in pregnancy if the mother wishes to confirm this		
Explains newborn bloodspot testing		
Explains importance of antenatal booking visit		
Identifies patient's ideas, concerns and expectations in an empathetic manner		
Summarises key points, checks understanding & avoids jargon		
Suggests follow up or take home information		
Completes station in a confident and professional manner		
Examiners Global Mark	/5	
Actors Global Mark	/5	
Total Station Mark	/30	

Learning points

It is useful to have a framework for explaining the inheritance patterns for autosomal recessive and dominant conditions. Remember you can use diagrams to help explain.

All newborn babies are offered a heel prick blood spot test 5-7 days after birth, but mothers may choose to undergo antenatal genetic screening and amniocentesis and chorionic villus sampling (CVS) are diagnostic in pregnancy.

Routine partner screening is offered to mothers who are known to be sickle cell carriers. If both parents are carriers they will be offered the chance to definitively test the fetus by chorionic villus sampling or Amniocentesis between 0-15 weeks gestation.

Case 20
Explaining try whooping cough vaccine

Task	Achieved	Not Achieved
Introduces self, washes hands		
Confirms name, age & occupation of patient		
Establishes reason for consultation		
Checks current knowledge of whooping cough and the vaccination, elicits concerns		
Explains what whooping cough/pertussis is and complications		
Discusses risk in young babies before immunisation, more likely to need admission		
Informs patient it is recommended nationally		
Discusses side effects of vaccine, no known contraindications		
Explains not a 'live' vaccine – therefore cannot get the disease from vaccination		
Explains when the vaccine is recommended in pregnancy (from 20 weeks up to 32 weeks)		
Explains it is less effective later in pregnancy, but can be give up until labour		
Advises that the baby still needs vaccination as part of their immunisation schedule after birth		
Advises she can make an informed decision		
Reassures patient that she will continue to be supported by staff regardless of her choice		
Advises patient to discuss this with her partner/support network/antenatal group		
Gives clear recommended advice in a non-judgemental and non-coercive manner		
Identifies patient's ideas, concerns and expectations in an empathetic manner		
Summarises key points, checks understanding & avoids jargon		
Suggests follow up or take home information		
Completes station in a confident and professional manner		
Examiners Global Mark	/5	
Actors Global Mark	/5	
Total Station Mark	/30	

Learning points

There is no known evidence to date that the vaccine is unsafe in pregnancy. It is important to confidently reiterate this to patients so that they can be assured that this is a national clinical recommendation and research to support this. Specifically, there was no increased risk in stillbirth seen in an observational study of over 20 000 women given the vaccine in pregnancy (*Donegan et al, 2014*).

In the UK there is no whooping cough-only vaccine, the vaccine you'll be given also protects against polio, diphtheria and tetanus. The vaccine is similar to the 4-in-1 vaccine – the pre-school booster that's routinely given to children before they start school.

Any discussions regarding pregnancy or childhood vaccinations can be difficult if parents have strong views against vaccines. As a health professional, it is important to given unbiased, factual information in order to allow patients to make an informed decision. Excellent patient information leaflets exist that should be given to parents so they can digest the facts in their own time in a less pressured environment. Follow up appointments should be made with their GPs to discuss it further.

Medicine

Case 1
Markscheme - Anaphylaxis

Task	Achieved	Not Achieved
Ensures personal safety (apron and gloves)		
Makes general end of the bed assessment		
Introduces self to patient		
Calls for help early		
Assesses airway		
Applies high flow oxygen (15L via a non-rebreathe mask)		
Assesses breathing (RR, Trachea, Percussion, Auscultation, sats)		
Assesses circulation (CRT, HR, BP)		
Cannulates patient		
Commences IV fluid challenge (500ml-100ml IV crystalloid)		
Assesses disability (Pupils, AVPU, Blood Sugar)		
Exposes patient (identifies rash, and antibiotic infusion)		
Stops antibiotic infusion		
Gives 500 micrograms of 1:1000 Adrenaline IM		
Reassesses patient using ABCDE approach		
Gives 200mg IV Hydrocortisone		
Gives 10mg IV Chlorphenamine		
Contacts senior (medical registrar, intensive care registrar)		
Maintains communication with patient throughout		
Able to discuss further management of patient (monitoring, steroids, change of antibiotics, incident report form, duty of candour etc.)		
Examiner's Global Mark	/5	
Actor's Global Mark	/5	
Total station Mark	/30	

Learning Points

Remember to stick to an ABCDE approach to assessment in your acute/ emergency OSCE stations. A systematic approach will prevent you from missing clinical points. After any intervention do remember to reassess the impact of your intervention.

Apply high flow oxygen and call for help early for any sick patient. Time flies in real life (and the OSCE) so putting out a call once you have ascertained the level of severity is essential.

The 1st line treatment of anaphylaxis includes imtra muscular (not intravenous) adrenaline, fluids and high flow oxygen. A second dose of IM adrenaline can be given after 5 minutes if there is an ongoing reaction. 2nd Line treatment includes hydrocortisone and chlorphenamine.

Case 2
Markscheme - Sepsis

Task	Achieved	Not Achieved
Ensures personal safety (apron and gloves)		
Makes general end of the bed assessment		
Introduces self to patient		
Calls for help		
Assesses airway		
Applies high flow oxygen (15L via a NRB Mask)		
Assesses breathing (RR, Trachea, Percussion, Auscultation, Saturations)		
Assesses circulation (CRT, HR, BP)		
Cannulates patient		
Takes bloods including lactate		
Takes blood cultures		
Commences IV fluid challenge (500ml-100ml IV crystalloid)		
Assesses disability (Pupils, AVPU, Blood Sugar)		
Requests temperature		
Exposes patient		
Commences appropriate broad-spectrum IV antibiotics		
Catheterises patient and monitors urine output		
Reassesses patient using ABCDE approach		
Able to list "Sepsis 6" Components		
Able to describe further management including close monitoring, ongoing IV antibiotics and ITU review if BP not responding to fluid resuscitation.		
Examiner's Global Mark	/5	
Actor's Global Mark	/5	
Total station Mark	/30	

Learning Points

Sepsis is a common presentation to both primary and secondary care. Sepsis management has evolved and early warning scores play a key part in knowing when and how to intervene. Red flag and Amber flag sepsis are two recent terms that have been validated. Red flag features include: Reduced conscious level to voice or pain only, new confusion, Systolic BP <90, HR >130, RR >25, Oxygen to keep saturations >92%, a non blanching rash, Anuria for >18 hours or recent chemotherapy.

The management of sepsis must be done efficiently. An easy way to do this is to think of the sepsis 6 as "3 in and 3 out";

IN	OUT
Oxygen	Blood Cultures
Fluids	Lactate
Antibiotics	Urine Output

Patients with a serum lactate >4mmol/L should be referred to critical care. As a junior doctor it is important to know the early pointers to stratifying how ill a patient is. Early escalation to seniors and specialists can reduce patient morbidity and mortality.

Case 3
Markscheme - GI Bleed

Task	Achieved	Not Achieved
Ensures personal safety (apron and gloves)		
Makes general end of the bed assessment		
Introduces self to patient		
Calls for Help		
Assesses airway		
Applies high flow oxygen (15L via a non-rebreathe mask)		
Assesses breathing (RR, Trachea, Percussion, Auscultation, Saturations)		
Assesses circulation (CRT, HR, BP)		
Cannulates patient using a large bore cannula		
Takes bloods including FBC, UE, LFTs, Clotting, Lactate, Group and Save)		
Requests 2nd large bore cannula		
Commences IV fluid challenge (500ml-100ml IV crystalloid)		
Assesses disability (Pupils, AVPU, Blood Sugar)		
Exposes patient		
Requests emergency blood/ activates Major haemorrhage transfusion protocol		
Reassesses patient using ABCDE approach		
Considers the use of broad spectrum antibiotics		
Considers the use of IV terlipressin		
Contacts the emergency endoscopist on-call		
Able to describe further management including close monitoring, transfusion, ITU review and endoscopy		
Examiner's Global Mark	/5	
Actor's Global Mark	/5	
Total station Mark	/30	

Learning Points

Have a high index of suspicion for a variceal bleed in patients with a history of liver disease and clinical signs of chronic liver disease.

"Replace like with like" and "switch off the tap". In the actively bleeding patient fluid resuscitation is a temporary measure; ultimately they will need blood. Endoscopy is required to identify a source of bleeding and provide definitive haemostasis.

In contrast to other patients with an upper GI Bleed, patients with known or suspected varices require the administration of prophylactic broad-spectrum antibiotics and terlipressin (a splanchnic vasoconstrictor that reduces portal hypertension).

Case 4
Markscheme - Respiratory examination

Task	Achieved	Not Achieved
Washes Hands		
Introduces themselves and clarifies the patient's details		
Gains consent to examine		
Asks the patient if they have any pain		
Exposes and positions the patient		
Inspects the patient and surrounding area from the end of the bed		
Examines hands and check for the presence of asterixis		
Checks pulse		
Counts respiratory rate		
Inspects the eyes and mouth		
Examines for cervical lymph nodes		
Palpates for tracheal position		
Inspects the chest wall		
Assesses chest expansion		
Performs percussion		
Auscultates		
Performs vocal resonance		
Examines for peripheral oedema		
Thanks the patient		
Presents findings		
Examiner's global mark	/5	
Actor's global mark	/5	
Total station mark	/30	

Learning Points

Stick to the structure; inspection, palpation, percussion, auscultation.

Remember to inspect, palpate, percuss and auscultate the anterior and posterior chest wall including the apices.

Clubbing in a respiratory patient may be caused by lung cancer, pulmonary fibrosis or chronic suppurative lung disease (empyema, cystic fibrosis, bronchiectasis)

Case 5
Markscheme - Abdominal examination

Task	Achieved	Not Achieved
Washes Hands		
Introduces themselves and clarifies the patient's details		
Gains consent to examine		
Asks the patient if they have any pain		
Exposes and positions the patient		
Inspects the patient and surrounding area from the end of the bed		
Examines hands and check for the presence of asterixis		
Checks the heart rate		
Inspects the eyes and mouth		
Inspects the abdomen		
Palpates all 4 quadrants of the abdomen (superficial and deep)		
Palpates the liver		
Percusses the liver		
Palpates the spleen		
Percusses the spleen		
Ballots the kidneys bilaterally		
Palpates the "mass" (renal transplant)		
Auscultates		
Thanks the patient		
Presents findings		
Examiner's global mark	/5	
Actor's global mark	/5	
Total station mark	/30	

Learning Points

Remember to lay the patient flat, and kneel whilst examining the abdomen. It is important to look at the patient's face whilst palpating to look for any signs of discomfort or pain.

Tenderness over a renal transplant graft may suggest that the graft is being rejected.

If the patient has a renal transplant look for evidence of previous renal replacement therapy (haemodialysis access or peritoneal dialysis access) and evidence of causes of end-stage renal failure such as diabetes or systemic lupus erythematosus (SLE).

Case 6
Markscheme - Cardiovascular examination

Task	Achieved	Not Achieved
Washes Hands		
Introduces themselves and clarifies the patient's details		
Gains consent to examine		
Asks the patient if they have any pain		
Exposes and positions the patient		
Inspects the patient and surrounding area from the end of the bed		
Examines hands		
Checks the radial pulse commenting on rate, rhythm, character		
Checks for a collapsing pulse		
Requests the blood pressure		
Inspects the face, eyes and mouth		
Assesses the JVP (and checks for hepatojugular reflux)		
Inspects the precordium		
Palpates apex beat		
Palpates for parasternal heave and thrills		
Auscultates in the aortic, pulmonary, tricuspid and mitral areas		
Auscultates the lung bases		
Examines for sacral and peripheral oedema		
Thanks the patient		
Presents findings		
Examiner's global mark	/5	
Actor's global mark	/5	
Total station mark	/30	

Learning Points

If you identify a murmur it is important to comment on the timing (systolic or diastolic), location and radiation.

The location of the apex beat may help you to differentiate between aortic stenosis and mitral regurgitation. In aortic stenosis the apex beat stays put. In mitral regurgitation the apex beat relocates.

The murmur of mitral regurgitation radiates into the axilla. The murmur of aortic stenosis radiates to the carotids. Utilising these clues can help you differentiate the murmurs with greater confidence.

Case 7
Markscheme - Cerebellar examination

Task	Achieved	Not Achieved
Washes Hands		
Introduces themselves and clarifies the patient's details		
Gains consent to examine		
Asks the patient if they have any pain		
Exposes and positions the patient		
Inspects the patient and surrounding area from the end of the bed		
Assesses eye movements and comments on the presence/absence of nystagmus		
Assesses speech for dysarthria		
Assesses for pronator drift		
Assesses for rebound phenomenon		
Assesses tone in the upper limb		
Assesses tone in the lower limb		
Assesses coordination in the lower limb		
Assesses for truncal ataxia		
Assesses coordination in the lower limb		
Performs Romberg's Test		
Observes the patient's gait		
Asks the patient to heel-toe walk		
Thanks the patient		
Presents findings		
Examiner's Global Mark	/5	
Actor/ Helper's Global Mark	/5	
Total station mark Mark	/30	

Learning Points

Romberg's test can help to differentiate between a cerebellar and a sensory ataxia. With a sensory ataxia the patient will become unsteady whilst standing with their eyes closed. With a cerebellar ataxia the patient will remain relatively steady whilst standing with their eyes closed.

Truncal ataxia can be tested by asking the patient to sit on the edge of the examination couch with their arms crossed across their chest.

If in doubt remember "DANISH"
Dysdiadokokinesis
Ataxia
Nystagmus
Intention tremor
Slurred/ Staccato speech
Hypotonia/ Heel-shin test

Case 8
Markscheme - Rheumatoid hand examination

Task	Achieved	Not Achieved
Washes Hands		
Introduces self and clarifies patient details		
Gains informed consent for examination		
Asks the patient if they have any pain		
Positions patient with hands resting on pillow		
Looks; inspects the hands on both sides (nail changes, skin changes, scars, muscle wasting, palmar thickening, deformities and joint swelling)		
Feels; temperature of both hands		
Feels; all joints for swelling and tenderness in a systematic manner (e.g. starting proximally at radial styloid, squeezing across MCP joints and going distally to interphalangeal joints)		
Feels; ulna and radial pulses bilaterally		
Move; asks patient to make prayer sign and reverse prayer sign.		
Move; demonstrates ulnar and radial deviation		
Move; demonstrates pronation and supination		
Checks power of radial, ulnar and medial nerves – finger extension, finger abduction, finger adduction, thumb abduction and adduction against resistance		
Briefly checks light touch sensation in distribution of radial, ulnar and median nerves		
Assesses function – power grip and pincer grip (e.g. hold pen, button, pick up coin)		
Checks elbows for scars, rheumatoid nodules and psoriasis		
Thanks patient		
Presents findings in a concise, logical manner.		
Correctly lists common hand features of rheumatoid arthritis		
Addresses patient's pain/attends to comfort		
Examiner's Global Mark	/5	
Actor / Helper's Global Mark	/5	
Total Station Mark	/30	

Learning Points

Always follow the principle LOOK, FEEL and MOVE in musculoskeletal examinations.

It is important to ask about pain, acknowledge pain and then pause to offer analgesia in any examination. Look at the patient's face whilst examining, as they may not volunteer this.

Rheumatoid arthritis and osteoarthritis are common exam cases and it is important you are confident with distinguishing between the different features of each:

Rheumatoid Arthritis	Osteoarthritis
Onset any age	Onset in old age
Autoimmune	Degenerative
Morning stiffness	Stiffness worse at end of day
Symmetrical pattern of joints affected	Asymmetrical
Classic deformities: Boutonnières, swan neck, Z-shaped thumb	Classic deformities: Bouchard's nodes (proximal), Heberden's node (distal), squaring of CMC joint of thumb
Extra-articular features e.g. rheumatoid nodules, pleural effusions, splenomegaly, nephrotic syndrome.	No systemic features. Large and small joints affected.

Case 9
Markscheme - Tremor

Task:	Achieved	Not Achieved
Washes hands		
Introduces self		
Confirms name and age of patient		
Explains examination and gets consent		
Exposes patient and asks patient to sit		
Asks about pain		
Inspects surroundings for walking aids etc.		
Examines patient from end of bed		
Inspects hands for resting tremor using distraction technique		
Assesses tone of upper limbs		
Assesses power of upper limbs		
Assesses co-ordination		
Assesses for bradykinesia		
Assesses face and eye movements		
Assesses speech		
Assesses motor function e.g. undoing a button		
Asks patient to write		
Observes gait		
Offers to test balance, complete full neurological examination, cerebellar examination, L/S BP, check drug chart, assess cognitive impairment.		
Summarises and gives at least 2 correct findings		
Examiner's Global Mark	/5	
Actor / Helper's Global Mark	/5	
Total Station Mark	/30	

Learning Points

It is likely that your patient in the exam will have real pathology. Ensure you practice with real Parkinson's patients before the exam so you feel confident and are easily able to recognise the typical features.

The three pathognomonic features of Parkinson's disease are; bradykinesia, resting pill-rolling tremor, increased tone (lead pipe rigidity).

Other typical positive finds are:
Cogwheel rigidity
Shuffling gait
Reduced arm swing
Stooped posture
Difficulty initiating movement
Hypophonia (quiet voice)
Hypomimia (expressionless face)
Small spidery handwriting (micrographia)

Signs such as impaired eye movements, cerebellar signs or cognitive impairment may suggest an alternative diagnosis such as one of the "Parkinson's Plus" Syndromes.

Case 10
Markscheme - ECG interpretation

Task	Achieved	Not Achieved
Identifies patient details		
Comments of the time and date of the ECG		
Comments on the reason for the ECG e.g. "chest pain"		
Checks that the ECG is calibrated correctly (25mm/second, 10m/milli-Volt)		
Comments on the rate		
Comments on the rhythm		
Comments on the axis		
Comments on P-wave morphology		
Comments on P-R interval		
Comments on QRS duration		
Comments on ST segments		
Identifies ST elevation and which territory is affected (inferior, lateral, septal, anterior)		
Comments on T-wave morphology		
Comments on the presence/ absence of Q waves		
Makes a diagnosis of STEMI		
States initial investigations would include bedside observations, bloods including troponin and a chest x-ray		
States they would assess the patient using an ABCDE approach		
States the management would include morphine, aspirin, oxygen and nitrates		
States the patient requires urgent PCI		
Able to identify the most-likely culprit vessel		
Examiner's global mark	/5	
Actor's global mark	/5	
Total station mark	/30	

Learning Points

A systematic approach to ECG interpretation will help you interpret almost any ECG. Even if there are obvious abnormalities sticking to the system will ensure you don't miss the other more subtle findings.

ST elevation in 2 or more consecutive ECG leads suggests an acute ST-elevation myocardial infarction. ST elevation must be more than 2 small squares in the chest leads, or more than 1 small square in the limb leads, to be significant.

Learn your leads;
Septal leads V1-V2
Anterior Leads V3-V4
Lateral Leads V5-V6
Inferior Leads II, III, aVF

Case 11
Markscheme - Chest X-Ray; pleural effusion

Task:	Achieved	Not Achieved
Interpretation/Presentation of chest x-ray		
Confirms patient details and date		
Comments on the position of the radiograph (AP/PA) film		
Comments on exposure		
Comments on rotation		
Comments on adequacy of field of view		
Comments on inspiratory effort		
Comments on trachea and mediastinum		
Comments on size of heart and cardiac borders		
Comments on costophrenic and cardiophrenic angles		
Comments on lung fields		
Identifies unilateral pleural effusion with meniscus and adjacent opacification.		
Comments on the presence of any extras; oxygen tubing, ECG leads, pacemakers, lines etc.		
Comments on soft tissue and bony abnormalities		
Explanation to patient		
Introduces self and role		
Explains the presence of a pleural effusion		
Briefly explains the likely cause and further management required		
Discussion with examiner		
Identifies parapneumonic effusion as most likely diagnosis		
Able to discuss differential diagnoses		
Identifies need for aspiration		
Adequate discussion on pleural fluid aspirate interpretation		
Examiner's Global Mark	/5	
Actor / Helper's Global Mark	/5	
Total Station Mark	/30	

Learning Points

When discussing the causes of a pleural effusion, remember to divide causes into transudate and exudate. On pleural fluid analysis, if protein < 25g/dl, the effusion is a transudate. If protein > 35g/dl, the effusion is an exudate. Light's criteria is applied if the protein content of the pleural fluid is between 25 – 35 g/dl to determine the nature of the fluid.

Case 12
Type 2 Respiratory Failure

Task:	Achieved	Not Achieved
Confirms patient details on printout are correct – name, date of birth and hospital number		
Confirms whether patient was on oxygen at time ABG taken		
Looks at the pH		
Identifies whether normal/ acidotic/ alkalotic		
Looks at pCO_2		
Identifies whether low/normal/high		
Looks at pO2		
Identifies whether low/normal/ high		
Looks at the bicarbonate		
Identifies whether low/normal/ high		
Looks at the BE		
Identifies whether low/normal/ high		
Looks at the lactate		
Identifies whether low/normal/ high		
Comments on electrolytes		
Comments on haemoglobin		
Presents findings in concise, logical manner		
Discusses management of patient		
Discusses causes of type 2 respiratory failure		
Discusses difference between type 1 and type 2 respiratory failure		
Examiner's Global Mark	/5	
Actor / Helper's Global Mark	/5	
Total Station Mark	/30	

Learning Points

Always double check patient identifiers first to make sure you are reviewing results of the right patient.

Check whether the patient was on oxygen or not (and how much) as this may affect your interpretation of the pO_2 and ABG.

Practice and develop a methodical approach to ABGs so you can recognize patterns quickly and present in a confident manner.

Look first at the pH
Then at the pCO_2
Then at the pO_2
Then at the bicarbonate and base excess
Then at the lactate

Case 13
Markscheme - Alcohol Excess

Task:	Achieved	Not achieved
Introduces self		
Checks name and DOB with patient		
Consents patient for discussion		
Checks understanding of why tests have been done		
Elicits any patient concerns		
Ask when bloods were last taken		
Explains that routine blood tests were taken to help determine the cause for his symptoms.		
Explains some of these results are abnormal, therefore you would like to ask a few further questions		
Checks for symptoms of alcohol excess/withdrawal		
Asks about past medical history, medications and allergies, family history and social history		
Explores cause: asks about alcohol intake and quantifies units		
CAGE questionnaire		
Explains that the blood tests show changes in particular affecting the markers for liver function		
Explains that these changes are likely due to excessive alcohol consumption and that bowel cancer is an unlikely cause		
Explains that the patient is experiencing withdrawal symptoms		
Explains that the patient will need to cut down on alcohol intake. Asks whether willing to do so and whether would require any help		
Explains that we will give medication to help with withdrawal symptoms and to replenish losses in any vitamins/minerals/fluids which commonly occurs with excess alcohol consumption		
Summarises discussion		
Checks understanding and answers any questions		
Thanks patient		
Examiner's Global Mark	/5	
Actor / Helper's Global Mark	/5	
Total Station Mark	/30	

Learning points

Use a structured approach when faced with data interpretation stations (e.g. Introduction, History, Explanation of Data, Management Plan)

A brief history from the patient in these stations as may give you clues about the cause if you are unclear from the results alone

Remember to explore the patient's concerns and reassure them where necessary

Case 14

Markscheme - Setting up a Syringe Driver

Task	Achieved	Not Achieved
Washes Hands		
Introduces self		
Confirms patient name, DOB and hospital number		
Explains procedure and gains consent		
Checks prescription on the drug chart		
Checks for drug allergies		
Checks water for injection with helper		
Draw up 20mls water for injection using a syringe and needle (non-touch technique)		
Takes vial of medication prescribed and checks drug, expiry date and concentration with helper (completing controlled drug book)		
Draws up diamorphine into syringe containing water for injection (non-touch technique)		
Places label on syringe (drug name, diluent, patient name, date and time infusion set up, signature)		
Attach the giving set to the syringe and prime the line		
Notes the amount of fluid in the syringe (ml or mm)		
Calculates rate of infusion over 24 hours		
Sets rate on pump		
Places syringe in pump		
Checks the butterfly needle is safe to use (surrounding area, date)		
Attaches syringe to butterfly needle		
Starts infusion		
Disposes of waste safely		
Examiner's global mark	/5	
Actor's global mark	/5	
Total station mark	/30	

Learning Points

When making drug calculations and using controlled drugs always make sure that you check your work with a second competent colleague.

There are many different brands of syringe driver and they all use different syringes. Familiarise yourself with the machines used in your trust, that are likely to be used in your exams, and ask the nursing staff to show you how they work.

A subcutaneous infusion can take 3-4 hours to establish a steady state drug level, therefore a stat dose of medication can be given prior to setting up the driver if the patient is symptomatic.

Case 15
Markscheme - ABPI

Task:	Achieved	Not achieved
Washes hands		
Introduces Self and clarifies patients' details		
Explains procedure and gains informed consent		
Establishes any contraindications to the procedure		
Asks the patient if they have any pain		
Positions patient lying down		
Assembles equipment (Continuous wave doppler unit, ultrasound gel, sphygmomanometer, calculator, non-sterile gloves)		
Places an appropriately sized cuff around the arm		
Locates the brachial pulse and applies ultrasound gel over the skin.		
Correctly holds the probe at a 45 degree angle in the direction of the blood flow in the artery and ensures a good signal		
Inflates the sphygmomanometer cuff until the signal disappears then slowly releases the pressure (22mmHg/second) until the signal returns. Records this value as the brachial systolic pressure.		
States would repeat the above on the other arm.		
Places the same sized cuff around the ankle above the malleoli		
Locates the dorsalis pedis pulse and applies ultrasound gel over the skin. Takes the ankle systolic pressure as described for the brachial and documents the result		
States they would repeat the above for the other ankle.		
Wipes the ultrasound gel from the skin and from the Doppler probe.		
Calculates the ABPI via the following equation: *ABPI= Highest Ankle Doppler pressure (for each leg)/Highest brachial Doppler pressure*		
Interprets the ABPI (>1.0-Normal, 0.4-0.8 Claudication, 0.1-0.4 Critical Ischaemia).		
Thanks patient		
Documents procedure clearly		
Examiner's Global Mark	/5	
Actor / Helper's Global Mark	/5	
Total Station Mark	/30	

Learning Points

The ratio of arm and ankle systolic pressure (the ABPI), which eliminates systolic pressure variation, is used to assess and monitor peripheral arterial disease. Remember that in patients with diabetes the ABPI can be falsely elevated, and therefore results in these patients should be interpreted with caution.

Practice co-ordinating inflating the cuff and keeping the Doppler probe in place, this can be tricky.

Learn the equation for calculating the ABPI and how to interpret the result obtained:

In a normal individual, the ABPI is between 0.92 and 1.3 with the majority of people having a ratio between 1 and 1.2.
An ABPI above 1.3 is usually indicative of non-compressible blood vessels.
An ABPI <0.9 indicates some arterial disease.
An ABPI >0.5 and <0.9 may be associated with intermittent claudication. Refer to a vascular surgeon if symptoms indicate.
An ABPI <0.5 indicates severe arterial disease and may be associated with rest pain, ischaemic ulceration or gangrene and may warrant urgent referral to a vascular surgeon.

Case 16
Markscheme - Putting up Blood

Task:	Achieved	Not Achieved
Introduces self		
Clarifies Identity of patient: Name		
Clarifies Identity of patient: Date of Birth		
Clarifies Identity of patient: Patient Number		
Cross-checks 3-point identity with prescription chart		
Cross-checks identity with blood product label		
Checks group of blood unit		
Checks expiry date of blood unit		
Performs two-person checks		
Reviews appropriate duration of administration		
Ensures suitable cannula in situ and functioning		
Ensures appropriate blood giving set available (filter giving set)		
Enquires about consent for receiving blood transfusion		
Checks for any allergies		
Visually inspects unit for damage/precipitants		
Requests / asks to review pre-transfusion observations (pulse rate, blood pressure, respiratory rate, temperature)		
Advises set of observations 15 minutes after start of transfusion		
Advises set of observations 60 minutes post-transfusion		
Aware of maximum time for blood to be out of fridge before return to blood bank when asked		
Maintains professional approach with patient and nursing staff		
Examiner's Global Mark	/5	
Actor / Helper's Global Mark	/5	
Total Station Mark	/30	

Learning Points

Patient identification is a crucial step in safe blood administration. Positive patient identification requires a minimum of 3 patient identifiers including full name, date of birth and unique identifier number (hospital unit number or NHS number).

The patient requires regular close observation during transfusion to monitor for the development of any transfusion-related complications. Guidance on the frequency of observations and the observation chart can usually be found on the blood prescription chart.

Packed red cells must be transfused within 4 hours of leaving the blood bank fridge to avoid waste. They can only be returned to the fridge if they have been out for less than 30 minutes.

Case 17
Markscheme - Blood Cultures

Task:	Achieved	Not achieved
Washes hands		
Introduces self		
Confirms patient name, DOB and hospital number		
Gains consent to take blood cultures		
Positions patient with forearm resting on cushion		
Selects the correct blood culture bottles and equipment, including sharps bin		
Removes tops from both blood culture bottles and cleans each with a separate alcohol wipe, and allows to dry.		
Applies tourniquet		
Selects appropriate vein		
Puts on gloves		
Cleans the area thoroughly with an alcohol wipe/ Chloroprep™		
Attaches needle to Vacutainer® correctly		
Warns patient to expect 'sharp scratch' or similar		
Retracts skin distally to stabilise vein and inserts needle correctly using aseptic non-touch technique		
Attaches blood culture bottles in the correct order (aerobic first) and withdraws 8-10mls of blood under vacuum		
Releases tourniquet		
Removes needle and immediately disposes of it in the sharps bin		
Applies pressure to venepuncture site and thanks patient		
Labels containers correctly by hand (or explains how to do so) and fills in the appropriate form		
Examiner's Global Mark	/5	
Actor / Helper's Global Mark	/5	
Total Station Mark	/30	

Learning points

Blood cultures provide valuable information about the aetiology of an infection and help guide management. They should be taken as soon as bacteraemia is suspected, ideally before antibiotic therapy has been commenced

It is important to maintain an Aseptic Non-Touch Technique (ANTT) whilst obtaining the blood sample as contamination can cause confusion and may lead to unnecessary investigations.

It is important that blood cultures are filled appropriately. The minimum sample required is 8-10mls of blood. This helps to improve the diagnostic yield of the sample.

Case 18

Markscheme - Shortness of Breath

Task	Achieved	Not Achieved
Washes hands		
Introduces self		
Confirms patient details (name, age, occupation)		
Gains consent to take history		
Starts consultation with open question		
Takes focussed dyspnoea history (onset, duration, severity, timing, precipitating factors, relieving factors)		
Enquires about exercise tolerance		
Elicits systems review (cough, chest pain, sweating, nausea, vomiting, palpitations, syncope, oedema, PND, orthopnoea)		
Elicits past medical history		
Elicits family history		
Elicits drug history and drug allergies		
Elicits social history		
Elicits alcohol history		
Elicits smoking history		
Enquires about patient's ideas, concerns and expectations		
Summarises back to patient		
Shows empathy and avoids jargon		
Presents findings in clear, concise manner		
Gives sensible differential diagnosis (e.g. heart failure, COPD, pulmonary fibrosis)		
Gives sensible management plan (e.g. examination, observations, bloods including BNP, ECG, CXR etc.)		
Examiner's Global Mark	/5	
Actor / Helper's Global Mark	/5	
Total Station Mark	/30	

Learning Points

Remember that shortness of breath may be due to respiratory, cardiac or metabolic causes.

Symptoms that are suggestive of heart failure include breathlessness on exertion, leg swelling, orthopnoea and paroxysmal nocturnal dyspnoea.

The New York Heart Association classification can be used to quantify patient's symptoms

No limitation of physical activity
Slight limitation of activity, comfortable at rest.
Marked limitation of activity, comfortable at rest.
Symptoms of heart failure at rest

Case 19
Markscheme - Diarrhoea

Task	Achieved	Not Achieved
Washes hands		
Introduces self		
Confirms patient details (name, age, occupation)		
Gains consent to take history		
Starts consultation with open question		
Establishes diarrhoea history (onset, frequency, pain, night-time symptoms, presence of blood, consistency, mucus, tenesmus)		
Elicits important additional symptoms (weight loss, fever, malaise, rashes, eye symptoms, appetite, nausea, vomiting)		
Asks about travel history and ill contacts		
Elicits systems review		
Elicits past medical and surgical history		
Elicits drug history and drug allergies (specifically asks about NSAIDs, steroids, anticoagulants)		
Elicits social history		
Elicits alcohol history		
Elicits smoking history		
Enquires about patient's ideas, concerns and expectations		
Summarises back to patient		
Shows empathy and avoids jargon		
Presents findings in clear, concise manner		
Gives sensible differential diagnosis (e.g. infective diarrhoea, inflammatory bowel disease)		
Gives sensible management plan (e.g. examination, observations, bloods including FBC, CRP, ESR, stool cultures, AXR etc.)		
Examiner's Global Mark	/5	
Actor / Helper's Global Mark	/5	
Total Station Mark	/30	

Learning points

It is essential to ask about foreign travel and unwell contacts. The majority of diarrhoea in young adults is infectious.

It is important to ask patients' the impact their condition is having on their job and social life. Listen to the patient and pick up on their non-verbal cues. Diarrhoea is affecting this patient's work and social life. It is important to pick up on this.

Diarrhoea red flags include weight loss, bleeding, night-time symptoms, family history of bowel cancer, abdominal masses and anaemia.

Case 20
Markscheme - Collapse

Task	Achieved	Not Achieved
Washes hands		
Introduces self		
Confirms patient details (name, age, occupation)		
Gains consent to take history		
Starts consultation with open question		
Establishes details prior to collapse (preceding symptoms, posture, prodrome, provoking factors)		
Elicits details during the collapse (duration, LOC, jerky movements, incontinence)		
Elicits details of behaviour after collapse (confusion/injuries/altered mental state)		
Elicits systems review		
Elicits past medical and surgical history		
Elicits drug history and drug allergies (specifically asks about anti-hypertensives, diuretics)		
Elicits social history		
Elicits alcohol history		
Elicits smoking history		
Enquires about patient's ideas, concerns and expectations		
Summarises back to patient		
Shows empathy and avoids jargon		
Presents findings in clear, concise manner		
Gives sensible differential diagnosis (e.g. postural hypotension, vasovagal syncope, carotid sinus hypersensitivity,cardiogenic)		
Gives sensible management plan (e.g. examination, observations, bloods, L/S BP, medication review, ECG)		
Examiner's Global Mark	/5	
Actor / Helper's Global Mark	/5	
Total Station Mark	/30	

Learning Points

When taking a syncope history think about the 3P's;
Posture
Prodrome
Provoking Factors

An eyewitness account may be crucial in determining whether an event was a transient loss of consciousness or seizure

TIA's do not cause loss of consciousness, and should not form part of the differential here.

Case 21
Markscheme - Weight loss

Task	Achieved	Not Achieved
Washes hands		
Introduces self		
Confirms patient details (name, age, occupation)		
Gains consent to take history		
Starts consultation with open question		
Establishes details of weight loss (duration, amount, loss of appetite, dietary intake)		
Screens for malignancy (dysphagia, abdominal distension, change in bowel habit, blood in stools)		
Elicits systems review in particular considers diabetes, hyperthyroidism, mood disorders,		
Elicits past medical and surgical history		
Elicits drug history and drug allergies (specifically asks about anti-hypertensives, diuretics)		
Elicits social history		
Elicits alcohol history		
Elicits smoking history		
Elicits family history in particular relating to cancer		
Enquires about patient's ideas, concerns and expectations		
Summarises back to patient		
Shows empathy and avoids jargon		
Presents findings in clear, concise manner		
Gives sensible differential diagnosis (e.g. malignancy, hyperthyroidism, malabsorption)		
Gives sensible management plan (e.g. examination, observations, bloods including coeliac screen, thyroid function, FBC, medication review, 2 week wait colonoscopy)		
Examiner's Global Mark	/5	
Actor / Helper's Global Mark	/5	
Total Station Mark	/30	

Learning Points

This is a difficult case. The differential diagnosis of weight loss is wide-ranging including endocrine disorders, malignancy, chronic disease, malabsorption, poor dentition, alcohol excess and depression.

Try to have a 'surgical sieve' as a template to use to create a list of differential diagnoses in your mind when taking a history. This will help guide your structure and questions you ask.

Red flags for weight loss include respiratory symptoms, bony pain, "B" symptoms, iron deficiency anaemia, increasing age amongst others.

Case 22

Explanation: Type 2 Diabetes

Task	Achieved	Not Achieved
Introduces self		
Confirms patient details (name, age, occupation)		
Gains consent for consultation		
Starts consultation with open question		
Takes a brief focussed history of prior events		
Asks about cardiovascular risk factors		
Gives a warning shot		
Informs patient of diagnosis		
Check's patient's understanding of condition		
Asks about patients ideas, concerns and expectations		
Explains the condition		
Explains the complications of the condition (e.g. ESRF, visual impairment, cardiovascular disease, amputation etc.)		
Explains the management of the condition (e.g. lifestyle, medications, insulin, smoking cessation etc.)		
Explains the prognosis of the condition (e.g. chronic but manageable)		
Signposts follow up and help available (e.g. diabetic nurse, patient groups, information leaflet)		
Ends consultation appropriately with summary.		
Gives patient adequate opportunities to ask questions and ensures patients' understanding of condition		
Elicits and addresses patient's concerns		
Demonstrates empathy and active listening.		
Clear structure to explanation, using jargon-free terms.		
Examiner's Global Mark	/5	
Actor / Helper's Global Mark	/5	
Total Station Mark	/30	

Learning Points

It is important to signpost patients to additional sources of support and information such as patient support groups, information leaflets, specialist nurses and reputable websites. Especially when diagnosing patients with a chronic condition.

In this case it is important to establish the patient's other cardiovascular risk factors as their management forms an important part of holistic care of the diabetic patient.

It can be useful to "safety-net" patients, so they know in which circumstances to consult further medical attention.

Case 23
Explaining a Procedure: Gastroscopy

Task	Achieved	Not Achieved
Introduces self and explains purpose of encounter.		
Confirms patient details (name, age, occupation).		
Check patient's existing knowledge of procedure.		
Provides brief summary of procedure, reason for doing it, and approximate length of procedure.		
Takes a brief drug history to check for drugs which may increase risk of bleeding, and checks patient allergies.		
Explains the need to fast 6 hours prior to procedure and ensures patient is able to do so.		
Explains that the back of the throat will be numbed with a local anaesthetic spray, and patient may be given sedation via a cannula.		
States position: left lateral, and mouthguard worn to prevent biting of scope		
Explains: breathing will not be affected, and heart rate/O2 saturations/blood pressure may be monitored throughout.		
Explains that the patient will be asked to swallow the scope, which will then be gently advanced down food pipe to visualize structures.		
Explains that biopsies may be taken if doctor feels it is necessary, and that this will be painless.		
Provides information on post-procedure care (eating and drinking, period of monitoring/ recovery)		
Advises patient not to drive/operate machinery 24 hours post-procedure, and for someone to collect patient post-procedure.		
Inform of when/where results available and follow up		
Advise to seek medical help if becomes unwell after procedure (e.g. fever, bleeding, significant pain).		
Ends consultation appropriately with summary.		
Gives patient adequate opportunities to ask questions and ensures patients' understanding of the procedure.		
Elicits and addresses patient's concerns regarding cancer and discomfort of procedure.		
Demonstrates empathy and active listening.		
Clear structure to explanation, using jargon-free terms.		
Examiner's Global Mark	/5	
Actor / Helper's Global Mark	/5	
Total Station Mark	/30	

Learning Points

Ensure that you elicit patient concerns and expectations early on, so you have plenty of time to address them during the consultation.

A systematic structure is key to ensuring you provide a clear, logical explanation. Think about explaining what happens before, during and after a procedure in order to structure this station

Familiarise yourself with common procedures that you may expected to explain, and think about how you may structure your explanation. Don't be afraid to admit that you don't know the minutiae but always offer to find out and get back to them.

Case 24
Markscheme - Dealing with a Complaint

Task	Achieved	Not Achieved
Introduces self		
Confirms patient details (name, age, occupation)		
Clarifies who they are speaking to and relationship to patient and gains consent to take collateral history		
Establishes relative's understanding of events		
Explains what happened		
Makes a sincere apology		
Establish relative's concerns		
Acknowledges relative's concerns		
Reassures relative that the patient will be thoroughly reviewed and checked for injuries		
Explains that this matter will be taken seriously		
Explains that an incident report will be completed		
Explains how incident will be investigated		
Offers to escalate to senior member of medical team or nursing team		
Acknowledges relative's right to contact PALs		
Signposts how they can contact PALs		
Checks relative is happy with explanation		
Summarises next steps and closes		
Remains impartial and does not apportion blame		
Is transparent and does not embellish facts		
Demonstrates empathy and active listening.		
Demonstrates appropriate use of body language		
Examiner's global mark	/5	
Actor/Helper's global mark	/5	
Total station mark	/30	

Learning Points

Offer an apology early on in the consultation. Remember that an apology is not an admission of guilt.

Showing empathy, respect and listening to the relative's concerns are often more important than the content of the conversation.

The complaint does not need to be resolved immediately. Do not try to embellish the facts. Acknowledge the unknowns and explain how the matter will be taken forward. It is sensible to arrange a follow up appointment and escalate to senior members of staff.

Case 25
Markscheme - Duty of Candour

Task	Achieved	Not Achieved
Introduces self		
Confirms patient details (name, age, occupation)		
Clarifies who they are speaking to and relationship to patient and gains consent to take collateral history		
Establishes relative's understanding of events		
Explains what happened		
Makes a sincere apology		
Establish relative's concerns		
Acknowledges relative's concerns		
Reassures relative that the patient is stable and being monitored in HDU		
Explains that this matter will be taken seriously		
Explains that an incident report will be completed		
Explains how incident will be investigated		
Offers to escalate to senior member of medical team or nursing team		
Acknowledges relative's right to contact PALs		
Signposts how they can contact PALs		
Checks relative is happy with explanation		
Summarises next steps and closes		
Remains impartial and does not apportion blame		
Is transparent and does not embellish facts		
Demonstrates empathy and active listening.		
Demonstrates appropriate use of body language		
Examiner's global mark	/5	
Actor/Helper's global mark	/5	
Total station mark	/30	

Learning points

Duty of Candour is a legal duty of healthcare trusts to inform and offer remedy (e.g. apology) to patients when a mistake is made or significant harm is done during provision of a healthcare service

Ensure detailed documentation of candid discussions is carried out including time and date of discussion, persons present, summary of the discussion and agreed next steps.

Reassure patients and their relatives that the matter will be thoroughly investigated, and that they will be kept informed on the course and outcome of this investigation.

Paediatrics

Case 1
History – Witnessed fit

Task	Achieved	Not Achieved
Introduces self		
Clarifies who they are speaking to and their relationship to child		
Elicits history from parent in a concise manner		
Elicits clear description of seizure		
Asks specifically about duration of seizure		
Asks about incontinence and tongue biting		
Establishes history of requiring medication to stop seizure		
Elicits history of being clumsy in the morning		
Asks about birth history		
Asks about past medical history		
Asks about drug history		
Establishes whether immunisations are up to date		
Asks about birth history		
Asks about developmental history		
Enquires about family history		
Elicits family history of epilepsy		
Asks about social history		
Responds appropriately to parental concerns about epilepsy		
Suggests appropriate investigations		
Summarises consultation & actions clearly		
Examiner's Global Mark	/5	
Actor / Helper's Global Mark	/5	
Total Station Mark	/30	

Learning Points

Take a clear chronological history when taking a collateral history regarding a possible witnessed seizure. Take a detailed account from the witness on what happened before, during and after the seizure. This will help clarify the type of seizure, and may inform your differential diagnoses for a non-traumatic loss of consciousness.

The importance of clear communication to reassure concerned parents especially after an episode of Status Epilepticus cannot be overstated. This also involves giving clear safety advice about minimizing risk of injury to the child in case of another seizure. Reassure parents that it is appropriate and important to call for an ambulance.

It is important to know how to investigate new or recurrent seizures. In this instance, basic blood tests and an ECG can be useful in ED to exclude non-neurological causes of loss of consciousness. Outpatient investigations such as EEG and MRI can be useful in determining the type or source of seizures. This can provide invaluable information with regards to treatment and prognosis.

Case 2
History – Shortness of breath

Task	Achieved	Not Achieved
Introduces self		
Clarifies who they are speaking to and relationship to child		
Elicits history from parent in a concise manner		
Elicits onset and duration of illness		
Elicits history of cough and coryza		
Asks about shortness of breath		
Elicits history of wheeze / noisy breathing		
Asks about feeding and fluid intake		
Asks about history of fever		
Asks about contact with other unwell children		
Asks about past medical history		
Asks about drug history		
Establishes whether immunisations are up to date		
Asks about birth history		
Asks about developmental history		
Enquires about family history		
Asks about social history		
Suggests diagnosis of bronchiolitis		
Suggests appropriate investigations		
Summarises history and management plan concisely		
Examiner's Global Mark	/5	
Actor / Helper's Global Mark	/5	
Total Station Mark	/30	

Learning Points

Bronchiolitis is a viral infection caused most commonly by Respiratory Syncytial Virus. It occurs most during the September to March period in the UK, affecting mostly children under 12-18 months. As it is viral in nature, it resolves without specific medical intervention in the vast majority of cases. Some children will need supportive treatment in the form of oxygen, fluid or feeding support, and in the most severe cases, ventilatory support in a high-dependency or intensive care unit.

Remember to ask about specific signs and symptoms when taking a paediatric respiratory history. When considering Bronchiolitis these should include coryzal symptoms, cough, increased work of breathing, poor feeding, reduced wet nappies and fever.

Know the clinical indicators of increased work of breathing in young children. These include tachypnoea, head-bobbing, nasal flaring, subcostal/intercostal recession and grunting. In severe cases children may have apnoeic episodes. Always remember to check oxygen saturations in case there is an oxygen requirement.

Case 3
History – Febrile convulsion

Task	Achieved	Not Achieved
Introduces self		
Clarifies who they are speaking to and relationship to child		
Elicits history from parent in a concise manner		
Elicits history of fever prior to episode		
Elicits clear description of seizure		
Asks specifically about duration		
Asks about incontinence and tongue biting		
Elicits 3 day history of tonsillitis		
Asks about fluid intake		
Asks about birth history		
Asks about past medical history		
Asks about drug history		
Establishes whether immunisations are up to date		
Asks about developmental history		
Enquires about family history		
Establishes past family history of febrile convulsion in mother and brother		
Asks about social history		
Responds appropriately to parental concerns about seizure		
Suggests likely diagnosis of febrile convulsion		
Summaries history and management plan concisely		
Examiner's Global Mark	/5	
Actor / Helper's Global Mark	/5	
Total Station Mark	/30	

Learning Points

A febrile convulsion is characterised as a seizure in the presence of a fever and is most common between the ages of 6 months and six years. Viral illnesses associated with febrile convulsions include tonsillitis, otitis media and gastroenteritis, but it is important to exclude serious bacterial infections such as urinary tract infections and meningitis. A thorough, clear history will help you identify the underlying cause.

Take a clear chronological history when taking a collateral history regarding a possible witnessed febrile convulsion. Take a detailed account from the witness on what happened before, during and after the seizure, as well as how long it lasted or whether any specific treatment was needed.

Febrile convulsions are twice as common in males than in females and occur between 2%-4% of children. Be aware that risk factors for repeat seizures include, younger age at first seizure, earlier in infection at first seizure, family history of febrile convulsions or any past medical history of focal neurology or developmental delay.

Case 4
History – Slow weight gain

Task	Achieved	Not Achieved
Introduces self		
Clarifies who they are speaking to and relationship to child		
Elicits history from mother in a concise manner		
Specifically asks about respiratory symptoms		
Specifically asks about GI symptoms, including diarrhoea and vomiting		
Specifically asks about infections		
Asks about feeding		
Asks about past medical history		
Asks about birth history		
Asks about family history		
Enquires about development		
Specifically asks whether the family is known to social services		
Identifies faltering growth from the growth chart		
Responds appropriately to parental concerns about growth		
Suggests appropriate differential diagnosis, including cystic fibrosis		
Suggests appropriate investigations, eg. baseline bloods, chest X-ray, urine dip, sputum culture, sweat test		
Summaries history and management plan concisely		
Management plan including MDT approach		
Suggests follow up to ensure weight gain improves		
Non-judgemental approach		
Examiner's Global Mark	/5	
Actor / Helper's Global Mark	/5	
Total Station Mark	/30	

Learning Points

Faltering growth (previously known as failure to thrive) is diagnosed when a child's weight crosses at least two centiles on the growth chart. It can helpful to think of causes of faltering growth as organic or non-organic, although there can be overlap. It is important to rule out organic causes, for example, coeliac disease, cow's milk protein intolerance, cystic fibrosis, hypothyroidism. You should also consider chronic or recurrent conditions, before considering non-organic causes, such as poor dietary intake, neglect, maternal mental health problems.

The multidisciplinary team is invaluable here. Consider the roles of the paediatrician, GP, health visitor, dietician, physiotherapist and others.

Remember to look for evidence of nutritional rickets, for example delayed dentition, frontal bossing, genu varum (bowed legs), developmental delay and cupping of epiphyses on X-ray.

Case 5
History – Unexplained injury

Task	Achieved	Not Achieved
Introduces self		
Clarifies who they are speaking to and relationship to child		
Elicits history from parent in a concise manner		
Clarifies the history around the burn		
Asks about birth and past medical history		
Asks about immunisations		
Asks about developmental milestones		
Enquires about home situation		
Enquires specifically about other children at home		
Enquires about involvement with social services		
Summarises history to parent and checks details		
Explains concerns to parent in non-accusatory way and in clear simple terms		
Identifies concerning features in this history: delay in presenting, burn in unusual place, story not consistent with developmental age, change in story		
States 'duty of care to child' as overarching priority		
Explains need for the paediatric senior team to review patient today, and for admission for further investigation		
States will call security/police if tries to leave		
Summarises history and management plan concisely		
Does not collude with parent		
Remains calm		
Non judgmental approach		
Examiner's Global Mark	/5	
Actor / Helper's Global Mark	/5	
Total Station Mark	/30	

Learning Points

Be aware of certain patterns of injury which suggest non-accidental injury, for example burn to the back of the hand, immersion scalds, spiral fracture of the humerus, bruising in an identifiable pattern, e.g. bite mark, finger prints.

Known your milestones – non-accidental injury may present with an injury which could not be sustained at that stage in development. Always remember that under 3 months of age that babies simply can not roll, and any family that bring their child to the ED having 'rolled off the bed' needs to be challenged.

Remember to remain professional and honest. Secrecy can cause a situation to escalate later on. A detailed social history is particularly important in this station, and it is important that it is taken sensitively. Do not be judgemental, but do not collude with the parents. Your first duty of care is to the child and by explaining that both you and the parents have a shared objective progress can be made.

Case 6
History – Weight loss in new born

Task	Achieved	Not Achieved
Introduces self		
Clarifies who they are speaking to and relationship to child		
Elicits history from mother in a concise manner		
Asks about feeding		
Asks specifically about urine output		
Asks about any other maternal concerns		
Asks about pregnancy and antenatal screening		
Asks about birth history		
Asks about risk factors for sepsis		
Asks about past medical history of child		
Asks about social history		
Identifies features which suggest that breastfeeding has not been successfully established		
Identifies that 12% weight loss in a newborn in concerning and required admission		
Explains that the baby needs to be admitted for investigations and feeding support		
Explains the need for additional feed in this case in clear, simple terms		
Reassures mother that formula is not harmful for her baby		
Responds appropriately to mother's concerns about feeding		
Summarises history and management plan concisely		
Suggests appropriate investigations: U&Es, bilirubin		
Empathetic approach towards mother		
Examiner's Global Mark	/5	
Actor / Helper's Global Mark	/5	
Total Station Mark	/30	

Learning Points

Many babies will lose some weight in the first week, but more than 10% weight loss is concerning and requires admission for investigation and feeding support. Don't forget to ask about the birth history, asking specifically about the presence of Group B Streptococcus, prolonged rupture of membranes, maternal fever or infection and prematurity – all place infants at risk of perinatal infection.

Remember the effects of poor feeding include not just weight loss, but dehydration, poor urine output, hypernatraemia, jaundice and hypoglycaemia.

Clear, empathetic communication in this case can help you to negotiate a management plan for the baby which the mother is happy with. It is important that she does not feel as though she has been forced to do something that she did not want to do.

Case 7
History - Deliberate self harm

Task	Achieved	Not Achieved
Introduces self		
Clarifies identity of patient		
Checks patient is still happy to talk without mother present		
Elicits what cuts were made with, when, and how		
Elicits intention of making cuts		
Asks about possible depressive symptoms (e.g. low mood, anhedonia, sleep, appetite)		
Asks about school; does she enjoy it? How is school performance? Does she find it stressful?		
Asks about friendship group / social support		
Ask about home life		
Clarifies that parents arguing does not pose any concern regarding abuse / domestic violence		
Asks specifically if she had suicidal intentions when self-harming		
Clarifies whether she has ever had suicidal ideation		
Uses age-appropriate language and terminology		
Responds empathetically to patient's emotional state		
Asks patient if there's anything that particularly worries her / that she thinks would help		
Summarises history back to patient		
Correctly assesses suicide risk as low		
Explains rationale for assigned suicide risk (e.g. intent, suicidal ideation, plans, protective factors)		
Demonstrates understanding of need to involve CAMHS and/or counselling services		
Demonstrates understanding of need to involve family (and possibly school) in future management		
Examiner's global mark	/5	
Actor's global mark	/5	
Total Station Mark	/30	

Learning Points

Speaking to the child without parents or guardians present can yield very important information. Feelings and emotions, home life, motives for self-harming actions, or other issues such as those surrounding boyfriends/girlfriends and/or sexual history can be very difficult for many children to discuss in front of the adults who care for them. In situations where it is important that the child fully discloses information about any of these areas, you should always attempt to speak to the child both with and without a parent or guardian present.

Stressors in childhood often arise from issues with home life, school, friendship group and relationships. To fully explore a self-harm history in a child you need ask specifically about these areas, as well as asking if there's anything else they are finding upsetting or stressful.

Child and Adolescent Mental Health Services (CAMHS) are integral in helping to support young children with self-harming behaviour and psychiatric conditions. However, when devising management plans it is important to involve all relevant parties – including school, and family – to ensure a holistic approach where the child is appropriately supported in all areas of their life.

Case 8
History – neonatal floppy episode

Task	Achieved	Not Achieved
Introduces self		
Clarifies who they are speaking to and relationship to child		
Elicits a clear history of floppy episode		
Clarifies whether any colour change during episode		
Clarifies resolution of episode (how long, what action was taken / needed)		
Elicits pregnancy and birth history		
Elicits any risk factors for sepsis (e.g. GBS, PROM, pyrexia)		
Takes a feeding history (e.g. how long, how often)		
Elicits past medical history, including appropriate weight gain		
Asks about other signs / symptoms of intercurrent illness (e.g. pyrexia, lethargy, not waking for feeds, cough / cold)		
Elicits family history (including consanguinity)		
Elicits social history		
Uses appropriate lay terminology		
Asks about mother's ideas / concerns / expectations		
Responds empathetically to mother's emotion and concerns		
Summarises history back to mother		
Considers sensible differential diagnosis (e.g. normal baby, reflux, sepsis, cardiac, metabolic, trauma, seizure)		
Is able to appropriately justify differential diagnoses offered		
Recognises importance of physical examination +/- prolonged observation to aid diagnosis and reassure parents		
Recognises need to discuss management with a senior		
Examiner's global mark	/5	
Actor's global mark	/5	
Total Station Mark	/30	

Learning Points

Sometimes it can be very difficult to determine exactly what causes a floppy episode in a baby, or whether it's anything to worry about. In a baby who seems well, but where the cause or the history isn't certain, a pragmatic management plan often involves simply admitting the baby and parent for observation. This may not offer any more information regarding the underlying cause of the episode, but can help parents to feel much less anxious about taking their baby home.

In babies of this age, sepsis is a significant cause for concern; they are still at risk of late Group B Streptococcal (GBS) sepsis, and have not yet started their programme of childhood immunisations. Because of this, we always make sure to ask about risk factors for infection being acquired around the time of labour:
Did the mother have prolonged rupture of membranes (PROM) of more than 24 hours?
Was she a known carrier of GBS (a positive swab or urine result during pregnancy, or a previous baby with invasive GBS disease)?
Did she have a pyrexia of 39°C or more during labour?
Were the obstetric team otherwise worried enough about infection in mother to give her IV antibiotics during labour?

In addition to sepsis, other pathologies that result in babies presenting to ED in the first few weeks of life – either actively unwell, or just 'not quite right' – are cardiac causes, particularly duct-dependent congenital heart defects, metabolic causes, and trauma / Non-accidental injury (NAI). You must consider all of these when taking a history about a child of this age.

Case 9
Examination – Newborn

Task:	Achieved	Not Achieved
Introduces self		
Clarifies who they are speaking to and relationship to child, gets consent for examination		
Conducts newborn exam in systematic manner with baby in a comfortable position and appropriately exposed		
Feel fontanelle and sutures and measure head circumference (say will plot on growth chart)		
Assess facial features, inspect ears and neck		
Check red reflexes		
Visually inspect palate using tongue depressor and torch		
Auscultate chest for heart sounds and over lung fields		
Palpate femoral pulses		
Palpate abdomen to identify any masses or liver enlargement		
Examines hips (Barlow and Ortolani tests)		
Inspect hands and feet		
Inspect genitalia and anus (check for bilateral descent of testes in male)		
Inspect spine and sacrum		
Test moro reflex and assess tone in ventral suspension (baby should briefly bring head to horizontal plane)		
Comment on skin (birthmarks/rashes)		
Summarises findings and presents succinctly		
Correctly suggest checking pre and post ductal saturations		
Advises mother about signs of heart failure in a newborn		
Suggests plotting growth parameters on growth chart		
Examiner's Global Mark	/5	
Actor / Helper's Global Mark	/5	
Total Station Mark	/30	

Learning Points

Heart murmurs are common in first few days of life but are frequently innocent. Common causes include patent ductus arteriousus (PDA) (should close within 24 hours), flow murmurs and small septal defects such as patent foramen ovale (PFO), atrial septal defect (ASD) and ventricular septal defect (VSD) although the latter are commonly not heard until the child is a few weeks of age.

Babies with a murmur audible after 24 hours of life should be screened using pre and post ductal saturations (a difference of more than 2% is significant and warrants further investigation). Four limb blood pressures are often performed to help identify children with coarctation in which case the lower limb blood pressures will be more than 20 mmHg *lower* than the upper limb blood pressures which is the reverse of normal.

Parents in infants with heart murmurs should be advised of the signs of heart failure in a newborn. These include breathlessness, especially with feeding, sweatiness, lethargy, pallor and cyanosis.

Case 10
Examination - Abdomen

Task:	Achieved	Not Achieved
Introduces self		
Washes hands		
Clarifies who they are speaking to and relationship to child, gains consent for examination		
Conducts exam in systematic manner within a comfortable position and child appropriately exposed		
Inspect from end of bed		
Inspect hands		
Inspect conjunctivae		
Inspect mouth		
Expose abdomen with child lying flat and relaxed		
Inspects abdomen more closely		
Superficial palpation of all quadrants		
Deep palpation of all 4 quadrants		
Palpate for liver and spleen		
Palpate for kidneys		
Palpate hernial orifices		
Briefly inspect genitalia		
Auscultate for bowel sounds		
Ask to plot height and weight for child on a growth chart		
Summarises findings and presents succinctly		
Correctly suggests possible diagnoses of abdominal migraine, constipation, coeliac disease, functional abdominal pain		
Examiner's Global Mark	/5	
Actor / Helper's Global Mark	/5	
Total Station Mark	/30	

Learning Points

Abdominal pain is a common complaint in the Paediatric Outpatient Department. It is frequently benign and self-limiting, but careful history and examination are required to identify the small number of children presenting with serious organic disease. Many children will have simple constipation and this should be identified in the history and treated appropriately.

Symptoms associated with a higher prevalence of organic disease include: weight loss, bleeding (upper or lower GI tract), severe, persistent diarrhoea or vomiting, persistent right upper quadrant or right lower quadrant pain, fever, family history of inflammatory bowel disease, jaundice, urinary symptoms and abnormal examination findings.

Investigations are rarely useful in the absence of alarm symptoms, however coeliac disease can present with non-specific abdominal symptoms and should always be excluded with a coeliac screen.

Case 11

Examination - Cardiovascular

Task:	Achieved	Not Achieved
Introduces self		
Washes hands		
Clarifies who they are speaking to and relationship to child, gets consent for examination		
Conducts exam in systematic manner within a comfortable position and child appropriately exposed		
Inspects from end of bed		
Inspects hands & nails		
Palpate radial pulse (radio-radial and radio-femoral delay)		
Inspects conjunctivae		
Inspects mouth		
Exposes chest and inspects for surgical scars/chest wall deformity/hyperdynamic praecordium		
Palpate for heaves/thrills		
Auscultate in aortic, pulmonary, mitral and tricuspid areas		
Listens for radiation of ejection systolic murmur appropriately (to interscapular region for coarctation)		
Listen to lung bases		
Palpate liver		
Palpate femoral pulses (if not already done)		
Summarises findings and presents succinctly		
Correctly suggests possible diagnosis of aortic coarctation		
Suggests performing 4 limb BP measurement and able to identify abnormal results		
Suggests plotting growth parameters on growth chart		
Examiner's Global Mark	/5	
Actor / Helper's Global Mark	/5	
Total Station Mark	/30	

Learning Points

Coarctation of the aorta may present in the neonatal period when the ductus arteriosus closes and adequate systemic blood flow cannot be maintained. Babies present in shock with poor perfusion, tachycardia, absent femoral pulses and a difference in pre and post ductal saturations (pre-ductal higher than post-ductal). This is a medical emergency requiring immediate treatment with prostaglandin.

Many children with juxta-ductal coarctation (constriction distal to the origin of the left subclavian artery) are asymptomatic and do not present until late in childhood, often because of an incidental finding of a murmur (classically ejection systolic with radiation to back) or raised BP. Lower limb blood pressures will be lower than upper limb pressures (normally lower limbs should be higher than upper limbs). Radio-femoral delay may also be present on examination and is due to formation of collateral blood vessels that supply the distal aorta.

Coarctation is surgically corrected or can be dilated via cardiac catheterisation. Complications include re-coarctation and residual hypertension which can lead to intracranial haemorrhage or encephalopathy if severe.

Case 12
Examination - Respiratory

Task:	Achieved	Not Achieved
Introduces self		
Clarifies who they are speaking to and relationship to child, gets consent for examination		
Washes hands		
Conducts exam in systematic manner within a comfortable position and child appropriately exposed		
Inspect from end of bed		
Note the presence of oxygen/inhalers/other medications at the bedside		
Inspect the hands (clubbing/cyanosis)		
Palpate radial pulse and count respiratory rate		
Looks for a BCG scar		
Inspect conjunctivae for pallor and tongue for central cyanosis		
Expose and inspect the chest		
Inspect chest from side during inspiration and expiration to look for increased antero-posterior diameter		
Palpate suprasternal notch for tracheal deviation		
Auscultate chest		
Percusses chest		
Palpates for tactile vocal fremitus		
Suggests plotting growth parameters on growth chart		
Ask to measure peak flow and oxygen saturations		
Summarises findings and presents succinctly		
Correctly suggests diagnosis of cystic fibrosis and identifies at least three people in MDT (doctor/nurse specialist/dietitian/physiotherapist/psychologist/pharmacist etc)		
Examiner's Global Mark	/5	
Actor / Helper's Global Mark	/5	
Total Station Mark	/30	

Learning Points

Cystic fibrosis is a genetic disease of exocrine gland function. There are numerous genetic mutations which give rise to the disease, the commonest in Northern Europe being the ΔF508 mutation which is present in up to 25% of cases. Abnormalities in chloride ion channel function lead to the production of thick, viscid secretions which have a number of effects.

Chronic production of mucus leads to airway plugging, inflammation and bronchiectasis as well as a pre-disposition to infection. Pancreatic exocrine function is affected, constipation is common and males are usually infertile. Patients can also have sinus involvement and eventually develop biliary obstruction and cirrhotic liver disease.

Management in a multi-disciplinary team is vital. Treatments for respiratory complications include regular chest physiotherapy and incentive spirometry, mucolytic drugs, regular prophylactic antibiotics and planned courses of intravenous antibiotics to prevent chest colonization and invasive infection. Pancreatic enzyme supplementation and dietetic support is necessary to achieve as near normal growth as possible and psychology input is important to help children adjust to living with a life-limiting disease.

Case 13
Examination - Upper limb

Task:	Achieved	Not Achieved
Introduces self		
Washes hands		
Clarifies who they are speaking to and relationship to child, gets consent for examination		
Appropriately exposes child		
Appropriately positions child		
Inspects patient from end of bed		
Inspect arms		
Assess tone in all muscle groups bilaterally		
Assess power in all muscle groups bilaterally (one arm at a time):		
Finger flexion (C8)		
Finger abduction (C8/T1)		
Wrist flexion/extension (C5/6)		
Elbow flexion(C5-6)/extension (C7/8)		
Abduction at shoulder (C5/6)		
Assess reflexes bilaterally (one arm at a time):		
Biceps (C5/6)		
Triceps (C6/7)		
Supinator (C5/6)		
Assess coordination (dysdiadochokinesis/past pointing/intention tremor)		
Summarises findings and presents succinctly		
Suggests upper motor neurone lesion		
Able to list differences between upper and lower motor neurone lesion findings		
Examiner's Global Mark	/5	
Actor / Helper's Global Mark	/5	
Total Station Mark	/30	

Learning Points

Remember to inspect the patient from the end of the bed. Taking note of the posture of the child's arms can reveal important features that will help your diagnosis. In this instance, the flexed posture of the arms are suggestive of increased muscle tone in an upper motor neurone lesion.

Remember to be gentle when examining a child with increased muscle tone. Sudden, forceful movements of stiff joints can be extremely painful and should be avoided. You may not need to fully extend the limb to establish that tone in increased!

Keep in mind the key differences in clinical findings that will help you differentiate upper and lower motor neurone lesions:

Upper Motor Neurone	Lower Motor Neurone
Flexed upper limb posture	Muscle wasting
Extended lower limb posture	Fasciculation
Increased tone	Reduced tone/flaccidity
Increased tendon reflexes	Reduced tendon reflexes

Case 14
Examination - Lower limb

Task:	Achieved	Not Achieved
Introduces self		
Washes hands		
Adequate exposure of the child		
General inspection of child		
Inspects legs for muscle wasting or hypertrophy		
Examines child's gait: to walk in line, test heel toe gait, walking on tip toes and heels		
Ask candidate to stand up from sitting on floor		
Positions child appropriately on bed		
Examines tone		
Examines power in hips and knees		
Examines power in ankles and big toe		
Examines knee jerk and ankle jerk reflexes		
Examines plantar reflexes		
Examines child's co-ordination: heel-shin test		
Examines fine sensation in both legs		
Offers to test pain sensation and proprioception		
States they would complete the examination by examining the upper limbs and cranial nerves		
Suggests plotting growth parameters on growth chart		
Summarise findings to examiner		
Gives appropriate differential diagnosis		
Examiner's Global Mark	/5	
Actor / Helper's Global Mark	/5	
Total Station Mark	/30	

Learning Points

Not all children will be able to follow all instructions so it is important to adapt it to make it fun for the child whilst covering all areas. Think about using toys to test the child's coordination, or can they jump or hop. If they can't walk can they crawl. It may be difficult to get a child to relax in order to elicit the tendon reflexes, so consider using reinforcement techniques. Ask the child to clench their teeth at the same time you elicit the reflex, or ask them to clench their hands together.

The type of gait may indicate the underlying condition:

Scissoring gait - spastic diplegia
Waddling gait - muscular dystrophy.
Antalgic gait -myositis or musculoskeletal pain
Circumducting gait- hemiplegia

Be aware of the primitive reflexes and the age you would expect them to disappear.

Reflex	Onset	Disappears
Moro	Birth	2-3 months, may persist to 6 months
Rooting	Birth	4 months
Palmar grasp	Birth	5-6 months age
Plantar reflex	Birth	1 year
Tonic neck reflex	1 month	4 months

Case 15
Communication – Explain asthma to older child

Task:	Achieved	Not Achieved
Introduces self to young person and parent		
Clarifies who they are speaking to and relationship to child/young person		
Explains that they have come to talk about the condition with young person and parent		
Asks the young person if anyone has spoken to them before about their condition		
Asks the young person what their current understanding asthma is		
Explains what asthma is in simple terms		
Asks about triggers for symptoms		
Explains that inhaler medication will improve symptoms		
Explains that the condition is lifelong and will require preventer medication to keep well		
Explains what different inhalers are for		
Advises to seek adult help If feeling very unwell and out of breath		
Advises to seek adult help if using reliever medication very frequently or more frequently than usual		
Main focus of communication is with the young person and not the parent.		
Explains underlying condition, and avoids use of medical terms or jargon		
If any medical terms used, explains what they mean		
Uses age appropriate language		
Summarises discussion concisely		
Clarifies understanding of explanation that has been given		
Asks if the child or parent has any further questions		
Offers information leaflet		
Examiner's Global Mark	/5	
Actor / Helper's Global Mark	/5	
Total Station Mark	/30	

Learning Points

Clarify with both young person what explanations may or may not have been given previously, and allow the young person to explain in their own words what they understand already.

Communication should be with the young person and not their parent. Asthma is being explained to the teenager, for them to understand. Use age appropriate language and not medical terms or words that may not be fully understood.

Ensure the young person knows when to seek advice from an adult as although they may be independently managing their condition on a day-to day basis, they need to be certain about when to seek help in order to avoid an undetected deterioration in their condition.

Case 16

Communication – Explain a febrile seizure to a parent

Task:	Achieved	Not Achieved
Introduces self to parent		
Clarifies who they are speaking to and relationship to child		
Explains that they have come to talk about the reason for admission to the hospital		
Asks if any explanation has been given previously by other members of staff		
Asks the parent to explain what their understanding is of the febrile convulsion		
Explains a febrile seizure is a fit/seizure caused by a fever		
Explains it is caused by a sudden increase in body temperature		
Explains fever itself is not harmful but a sign the body is fighting infection		
Explains it is common in young children		
Explains febrile seizure is most common between 6 months and 6 years		
Explains most children will only have 1 febrile convulsion but some do have them again at times of high fever		
Clarifies that with simple febrile convulsions, there is no increase in risk of epilepsy		
Reassures parent the febrile convulsion is not harmful to the child (e.g not associated with brain damage)		
Explains common signs of a convulsion		
Explains what to do if Ben has a further convulsion (stay calm, place child on side, call ambulance)		
Appropriate use of language with explanation of any medical terms used		
Clarifies understanding of explanation that has been given		
Summarises consultation		
Asks if the child or parent has any further questions		
Offers information leaflet		
Examiner's Global Mark	/5	
Actor / Helper's Global Mark	/5	
Total Station Mark	/30	

Learning Points

Febrile convulsions can be very frightening for parents to witness, so it is important to have an empathetic approach, and acknowledge and address their questions.

There is often concern that febrile convulsions will lead to epilepsy and it is important that you explain this is not the case, as this is often a major cause of anxiety.

Ensure you explain to parents what to do should it happen again. This should include removing objects that a child may injure themselves on in the middle of a seizure, and simple advice regarding not overheating or rapidly cooling a child who is likely to have a fever. Most ED departments have an information leaflet that can be given to people to take home for reference.

Case 17
Communication – Discuss use of antibiotics in a viral illness

Task:	Achieved	Not Achieved
Introduces self		
Clarifies who they are speaking to and relationship to child		
Seeks clarification about what has been explained so far		
Elicits parents understanding of the role of antibiotics		
Elicits parental concerns		
Elicits brief history of viral symptoms		
Explains that antibiotics not effective in treatment of viral infection		
Explains risk of side effects of antibiotics when used inappropriately: diarrhoea, resistance		
Explains usual course of viral infections		
Ensures parent satisfied with explanation of viral infection		
Asks if the parent has any further questions		
Empathetic approach to parent		
Uses appropriate language		
Explains any medical terms used		
Offers to discuss with senior if needed		
Does not offer antibiotics as treatment for the viral infection		
Summarises consultation		
Advises parent to return for review if child deteriorates or does not improve		
Offers information leaflet		
Non-judgemental approach		
Examiner's Global Mark	/5	
Actor / Helper's Global Mark	/5	
Total Station Mark	/30	

Learning Points

When providing additional information to a patient/parent who has been seen by another professional, you should always clarify what has already been explained in order to minimize any misunderstanding or miscommunication.

Do not dismiss the concerns of a patient or parent, however unfounded you may feel they are. They often have good reasons that you may be unaware of unless you explore the situation in more detail.

Antibiotics are not effective in the treatment of viral infections and should not be prescribed. Viral infections require symptomatic treatment only and will resolve with time. As differentiating between a bacterial and viral infection can be clinically challenging, the child should be brought back for re-evaluation if symptoms are worsening or not settling. This is termed "safety netting".

Case 18
Communication – Counselling for impending preterm delivery

Task:	Achieved	Not Achieved
Introduces self		
Clarifies who they are speaking to		
Sets the agenda and explain purpose of discussion		
Establishes current understanding of preterm birth and consequences for babies		
Explains that premature baby is unable to survive without support and may need resuscitation		
Explains that paediatric team will be present at delivery		
Explains that baby will be assessed and supported with breathing and circulation as required		
Explains that baby will be shown to mother and admitted to neonatal unit for treatment		
Explains that prematurity is directly linked with morbidity and mortality		
Explains that baby will need breathing support either by intubation or non-invasive methods		
Explains that baby will have brain scans and development will be monitored long term		
Explains that baby will initially be unable to feed independently and will need TPN		
Emphasises importance of breast milk as protector against gut disease and encourages mother to express		
Explains that baby will need surveillance eg ROP screen to identify and address problems early		
Reassure mother that all steps will be taken to optimise outcome for the baby once born		
Asks parent if they have any further questions		
Summarises consultation & actions from here on		
Offers to come back to speak to the mother again later if she wishes		
Uses appropriate language and explains medical jargon		
Offers information leaflet		
Examiner's Global Mark	/5	
Actor / Helper's Global Mark	/5	
Total Station Mark	/30	

Learning Points

Care of the preterm infant is a developing field as new evidence becomes available that helps tailor interventions and optimises outcome.

Morbidity and mortality rates are directly linked to the degree of prematurity in infants. The EPICure series of studies of survival and later health among babies and young people who were born at extremely low gestations offers data than can be useful when discussing prognosis with parents (EPICure 2006)

In addition to long term outcomes it is also important to discuss the process of resuscitation. Most parents do not expect the interventions and resuscitation performed during the delivery of an extremely premature infant and can find the experience quite traumatic. Briefing them before the delivery on what is going to happen helps them cope with this better.

Case 19
Communication – Explain need for transfer to tertiary unit for acute condition

Task:	Achieved	Not Achieved
Introduces self		
Clarifies who they are speaking to and relationship to child, ask for child's name		
Sets the agenda and explain purpose of discussion		
Clarifies parent's understanding of events so far		
Reiterates that baby was deprived of oxygen at birth which is the cause of its current condition		
Explain that baby had a seizure that was treated with medication and baby is now stable		
Explain that seizure shows that brain has been affected and treatment is needed to protect it from further damage		
Explain that cooling treatment can be given at a tertiary centre but passive cooling already started		
Explain that baby will be transferred safely by the transport team		
Explain that further tests eg MRI and EEG will be performed to better define prognosis		
Explain that it is too soon to determine prognosis but all steps are taken to optimise it		
Explain that length of stay at tertiary centre will depend on baby's progress.		
Explain baby will be nil by mouth for now but milk can be expressed and given to baby later.		
Explain that long term surveillance will be required		
Explain that 24 hour access to the baby will be facilitated for the parents by receiving hospital		
Asks parent if they have any further questions		
Summarises consultation & actions from here on		
Offers to come back and update parents again later		
Uses appropriate language & explains any jargon		
Offers information leaflet		
Examiner's Global Mark	/5	
Actor / Helper's Global Mark	/5	
Total Station Mark	/30	

Learning Points

In developed countries, hypoxic ischaemic encephalopathy (HIE) affects 3–5 infants per 1000 live births, and is an important cause of cerebral palsy and developmental difficulties. Diagnosis and severity of HIE can be determined using the Sarnat & Sarnat staging method (Sarnat & Sarnat 1976).

Whilst damage from the primary insult cannot be repaired, moderate cooling of the body (to between 32 and 34 degrees Celsius) has been shown to prevent further brain damage and death in asphyxiated newborn infants, and is now a standard of care in neonatology. Criteria for therapeutic hypothermia can be found at the TOBY Cooling Register Clinician's Handbook (National Perinatal Epidemiology Unit 2010)

The prognosis in this case is difficult to determine and further investigations (MRI, EEG) can help in defining outcome. Long term neurological surveillance and examination is indicated in babies who have suffered moderate or severe HIE.

Case 20

Communication – Explanation of bronchiolitis

Task:	Achieved	Not Achieved
Introduces self		
Clarifies who they are speaking to and their relationship to child		
Sets the agenda and explains purpose of discussion		
Establishes current understanding		
Explains that symptoms are likely due to bronchiolitis		
Explains that it is viral illness causing airway inflammation		
Explains that it is not asthma although some children develop asthma later when older		
Explains that severity can vary and children can get worse before they get better		
Explains that treatment is supportive with oxygen and hydration (IV or enteral)		
Explains use of oxygen as supportive treatment		
Explains that baby needs to be admitted in view of oxygen requirement and poor feeding		
Explains that symptoms can last for up to two weeks		
Explains that once there is no further need for oxygen and feeding is better, the child can go home		
Explain there is no need for antibiotics unless evidence of underlying bacterial infection		
Give advice on bronchiolitis prevention eg through good hygiene		
Asks parent if they have any further questions		
Summarises consultation & actions from here on		
Empathetic approach		
Uses appropriate language & explains any jargon		
Offers information leaflet		
Examiner's Global Mark	/5	
Actor / Helper's Global Mark	/5	
Total Station Mark	/30	

Learning Points

Bronchiolitis is a very common condition and in most cases it is benign and resolves spontaneously. However, there is a large range of severity and the condition can become life threatening.

Additional oxygen requirement and poor hydration are the two main determinants of whether a child needs to be admitted to hospital for bronchiolitis.

Most bronchiolitis is caused by viral infection but bacterial secondary infection is a possibility. In severe cases consider investigations such as chest radiography and antibiotics if there is an obvious bacterial focus. However, most bronchiolitis treatment is supportive and investigations are not required.

Case 21

Communication – Demonstrate use of inhaler and spacer

Task	Achieved	Not achieved
Introduces self with name and position		
Clarifies who they are speaking to		
Establishes previous knowledge of inhaler/spacer usage		
Acknowledges parent's concerns		
Explains when inhaler/spacer should be used		
Explains that inhaler with spacer is a very effective way of delivering salbutamol in children		
Demonstrates need to shake inhaler for 5 seconds (this helps mix medicine with propellant) and then place into spacer		
Shows how to position / hold child (cuddles child on your lap facing away from them)		
Demonstrates how to put mask on face to get good seal and avoid eye area		
Shows how to press once on canister to release one dose/puff of medication		
Shows ned to allow child to breathe normally for 10 seconds with mask in place		
Removes mask and waits approximately one minute before repeating dose if required		
Explains need to clean monthly or if visibly dirty		
Shows how to clean with lukewarm water and mild soap		
Explains need to allow to drip dry		
Summarises discussion		
Offers written information (wheeze management plan)		
Suggests reputable websites for further information e.g. Asthma UK		
Asks if mother has any other questions now		
Offers to come back and discuss again later if parent has more questions		
Examiner's global mark	/5	
Actor's / Helper's global mark	/5	
Total station mark	/30	

Learning points:

The inhaler and spacer (+ mask) is a very effective technique at delivering medicine. The medicine gets straight into the lungs where it is needed and quickly too. In addition there are less side effects as not much medicine is absorbed to the rest of body. MDIs with a spacer are easier to use as the spacer collects the medicine inside them, so the parent does not have to worry about pressing the inhaler and child having to breathe in at exactly the same time.

Many children with asthma are prescribed two different types of asthma inhaler: a daily preventer inhaler to help protect their airways and reduce the chance of triggers causing asthma symptoms and a reliever inhaler for immediate relief of symptoms. As the child gets bigger inhalers and spacers might need to change. The child should see the asthma nurse or GP every 6 months for an asthma review.

When teaching a parent/patient a new technique it is important to initially demonstrate that technique yourself. Allow enough time for the parent (patient) to practice with you helping them and then ask them to demonstrate to you the technique or repeat the instructions back to you.

Case 22
Communication – Explain diagnosis of trisomy 21 to a parent

Task	Achieved	Not achieved
Introduces self with name and position		
Clarifies who they are speaking to & how they can help		
Allows mother time and space to talk when tearful		
Empathises with mother as to why she is feeling anxious		
Establishes current understanding of Trisomy 21		
Explains that antenatal scan may not always show signs of Down's		
Explains concisely Down Syndrome is – genetic condition with extra chromosome		
Explains what immediate management goals are while inpatient – establish feeding, blood tests (TSH) to detect hypothyroidism, echocardiogram to rule out congenital anomalies.		
Explains referral to community paediatrics will occur		
Explains involvement of a MDT (SALT, Physio, OT, dietician)		
Explains some potential long term problems – developmental delay, learning difficulties, hearing and visual problems		
Explains some people with Down Syndrome go to mainstream school, have employment, live independently.		
Explains there will be planned regular reviews		
Offers to chase up genetic test result		
Offers seniors to return to discuss with parents		
Offers written information		
Directs mother to patient support group		
Asks if mother has any other questions now		
Summarises discussion		
Offers to come back and discuss again later if parent has more questions		
Examiner's global mark	/5	
Actor's / Helper's global mark	/5	
Total station mark	/30	

Learning points:

Down syndrome is not preventable but can be screened for antenatally. The screening involves blood tests and measurements from ultrasound to work out the chance of a baby being born with Down's Syndrome. The combined test is offered in early pregnancy (10-14 weeks) and the quad test is offered later (14-20 weeks). Diagnostic tests include CVS and Amniocentesis.

It is important to be honest when giving parents a diagnosis. If you can't answer their questions say you will find out and get back to them or that you will get a senior to talk to them. Try not to overload them with too much information.

When giving a new diagnosis to a patient / parents there are a number of key points to always follow: arrange for further discussion another time, give written information if available and direct them to patient support groups.

Case 23
Clinical skills – Intramuscular injection

Task	Achieved	Not Achieved
Introduces self		
Clarifies who they are speaking to and relationship to child		
Establishes current understanding of procedure		
Explains intramuscular injections provide a depot for the drug / vaccine to dissipate through the body over a longer time		
Lists complications: Common - tenderness at local site. Rare - bleeding, infection, inadvertent iv administration		
Explains fever and malaise common after immunisations – manage with paracetamol, needs clinical review or antibiotics if other additional symptoms		
Asks if parent has any other concerns or questions		
Obtains verbal consent		
Assembles equipment (appropriate gauge needle, syringe, plaster, 70% alcohol wipe)		
Confirms name and DOB of baby on ID band and with mother		
Confirms allergy status		
Checks drug dose and expiry date with colleague		
Appropriate decontamination of hands and puts on gloves		
Does not recontaminate		
Appropriate site (middle third of thigh preferred, can also use deltoid muscle)		
Takes secure hold of child's limb		
Inserts needle at 90 degree angle to skin		
Aspirates prior to injecting		
Discards needle into sharps bin safely		
Appropriate post procedure care (check for bleeding, apply plaster, ensures child is comfortable)		
Examiner's Global Mark	/5	
Actor / Helper's Global Mark	/5	
Total Station Mark	/30	

Learning points

The middle third of the thigh is the best place for intramuscular injections in babies as this is the location of largest muscle mass. The deltoid muscle can also be used. Each injection should be at a different site.

Remember to anticipate a struggle and secure the limb well before you start to minimize risk of needlestick injury to yourself and distress to the child.

If administering vaccinations in a hospital setting, details of the immunisation (brand, lot, expiry, site and date) should be recorded in the drug chart, the hospital notes and the red book.

Case 24
Clinical skills – Cardiac arrest

Task:	Achieved	Not Achieved
Introduces self		
Assesses response by gently shaking and calling patient's name		
Manually opens airway (Head tilt, chin lift)		
Checks if patient is breathing for 10 seconds		
Gives 5 rescue breaths using bag-valve mask		
Assesses for signs of life		
Palpates central pulse for 10 seconds		
Recognises cardiac arrest and commences CPR at rate of 100-120 per minute		
Asks team member to put out paediatric cardiac arrest call		
Asks team member (once available) to manage airway then instigates compression:ventilation ratio of 15:2		
Asks team member to attach defibrillation pads and then stops CPR to assess rhythm		
Correctly gives adrenaline (0.1ml/kg of 1:10,000) as Pulseless Electrical Activity (PEA) identified		
Continues CPR for 2 minute cycle and then re-assesses rhythm		
Recommences CPR as still PEA		
Considers reversible causes (4Hs and 4Ts)		
Re-assesses rhythm after 2 minute cycle		
Recognises 'shockable rhythm' and appropriately deliver shock. Recommences CPR immediately		
Recognises return of spontaneous circulation and states will commence 'post cardiac arrest treatment'		
Allocates staff member to support parents		
Systematic approach to cardiac arrest in the child		
Examiner's Global Mark	/5	
Actor / Helper's Global Mark	/5	
Total Station Mark	/30	

Learning Points

'Non-shockable rhythms' (asystole or PEA) are a more common finding in children in cardiac arrest compared with 'shockable rhythms' (VF or pulseless VT). It is important you know how to manage the sequence of events for both pathways and also when to give cardiac drugs.

Drug	Dose	Route	Given
Adrenaline	10micrograms/kg 0.1ml/kg	IV/IO	Immediately with PEA/Asystole then every 4 minutes After 3rd shock if VF/pulseless VT, then after every alternate shock
Amiodarone	5mg/kg	IV/IO	After 3rd and 5th DC shock only
Lidocaine (alternative to amiodarone if unavailable)	1mg/kg	IV/IO	After 3rd and 5th DC shock only
Magnesium	25-50mg/kg	IV/IO	Polymorphic VT (torsades de pointes)

Be able to list the reversible causes for cardiac arrest (4Hs and 4Ts) but remember the most common causes in children are hypoxia and hypovolaemia.

'4Hs'	'4Ts'
Hypoxia	Thromboembolism (pulmonary or coronary)
Hypovolaemia	Tension pneumothorax
Hyper/hypokalaemia, and other Metabolic disturbances	Tamponade (cardiac)
Hypothermia	Toxic/therapeutic disturbance

It is very uncommon for children to have a cardiac arrest, but when it does happen it can be very upsetting for all the team involved. Ensure you make the time for a debrief session and seek the support you need. Further information is available from the Resuscitation Council UK website (Resuscitation Council UK 2015)

Case 25
Clinical skills – Interpreting a fracture

Task:	Achieved	Not Achieved
Introduces self to medical student		
Clarifies student's current level of knowledge of reporting fractures		
Checks radiograph has correct patient name		
Checks radiograph has correct date of birth		
Checks radiograph has correct hospital number		
Ensures correct date on the radiograph		
States that they are AP and lateral films of the radius and ulna, including the wrist and elbow joints.		
States the type of bone (i.e. radius)		
States the segment of bone (i.e. distal)		
States the pattern of the fracture (i.e. transverse)		
States that there is bone deformity (i.e. angulation)		
Suggests fracture may be caused by trauma eg., fall		
Suggests fracture may be a result of NAI		
Suggests giving analgesia		
Suggests senior ED / Orthopaedic review		
Suggests appropriate manipulation / casting of fracture		
States would ensure child had safeguarding check		
Summarises fracture and management plan concisely		
Systematic approach to radiograph interpretation		
Answers questions from medical student		
Examiner's Global Mark	/5	
Actor / Helper's Global Mark	/5	
Total Station Mark	/30	

Learning Points

Being able to have a systematic approach to interpreting fractures is crucial and will ensure you do not miss key features. Remember to report the date, name and type of film.

Developmental milestones are important when thinking of differential causes, as it is essential that the fracture be in keeping with the history for a child of that age. If you are not sure ALWAYS discuss with a senior for a child of any age and ensure a safeguarding check is completed.

All long bone fractures in a child <18 months should be highly suspicious for 'non accidental injury' and be discussed with an Emergency department or Paediatric consultant (Cardiff Child Protection Systematic Reviews 2016).

General Practice

Case 1
Mark Scheme: Hypertension management

Task	Achieved	Not Achieved
Introduces himself / herself		
Confirms patient details and purpose of consultation		
Takes a brief history, establishing lack of symptoms.		
Asks about past medical history- asking specifically about cardiac history, diabetes, high cholesterol.		
Asks about medications and allergies		
Asks about family history & social history including alcohol and smoking		
Elicits other risk factors - diet, exercise, weight gain.		
Summarises findings concisely		
Able to identify that this patient may have Hypertension		
Plans to examine or asks for examination findings		
Suggests appropriate investigations		
Blood tests - cholesterol, HbA1c, renal function		
Urine dip - assess for end organ damage		
Appropriate management plan & follow-up		
Monitor blood pressure at home		
Initiates antihypertensive according to guidelines		
Follow up in 2 weeks with blood pressure diary		
Explains probable diagnosis is hypertension and explains what this in lay terms for patient.		
Explains need for ambulatory blood pressure monitoring to confirm diagnosis.		
Discusses need for low salt-diet and change to exercise regime		
Discusses smoking cessation		
Offers at least one resource or community intervention.		
Discusses possibly needing to start medication and explains the side effects		
Acknowledges & addresses patient's ideas, concerns and expectations		
Gives patient opportunity to ask questions		
Examiner's Global Mark	/5	
Actor / Helper's Global Mark	/5	
Total Station Mark	/30	

Learning Points

It is important to always start with lifestyle interventions to help the patient take ownership of their disease. Offer them different community resources and interventions to help e.g. smoking cessation nurses, dieticians and group exercise classes.

With a new diagnosis of hypertension it is important to think of other cardiovascular risk factors and how to assess for end-organ damage.

With management stations spend less time on the history and focus on a simple explanation of the diagnosis and the upcoming management rationale.

Case 2
Mark Scheme: Palpitations

Task	Achieved	Not Achieved
Introduces himself / herself		
Confirms patient details and purpose of consultation		
Established the main presenting complaint		
Elicits palpitations and their length and pattern		
Elicits lack of prior warning		
Elicits associated chest pain & shortness of breath		
Asks about pre-syncopal symptoms		
Asks about thyroid related symptoms: sweating and temperature control, weight changes		
Asks about headache.		
Asks about social history including caffeine, alcohol & smoking		
Asks about past medical history		
Asks about medications and allergies		
Asks about family history		
Plans to examine or asks for examination findings		
Summarises findings concisely		
Able to provide appropriate differential diagnoses Atrial Fibrillation Sinus Tachycardia - ?anxiety related or normal variant Other arrhythmia		
Suggests appropriate investigations Basic Bloods: FBC - to exclude anaemia, TFTs - to exclude thyroid related atrial fibrillation ECG 24hr tape or 7day monitor		
Appropriate management plan & follow-up Follow up after the investigations Consider alternative causes e.g. Hyperthyroidism Consider medical treatment using rhythm control as <65yrs Consider anticoagulation using the CHA2DS2VAS Score Seek expert advice		
Acknowledge & addresses patient's ideas, concerns and expectations		
Gives patient opportunity to ask questions		
Examiner's Global Mark	/5	
Actor / Helper's Global Mark	/5	
Total Station Mark	/30	

Learning Points

Palpitations are a common complaint in general practice and it is important to realize how concerning they can be for the patient. Therefore you must take into consideration the impact these symptoms are having on activities of daily living.

It is important to think about the likely causes in different groups of patients i.e age, thryrotoxicosis, alcohol, caffeine and recreational drugs

A normal ECG does not preclude AF/arrhythmia and if the palpitations are occasional longer monitoring should be considered to help pick any underlying rhythm.

Case 3
Mark Scheme: Chronic Obstructive Pulmonary Disease

Task:	Achieved	Not Achieved
Introduces himself / herself		
Confirms patient details and purpose of consultation		
Established the main presenting complaint		
Explores symptom of worsened breathlessness - duration, onset (sudden / gradual), timing, exacerbating and relieving factors, exercise tolerance, use of inhalers- and compares to baseline		
Explores symptom of cough - duration, whether cough is productive, coryzal symptoms - and compares to baseline		
Asks about red flags – weight loss, change in appetite, haemoptysis, night sweats		
Asks about chest pain and leg swelling		
Asks about past medical history specifically previous history of respiratory and cardiac disease and venous thrombo-embolism		
Establishes history of COPD - age at diagnosis, nature of symptoms, admissions to hospital / intensive care		
Asks about medications and allergies		
Asks about family history & social history including alcohol and smoking		
Checks inhaler technique (candidate informed that it is adequate)		
Checks adherence to medication (and that medication is in date)		
Plans to examine or asks for examination findings		
Summarises findings concisely		
Able to provide appropriate differential diagnoses Acute Non Infective Exacerbation of COPD, Acute infective exacerbation of COPD, Heart Failure, Pulmonary Embolism, Lung Cancer		
Suggests appropriate investigations - Blood test, Chest x-ray, Spirometry to assess worsening COPD, Carbon monoxide monitoring		
Appropriate management plan & follow-up 5-7 day course of oral prednisolone, arrange a rescue pack of antibiotics to take away and be used in case infection develops Review in 6 weeks +/- chest x-ray, Consider adjunct treatment such as mucolytic, dietary supplements, psychological support, Pulmonary rehabilitation		
Acknowledges & addresses patient's ideas, concerns and expectations		
Gives patient opportunity to ask questions		
Examiner's Global Mark	/5	
Actor / Helper's Global Mark	/5	
Total Station Mark	/30	

Learning Points

Even if you know that a patient has a chronic condition such as COPD from the outset, which in this case you do not, it's important to take the history of the presenting symptoms with an open mind. Not every patient with COPD who comes in with increased shortness of breath is going to have an exacerbation of their COPD. Think about the differential diagnosis systematically.

When taking a history of breathlessness always establish level of function and compare to *their* baseline. This could be referenced from the distance walked or the activities carried out at home.

It is important to be aware of the holistic and multidisciplinary care provided in the community for COPD including smoking cessation and pulmonary rehabilitation.

Case 4
Mark Scheme: Chronic Cough

Task:	Achieved	Not Achieved
Introduces himself / herself		
Confirms patient details and purpose of consultation		
Established the main presenting complaint		
Explores symptom of cough - duration, whether cough is productive, coryzal symptoms		
Asks about red flags – weight loss, change in appetite, haemoptysis, night sweats		
Identify any exacerbating factors (e.g. dust, pets)		
Asks about associated features- chest pain and shortness of breath		
Exclude symptoms of heart failure, pulmonary embolism, infection		
Asks about past medical history specifically respiratory, cardiovascular problems, infections or causes of immunosuppression.		
Asks specifically about exposure to tuberculosis		
Asks about medications and allergies		
Asks about family history of lung cancer		
Asks about social history including alcohol and smoking		
Plans to examine or asks for examination findings		
Summarises findings concisely		
Able to provide appropriate differential diagnoses Lung cancer + Tuberculosis		
Suggests appropriate investigations Routine blood tests - FBC - to check anaemia or other infection or immunosuppression, Blood film, CXR Sputum Culture Mantoux		
Appropriate management plan & follow-up 2 week referral pathway as per NICE guidelines May require support at home, can refer to community services for carers for wife.		
Acknowledges & addresses patient's ideas, concerns and expectations		
Gives patient opportunity to ask questions		
Examiner's Global Mark	/5	
Actor / Helper's Global Mark	/5	
Total Station Mark	/30	

Learning Points

Lung cancer has a number of different presentations, it does not only occur in patients who have an extensive smoking history. In addition there are local and paraneoplastic complications associated with lung cancer, and complications related to metastases.

It is essential to know and make a point of excluding red flag symptoms for lung cancer but try to avoid fixation error (focusing on one differential to the extent of being blind to alternative diagnoses). Think systematically and consider what other pathologies could cause the presenting symptoms.

It is advisable to start with open questions, to allow the patient to tell you the story in their own words, but do push them to be specific on important points in your closed questioning.

Case 5
Mark Scheme: Headache

Task:	Achieved	Not Achieved
Introduces himself / herself		
Confirms patient details and purpose of consultation		
Established the main presenting complaint		
Asks about site, radiation of headache and character and severity of the pain.		
Asks about timing of the headache. How quick is the onset? How long does it last for? How frequently do they have them?		
Asks if there has been any recent trauma, nausea or vomiting.		
Asks about aura or any preceding symptoms.		
Asks if they have any visual symptoms including photophobia and whether they have had a recent eye test.		
Asks about red flag symptoms including fever, neck stiffness, rash, seizures, limb weakness, weight loss		
Asks about triggers or anything that makes the headache worse or if anything improves the headache including lying in a dark room or analgesia		
Asks about medication and allergies, enquiring specifically about what analgesia they have been taking including dose and frequency.		
Asks about past medical history and family history		
Asks about social history, enquiring specifically about work, stress, alcohol, smoking and recreational drug use.		
Plans to examine or asks for examination findings		
Summarises findings concisely		
Able to provide appropriate differential diagnoses Migraine with aura, tension headaches, cluster headaches, drug related headaches (caffeine or analgesia), raised intracranial pressure secondary to space occupying lesion. Exclude acute causes: Meningitis, Vascular (Subarachnoid haemorrhage)		
Suggests appropriate investigations Routine Bloods: FBC- identify markers of infection Imaging: CT scan		
Appropriate management plan & follow-up Avoid triggers Analgesia -working along the WHO Pain Ladder. Has considered that patient may have to use a different form of contraception to the oral contraceptive pill. Acknowledges & addresses patient's ideas, concerns and expectations		
Gives patient opportunity to ask questions		
Examiner's Global Mark	/5	
Actor / Helper's Global Mark	/5	
Total Station Mark	/30	

Learning Points

Always consider red flag symptoms in any pain presentation. Are there any features that make this an acute emergency or make you suspect a malignancy?

Don't be afraid to ask if anyone feels stressed or under pressure at home or work. You do not need to go into details or solve all their problems but it helps to get an idea of the bigger picture and may help explain their symptoms or behaviour. Make sure to do it sensitively and react compassionately.

In any pain presentation make sure to take a thorough history of exactly which analgesia a patient has taken, at which dose and how frequently. This can give you an idea of the severity of the pain, if they are taking appropriate pain relief, whether they are taking therapeutic levels of a drug and also spot staggered overdoses.

Case 6
Mark Scheme: Memory Loss

Task:	Achieved	Not Achieved
Introduces himself / herself		
Confirms patient details and purpose of consultation		
Established the main presenting complaint and chronicity		
Elicits sleep disturbances and behavioural disturbances		
Establishes lack of hallucinations		
Establishes lack of fluctuance throughout day.		
Establishes lack of stepwise decline		
Establishes lack of recent trigger (infection)		
Discusses impact on ADL's (cleaning, washing, toileting)		
Establishes dangerous symptoms and safety issues (regarding gas cooker and wandering)		
Asks about past medical history		
Asks about medications and allergies		
Asks about family history & social history including prior occupation, alcohol and smoking.		
Asks about support from family and friends		
Summarises findings concisely		
Able to provide appropriate differential diagnoses Alzheimer's Disease Vascular Dementia Lewy Body Dementia		
Suggests appropriate investigations Routine bloods: FBC: review inflammatory markers, B12/folate, Thyroid function, Renal function. Urine dip Blood sugar Imaging: CT head		
Appropriate management plan & follow-up Offers a review appointment to see how they are managing and also to formally examine Mr Collier Referral to memory clinic Referral to community services for potential carers to help at home e.g. physiotherapy and occupational health		
Acknowledges & addresses patient's ideas, concerns and expectations		
Gives patient opportunity to ask questions		
Examiner's Global Mark	/5	
Actor / Helper's Global Mark	/5	
Total Station Mark	/30	

Learning Points

There are subtle differences within dementia. A good way to separate Alzheimer's Disease, vascular dementia and Lewy-Body Dementia is to think about the temporal pattern of the disease (progressive, step-wise and fluctuating deterioration respectively).

It is important to be aware of the effect dementia has on family members who are often the principal carers. With an aging population the role of families to deliver care has increased. There is now a need for clinicians to consider the wellbeing of the patient's relatives and the mental and physical effects of the illness on their own health.

Within the community it is important to be aware of community geriatric and memory services and the role the MDT can play. The memory teams can consist of geriatricians, nurse specialists, psychaitrists and pyschologists.

Case 7
Mark Scheme: Multiple Sclerosis

Task	Achieved	Not Achieved
Introduces himself / herself		
Confirms patient details and purpose of consultation		
Established the main presenting complaint		
Elicits her symptoms		
Asks about past medical history		
Asks about medications and allergies		
Asks about family history & social history including alcohol and smoking		
Plans to examine or asks for examination findings		
Explains that her symptoms sound like an upper respiratory tract infection and are unlikely to be related to her multiple sclerosis		
Acknowledges & addresses patient's ideas, concerns and expectations		
Briefly gives an explanation of what multiple sclerosis is.		
Asks the patient what symptoms she has experienced and explains what other symptoms to look out for- eye symptoms, motor/sensory problems, incontinence		
Explains to the patient that she should contact either her GP or MS nurse if she has any further symptoms. However, it tends to be your neurologist who decided on medications.		
Explained that although some symptoms of MS resolve completely some can remain.		
Explains to the patient that it should be possible to make arrangements at work help her (for example- teaching all her classes in the same classroom). Suggest making an appointment with headteacher or if possible disability officer to talk about her MS and to see what arrangements are possible.		
Addresses patient's social support: mentions a support service such as the multiple sclerosis trust who can provide individual support and further information.		
Appropriate management plan & follow-up. Offers a review appointment to see how they are managing. Review of her sleep and symptoms of depression at the next consultation		
Summarises the consultation to the patient concisely		
Assesses patient's understanding of the information given to her		
Gives patient opportunity to ask questions		
Examiner's Global Mark	/5	
Actor / Helper's Global Mark	/5	
Total Station Mark	/30	

Learning Points

If you are asked to discuss a patient's condition or new diagnosis, it is essential to start is by establishing what they know so far and what they would like to know. This can help provide a structure for you explanation and help fill the gaps in their knowledge.

A new diagnosis of a progressive or chronic condition can be terrifying. Showing empathy and kindness are key. You won't be able to answer all their questions about the future in a short consultation but reassuring them of the support they have and making them aware of the team available will help address their fears.

When providing a lot of information in a single consultation it can be useful to offer them a further appointment in a few weeks to check in and see how they are getting along. Also remember patients with chronic conditions are at a higher risk of developing depression so it is good to review their mood regularly.

Case 8

Mark Scheme: Alcoholic Liver disease

Task	Achieved	Not Achieved
Introduces himself / herself		
Confirms patient details and purpose of consultation		
Established the main presenting complaint		
Finds out how long he has had a drinking problem		
Enquires about triggers for increasing alcohol use		
Asks about what/how much he drinks		
Uses the CAGE questionnaire, or another tool to assess if there is an alcohol problem Asks if they feel they should cut down on their drinking Asks if they have been annoyed by other people criticizing their drinking Asks if they feel guilty about their drinking Asks if they have had to drink first thing in the morning		
Asks if they have missed work or other responsibilities because of alcohol		
Asks if alcohol has put strain on personal relationships		
Enquires about other drugs & smoking		
Enquires about problems with legal authorities		
Asks about their motivation to stop drinking alcohol		
Asks about alcohol related symptoms: gastritis, peripheral sensory neuropathy, memory problems, palpitations.		
Asks about past medical history, medications and allergies, family history.		
Plans to examine or asks for examination findings		
Summarises findings concisely		
Appropriate management plan & follow-up States wants to make follow up appointment to discuss this further Signposts to written/online advice about alcohol misuse in the meantime		
Remains non-judgemental		
Acknowledges & addresses patient's ideas, concerns and expectations		
Gives patient opportunity to ask questions		
Examiner's Global Mark	/5	
Actor / Helper's Global Mark	/5	
Total Station Mark	/30	

Learning Points

The CAGE questionnaire is a quick and easy tool to identify if a person has a significant alcohol problem. There are other tools, such as the AUDIT tool, however this takes several minutes to complete.

Offering advice about alcohol misuse will require much more than a single appointment, so it is imperative to take a full history and make follow up appointments to further discuss.

It is important to remain non-judgemental when discussing such sensitive topics. However, you must also establish a clear history and will need to ask sensitive questions.

Case 9
Mark Scheme: Rectal Bleeding

Task	Achieved	Not Achieved
Introduces himself / herself		
Confirms patient details and purpose of consultation		
Established the main presenting complaint		
Asks about straining		
Asks about pain on passing stools		
Asks about anal itch		
Asks about abdominal pain		
Asks about red flag symptoms - weight loss, loss of appetite, lethargy, night sweats, fevers, change in bowel habit		
Asks patient about fibre & fluid intake		
Asks about past medical history		
Asks about medications and allergies		
Asks about family history & social history including alcohol and smoking		
Plans to examine or asks for examination findings		
Summarises findings concisely		
Able to provide appropriate differential diagnoses Haemorrhoids Anal Fissure Inflammatory Bowel disease		
Suggests appropriate investigations Bloods - exclude IBD Imaging - Rigid sigmoidoscopy		
Offers lifestyle advice Drinking plenty of water. Eating lots of fibre rich foods. Wiping hard makes haemorrhoids wors. Warm baths can help.		
Appropriate management plan & follow-up Explains need for soft stool to allow haemorrhoids to heal Offers topical creams/suppositories for symptom relief Offers a review appointment to see how they are managing.		
Acknowledges & addresses patient's ideas, concerns and expectations		
Gives patient opportunity to ask questions		
Examiner's Global Mark	/5	
Actor / Helper's Global Mark	/5	
Total Station Mark	/30	

Learning Points

Remember to consider that many different factors can lead to haemorrhoids, not just constipation and straining when opening bowels, including age, raised intra-abdominal pressure (pregnancy, ascites, pelvic mass), chronic cough, heavy lifting, low fibre diet.

Management of haemorrhoids is predominantly lifestyle advice, such as dietary advice, and it is important to emphasize to the patient that these changes will be long-term to reduce recurrence of haemorrhoids.

It is important to ask about red flag symptoms for lower gastrointestinal cancers to ensure you do not miss something sinister, even if they fall outside the typical age group. Urgent referral via the 2 week wait cancer pathway is recommended for patients aged 40 and over who present with rectal bleeding with a change of bowel habit with looser stools and/or increased stool frequency that has been present for six weeks or more.

Case 10
Mark Scheme: Lump in the breast

Task	Achieved	Not Achieved
Introduces himself / herself		
Confirms patient details and purpose of consultation		
Established the main presenting complaint		
Asks about the lump - size, site, shape		
Asks if the lump is painful, if it is mobile or fixed to the skin		
Ask about nipple changes - discharge or bleeding, or change in shape/inversion		
Asks about overlying skin changes (eg. peau d' orange)		
Asks about red flag symptoms - weight loss, loss of appetite, lethargy, night sweats, fevers		
Asks about bony pain or swelling elsewhere (e.g. lymph nodes)		
Asks about recent trauma and breastfeeding		
Asks about past medical history		
Asks about medications and allergies specifically about hormone replacement therapy		
Asks about family history of cancer & social history including alcohol and smoking		
Plans to examine or asks for examination findings		
Summarises findings concisely		
Able to provide appropriate differential diagnoses Breast carcinoma Duct Ectasia Cystic disease Benign mammary dysplasia		
Suggests appropriate investigations Triple assessment History and examination Imaging - mammography/USS Fine needle aspiration (biopsy)		
Appropriate management plan & follow-up 2 week wait referral to breast surgeons Offers a review appointment to see how they are managing.		
Acknowledges & addresses patient's ideas, concerns and expectations		
Gives patient opportunity to ask questions		
Examiner's global mark	/5	
Actor/helper's global mark	/5	
Total station mark	/30	

Learning Points

Breast lumps are a cause for concern amongst women (and men) but fortunately, most are benign—caused by fibroadenomas. These typically present in younger women of childbearing age, with non-tender, highly mobile masses that come and go as related to hormonal changes in the body.

The key things to look out for in the presentation that suggests malignancy include a hard/irregular lump, tethering to bone or skin, bloody discharge and lymphadenopathy. These patients should be referred under the "two week rule" to secondary care.

In the general practice setting you should have a low threshold for referring patients of any age with a family history of breast or uterine cancer, due to its potential heritability (with mutations of the BRCA1/2 tumour suppressor genes).

Case 11
Mark Scheme: Haematuria

Task:	Achieved	Not Achieved
Introduces himself / herself		
Confirms patient details and purpose of consultation		
Established the main presenting complaint		
Asks about nature of haematuria: duration, intermittent or continuous and progression		
Asks about the blood - colour (fresh red, dark) and amount of bleeding.		
Asks about red flag symptoms - weight loss, loss of appetite, lethargy, night sweats, fevers		
Asks about symptoms of anaemia—tiredness, breathlessness		
Lower Urinary Tract Symptoms associated with storage (volume, urgency, frequency, nocturia)		
Lower Urinary Tract Symptoms associated with voiding (terminal dribbling, poor flow, hesitancy, sensation of incomplete voiding)		
Lower Urinary Tract Symptoms associated with infection (dysuria)		
Asks about past medical history		
Asks about medications and allergies		
Asks about family history & social history including occupation, alcohol and smoking		
Plans to examine or asks for examination findings		
Summarises findings concisely		
Able to provide appropriate differential diagnoses Bladder transitional cell carcinoma Other malignancies of the renal tract Urinary tract infection Glomerulonephritis Prostate cancer / BPH Drug reaction e.g. rifampicin,		
Appropriate management plan & follow-up 2 week wait referral to urology Offers a review appointment to see how they are managing.		
Acknowledges & addresses patient's ideas, concerns and expectations		
Gives patient opportunity to ask questions		
Examiner's global mark	/5	
Actor/helper's global mark	/5	
Total station mark	/35	

Learning Points

In the general practice setting, anybody over the age of forty-five years with visible haematuria, or over sixty with microscopic haematuria, in the absence of a urinary tract infection, should be referred for urgent urological assessment to rule out cancer.

Risk factors for bladder cancer in the Western world revolve around the exposure to polycyclic aromatic hydrocarbons—in other words, tobacco smokers, and those with occupational exposure (industrial workers in regular contact with metalwork, paint, petroleum, dyes and solvents).

Operative management of bladder cancer, or complications from the cancer itself (e.g. clot retention) can necessitate the use of a catheter, which can cause a patient distress, embarrassment or inconvenience—particularly on day to day life when used long term. Be mindful of this when counselling your patients!

Case 12
Mark Scheme: Lower Urinary Tract Infection

Task:	Achieved	Not Achieved
Introduces himself / herself		
Confirms patient details and purpose of consultation		
Established the main presenting complaint		
Asks specifically about the nature of her pain, frequency and urgency, haematuria.		
Asks if she has had any fevers or loin pain		
Sensitively screens for a sexually transmitted infection.		
Asks about her past medical history including previous urinary tract infections		
Ask if she or any family members have any renal tract abnormalities or known impaired renal function.		
Asks about medications, allergies and social history including alcohol and smoking		
Plans to examine or asks for examination findings		
Summarises findings concisely		
Able to provide appropriate differential diagnoses Likely urinary tract infection Exclude pyelonephritis		
Suggests appropriate investigations Urine dip and culture		
Appropriate management plan & follow-up Antibiotics therapy according to guidelines - trimethoprim or nitrofurantoin. Suitable pain relief with paracetamol Offers a review appointment to see how they are managing.		
Acknowledges & addresses patient's ideas, concerns and expectations		
Gives patient opportunity to ask questions		
Explains diagnosis and management to the patient.		
Provides safety netting advice to return if she develops a fever or loin pain or if her symptoms do not improve.		
Addresses the complex questions that the patient has and suggests alternative to medical textbook, patient friendly resources.		
Explains clearly to the patient how to take a mid-stream urine.		
Examiner's Global Mark	/5	
Actor / Helper's Global Mark	/5	
Total Station Mark	/30	

Learning Points

A recurrent UTI refers to 2 or more infections in 6 months or 3 or more infections in 1 year. A recurrent UTI can either be due to relapse or reinfection. Relapse is a recurrent UTI with the same strain of organism. Relapse is a likely cause if infection recurs shortly after treatment. Reinfection is a recurrent UTI with a different strain or species of organism. It is the likely cause of recurrent infection more than two weeks after the initial treatment.

It is important to clearly explain to a patient how to take a mid-stream urine: Firstly the peri-urethral area should be cleaned. About 10ml of urine should be collected at mid-stream- the middle point of urination, without interrupting urine flow to start or stop the collection. It must be collected into a sterile container.

Patients will often come into your consultation room and know what is wrong with them, listen to what their thoughts are and work together with them to build a rapport. Some patients will do excessive research but find it difficult to understand or interpret their research, point them in the right direction for resources more suited for their understanding.

Case 13
Mark Scheme: Diabetic Management

Task	Achieved	Not Achieved
Introduces himself / herself		
Confirms patient details and purpose of consultation		
Established the main presenting complaint		
Elicits duration of current management		
Asks about current monitoring : BP, Urine, Feet, Eyes		
Asks about last HbA1c result, date of test and interprets correctly		
Asks about past medical history specifically Ischaemic heart disease/heart failure , osteoporosis, bladder Ca (ie risks of glitazones), renal failure, stroke		
Asks about medications and allergies		
Asks about family history & social history including alcohol and smoking		
Asks about diet and exercise		
Elicits symptoms of Hypoglycaemia - dizziness, sweating, improved with eating		
Safety net for Hypoglycaemia in future (patient leaflet) considering occupation.		
Checks understanding		
Plans to examine or asks for examination findings		
Summarises findings concisely		
Able to provide appropriate differential diagnoses Hypoglycaemia secondary to gliclazide		
Suggests appropriate investigations Routine Bloods -HbA1c in 3-4 months Urine for dipstick and/or Albumin:Creatinine ratio Examining the feet and eye tests annually.		
Appropriate management plan & follow-up Switching Gliclazide to alternative therapy Provides appropriate alternate agent – glitazone/gliptin. Insulin NOT an option. Offers a review appointment to see how they are managing.		
Acknowledges & addresses patient's ideas, concerns and expectations		
Gives patient opportunity to ask questions		
Examiner's Global Mark	/5	
Actor / Helper's Global Mark	/5	
Total Station Mark	/30	

Learning points

Sulphonylureas such as Gliclazide are known to cause Hypoglycaemia, which is highly significant in this scenario as the patient is about to drive HGVs which can predispose not only him but also others on the road to accidents.

Patients often have concerns when their established medical regime requires change. Elicit and address their concerns and explain to them why the change is necessary. If at all possible never change multiple drugs at the same time as this can lead to confusion and errors and make interpretation of approval or deterioration difficult for the clinician.

Be aware of the adverse effects of common medications such as Metformin, Gliclazide, Pioglitazone and Insulin.

Case 14
Mark Scheme: Skin Rash

Task	Achieved	Not Achieved
Introduces himself / herself		
Confirms patient details and purpose of consultation		
Established the main presenting complaint		
Asks about duration, evolution (growth, itching, pain, any bleeding or pus), any other lesions on body		
Assesses relieving factors (sunshine, creams), exacerbating factors (smoking, alcohol, stress, trauma, drugs)		
Assesses joint pain, swelling, stiffness, oral ulcers, bowel motions, urinary habits and recent infections		
Asks about red flag symptoms - weight loss, loss of appetite, lethargy, night sweats, fevers		
Asks about past medical history, medications and allergies		
Asks about family history & social history including alcohol and smoking		
Atopy: hayfever, asthma, allergies, eczema		
Plans to examine or asks for examination findings		
Examines rash: site, size, shape, colour, described as a plaque		
Assesses demarcation (well defined vs poor), temperature, tenderness, blood/pus, blister formation		
Asks to pain/stiffness/ range of motion in joint and other areas of the body for similar rashes - hands/ears		
Summarises findings concisely		
Able to provide appropriate differential diagnoses Psoriasis Dermatitis/eczema Lichen Planus Discoid Lupus		
Appropriate management plan & follow-up Starts a weak steroid cream / Vitamin D analogue or combination Offers a review appointment to see how they are managing.		
Acknowledges & addresses patient's ideas, concerns and expectations		
Explains why Methotrexate is not appropriate at this stage (Side effects: neutropenia, pulmonary fibrosis, cirrhosis)		
Gives patient opportunity to ask questions		
Examiner's Global Mark	/5	
Actor / Helper's Global Mark	/5	
Total Station Mark	/30	

Learning points

Remember the classic exacerbating and relieving factors of Psoriasis as in this scenario as it can greatly aid in the diagnosis of the rash.

Know the stages of management of Psoriasis (emollients, steroid cream, vitamin D analogues, UV therapy, systemic agents like Methotrexate) and the common adverse effects of Methotrexate.

The patient may already have an agenda of their own and want a specific treatment. It is only after finding out why they want it and addressing their concerns with full explanations that you will be able to reassure them.

Case 15
Mark Scheme: Skin mole

Task:	Achieved	Not Achieved
Introduces himself / herself		
Confirms patient details and purpose of consultation		
Established the main presenting complaint		
Asks about duration, evolution (growth, itching, pain, any bleeding or pus), any other lesions on body		
Assesses risk factors for sun exposure: travel abroad, sunbathing, use of sun bed, use of protective sun creams		
Asks about red flag symptoms - weight loss, loss of appetite, lethargy, night sweats, fevers		
Asks about past medical history		
Asks about medications and allergies		
Asks about family history & social history including alcohol and smoking		
Plans to examine or asks for examination findings		
Examines mole: site, size, shape, colour/pigmentation		
Assesses ABCDE (asymmetry, border, colour, diameter, evolution)		
Assesses demarcation (well defined vs poor), temperature, tenderness, blood/pus, blister formation		
Asks to examine lymph nodes and other areas of the body for similar moles.		
Summarises findings concisely		
Able to provide appropriate differential diagnoses Malignant melanoma Basal cell carcinoma Squamous cell carcinoma Benign melanocytic lesion		
Suggests appropriate investigations Clinical diagnosis, however is sent for biopsy following excision		
Appropriate management plan & follow-up Monitoring lesion (photos/measuring) Urgent 2 week wait referral to Dermatology services Offers a review appointment to see how they are managing.		
Acknowledges & addresses patient's ideas, concerns and expectations		
Gives patient opportunity to ask questions		
Examiner's Global Mark	/5	
Actor / Helper's Global Mark	/5	
Total Station Mark	/30	

Learning points

Always remember to assess pigmented lesions with a suspicion of a possible Malignant Melanoma and use the ABCDE approach: A – asymmetry, B – border (even/uneven), C- colour (uniform or not), D – diameter (greater than 6mm), E – evolution (change of lesion over time/bleeding).

It is vital to ask about sun exposure and family history in this scenario and any lesion with a suspected malignant nature such as Squamous cell carcinoma of the skin.

Not everyone is concerned about a "mole" and it is important to explain the reason behind actions such as 2 week wait referral to ensure they follow this through and receive appropriate treatment.

Printed in Great Britain
by Amazon